W0043272

Current Topics in Pathology
73

Editors

C.L. Berry   E. Grundmann   W.H. Kirsten

Advisory Board

H.-W. Altmann, K. Benirschke, A. Bohle, H. Cottier
M. Eder, P. Gedigk, Chr. Hedinger, S. Iijima
J.L. Van Lancker, K. Lennert, H. Meessen, B. Morson
W. Sandritter, G. Seifert, S. Sell, T. Takeuchi
H.U. Zollinger

Pulmonary Diseases

Clinicopathological Correlations

Contributors

P. Dalquen · D. Francis · S.G. Haworth
M. Jacobsen · W. Kißler · G. Müller · K.-M. Müller
M. Oberholzer · H.-E. Schaefer · W. Wierich

Editor

K.-M. Müller

With 124 Figures

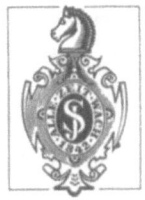

Springer-Verlag
Berlin Heidelberg GmbH 1983

K.-M. Müller, Professor Dr., Leiter des Instituts für Pathologie der Berufsgenossenschaftlichen Krankenanstalten "Bergmannsheil", Universitätsklinik Bochum, Hunscheidtstraße 1, D-4630 Bochum 1

C.L. Berry, Professor Dr., Department of Morbid Anatomy. The London
Hospital Medical College, GB-London E1 1BB

E. Grundmann, Professor Dr., Pathologisches Institut der Universität,
Domagkstraße 17, D-4400 Münster/Westfalen

W.H. Kirsten, Professor Dr., Department of Pathology, The University
of Chicago, 950 East 59th Street, Chicago, IL 60637, USA

ISBN 978-3-642-69136-2   ISBN 978-3-642-69134-8 (eBook)
DOI 10.1007/978-3-642-69134-8

Library of Congress Cataloging in Publication Data. Pulmonary diseases – clinicopathological
correlations. (Current topics in pathology; 73) Bibliography: p. Includes index. 1. Lungs –
Diseases – Addresses, essays, lectures. I. Dalquen, P. II. Müller, K.-M. (Klaus-Michael), 1940–.
III. Series. [DNLM: 1. Lung diseases – Pathology. W1 CU821H v. 73/WF 600 P9834302]
RBl.E6 vol. 73 [RC756] 616.07s [616.2′4] 83-6794

This work is subject to copyright. All rights are reserved, whether the whole or part of the
material is concerned, specifically those of translation, reprinting, re-use of illustrations, broad-
casting, reproduction by photocopying machine or similar means, and storage in data banks.

Under § 54 of the German Copyright Law where copies are made for other than private use,
a fee is payable to "Verwertungsgesellschaft Wort", Munich.

© by Springer-Verlag Berlin Heidelberg 1983
Softcover reprint of the hardcover 1st edition 1983

The use of registered names, trademarks, etc. in this publication does not imply, even in the
absence of a specific statement, that such names are exempt from the relevant protective laws
and regulations and therefore free for general use.

Product Liability: The publisher can give no guarantee for information about drug dosage
and application thereof contained in this book. In every individual case the respective user
must check its accuracy by consulting other pharmaceutical literature.

2122/3130-543210

List of Contributors

Dalquen, Priv.-Doz.
Dr. P.

Institut für Pathologie, Schönbeinstraße 40,
CH-4056 Basel

Francis, Dr. Dorthe

Department of Pulmonary Pathology, Bispebjerg
Hospital, Bispebjerg Bakke 23, DK-2400
Copenhagen NV

Haworth, Dr. Sheila G.

Reader in Paediatric Cardiology, Department of
Paediatric Cardiology, Institute of Child Health,
University of London, The Hospital for Sick
Children, Great Ormond Street, GB-London
WC1N 3JH

Jacobsen, Dr. Marianne

Department of Pulmonary Pathology, Bispebjerg
Hospital, Bispebjerg Bakke 23, DK-2400
Copenhagen NV

Kißler, Prof. Dr. W.

Institut für Pathologie der Ruhr-Universität
Bochum, Universitätsstraße 150, D-4630
Bochum-Querenburg

Müller, Dr. G.

Institut für Pathologie der Universität Münster,
Domagkstraße 17, D-4400 Münster/Westf.

Müller, Prof. Dr. K.-M.

Direktor des Instituts für Pathologie der
Berufsgenossenschaftlichen Krankenanstalten
,,Bergmannsheil", Universitätsklinik Bochum,
Hunscheidtstraße 1, D-4360 Bochum 1

Oberholzer, Dr. M.

Institut für Pathologie, Schönbeinstraße 40,
CH-4056 Basel

Schaefer, Prof. Dr. H.-E.

Pathologisches Institut der Universität, Joseph-
Stelzmann-Straße 9, D–5000 Köln 41

Wierich, Priv.-Doz. Dr. W.

Leitender Arzt des Pathologischen Instituts am
Prosper-Hospital, Mühlenstraße 27,
D-4350 Recklinghausen

List of Contributors

Preface

The extension of clinical, endoscopic, and bioptic lung examination procedures and function analyses has resulted in more detailed knowledge of the pathology and pathogenetic factors of numerous bronchopulmonary diseases. Morphometric, histochemical, ultrastructural, and immunologic examination methods are now constituent parts of lung pathology.

This volume, written by numerous experts treats the special subjects of bronchial system pathology, pulmonary circulation, inflammatory and fibrous lung tissue diseases, and borderline areas of lung tumors. With regard to the results, some of which have been obtained experimentally, great importance has been attached to the presentation of the applied morphometric, histochemical, immunologic, and ultrastructural investigation methods. The book is intended to improve and extend the discussion between clinicians and morphologists. For the majority of lung diseases, which are discussed in detail in chapters dedicated to the morphological aspects, definitive categorization and assessment of the findings are only possible if clinical picture and disease progress are known. Furthermore, the findings documented here, which can be grasped morphologically, provide important indications for the evaluation and classification of syndromes and for prophylactic clinical measures.

I would like to thank Professor Grundmann, who initiated this volume, and the contributing authors. Special appreciation and recognition are due the staff of Springer-Verlag for their cooperation and for the organization, printing, and perfect illustration of the contributions.

Bochum   *K.-M. Müller*

Contents

Indexed in ISR

Methods and Results of Postmortem Studies of Airway Dynamics in Normal Lungs and Lungs with Minimal Obstruction*

W. WIERICH

I. Introduction

Simple postmortem investigations of airway dynamics were first communicated by *Carson* (1820). These investigations and numerous subsequent studies provided the first information on the elastic properties of lungs (*Hutchinson* 1846; *Donders* 1853; *Liebermeister* 1907; *Jaquet* 1908; *Bönninger* 1909; *Cloetta* 1913).

The investigations by *von Neergard* (1929), which were taken up again by a great many researchers after 1955, demonstrated that the surface tension forces at the alveolar interface substantially influence the elastic recoil force of the lungs (*Pattle* 1955). It was shown by numerous authors that especially in newborns, a lining of the alveoli by a surface-active substance, the "surfactant," is of great importance for normal function of the lungs (*Gruenwald* 1958; *Kluge* 1967; *Scarpelli* 1968; *Schoedel* 1971; *Avery* and *Fletcher* 1974; *Wierich* 1977). *Weibel* and *Gil* (1968) were able to demonstrate the presence of the surfactant for the first time by electron-microscopic studies.

Investigations on the flow resistance in the lungs and its distribution in the various parts of the bronchial systems were first undertaken by *von Recklinghausen* (1869) using a very simplified tube model with regular dichotomous branching. The concepts of airway dynamics, which even today are still valid in many points, go back to the investigations and theoretical reflections of *Rohrer* (1915, 1925). In his studies *Rohrer* successively measured the diameters and the lengths of all bronchi and bronchioli down to a diameter of 1 mm in a collapsed human lung. The number of bronchus generations and their lengths, as well as numerous mean lengths and volumes in various bronchus regions, were calculated from these values with remarkable meticulousness.

* Supported in part by the Ministerium für Wissenschaft und Forschung des Landes Nordrhein-Westfalen

Using these data, *Rohrer* calculated the decrease in pressure as well as the flow rate distribution, the distribution of flow resistances in the bronchial system down to the alveoli, and also the elastic retractive forces of the lungs. The exceedingly voluminous data from *Rohrer's* investigations were the basis for the reflections and calculations of *Rahn* et al. (1946) on the pressure-volume relationships of the lungs and the thorax, which are also fundamental for clinical problems.

II. Investigation Materials

Successful postmortem investigations of airway dynamics were performed on a total of 226 lungs obtained from autopsy material from the Institute of Pathology, Ruhr University in Bochum. Besides normal lungs, lungs with very diverse pathological changes were included. After meticulous histological control, 68 lungs from between the second and ninth decades of life were found which could be regarded as normal. Despite systematic changes due to age, the functional parameters showed a high degree of agreement (*Wierich* and *Hartung* 1979). The following morphological alterations did not reveal any significant effects on the parameters of airway dynamics: slight hypostatic pulmonary edema, focal alveolar hemorrhages, circumscribed reversible atelectasis, occasional small tumor metastases, and moderate inflammatory changes in large and intermediate bronchi, in some cases with epithelial metaplasia.

There were nonlinear relationships between the age of the person and most parameters of normal lungs, represented by equations of higher order ($Y = a + b \times$ age $+ c \times$ age^2). This nonlinear dependence for the overall group of 68 normal lungs is shown in Fig. 1a by the example of total airways resistance (Rt). This age dependence of the resistance could be partially explained by the result of the morphometric investigations by *Niewoehner* and *Kleinerman* (1974). These authors found a significant positive correlation between age and mean bronchiolar diameter (MBD), from the second to the third decade of life. Beyond the third decade, there was a significant negative correlation between age and MBD (Fig. 1b). Further measurements have revealed that the relationship between age and MBD can likewise be represented by a higher order function (*Niewoehner* et al. 1977).

In the present study, rather than compare the measurements of normal lungs with the corresponding values from lungs with different degrees of airways obstruction and various pathological alterations, it appeared to be meaningful to compare the results from normal lungs with those from a large number of lungs having the same kind of pathological alterations. In order also to consider a current clinical problem, the results from lungs with very slight obstruction are reported, and the interactions between morphology and airway dynamics are discussed.

Parameters of airway dynamics in lungs with slight obstruction could not be compared with those in the 68 normal lungs, because a sufficient number of lungs with the same age distribution and pathologically altered in the same way were not available for investigation. The problem of a systematic statistical comparison between normal lungs and lungs with mild airways obstruction was solved by restricting the study to a certain age range. The period between the 35th and 55th years of life was chosen because

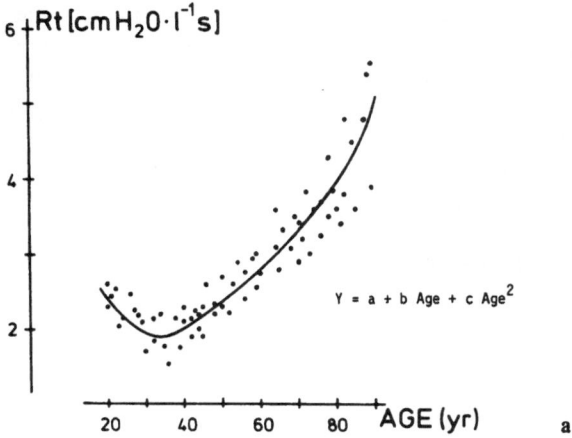

$$Y = a + b\ Age + c\ Age^2$$

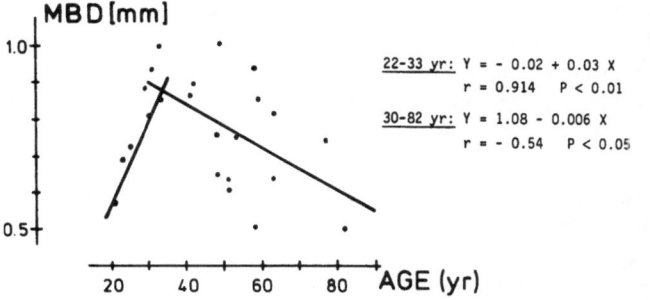

22-33 yr: Y = - 0.02 + 0.03 X
r = 0.914 P < 0.01

30-82 yr: Y = 1.08 - 0.006 X
r = - 0.54 P < 0.05

Fig. 1a. Total airways resistance *(Rt)* plotted against age. Results of postmortem measurements in 68 normal lungs. See text for explanation. **b** Correlations between mean bronchiole diameter *(MBD)* and age. Original values according to *Niewoehner* and *Kleinerman* (1974). Reproduced with permission of the authors and the American Physiological Society

there is an almost linear correlation between age and functional parameters in this age group, and a sufficient numer of lungs with minimal obstruction could be investigated. On account of sex differences, only the lungs of male subjects were chosen for this comparative investigation. The group of normal lungs comprised 18 cases (N group). The mean age was 44.2 years (SD ± 6.5 years); the average weight was 374 ± 33.1 g. In the group with slight obstruction, there were 14 lungs from the same age range (B group), with a mean age of 43.8 ± 6.9 years and a mean weight of 377.0 ± 28.4 g. The differences between the groups were not significant.

By definition, obstructive changes in the lungs are characterized primarily by an increase in resistance. A minimal obstruction was assumed when the total airways resistance as well as its peripheral component was significantly above the corresponding values in normal lungs during ventilation in an artifical thorax (especially at high frequency). Moreover, very uniform morphological alterations were found in lungs which showed signs of chronic bronchiolitis. The structure of the bronchioli and of the peribronchiolar tissue was preserved throughout in these lungs and did not show any deviations from that of normal lungs. Pulmonary emphysema was not present in any of the cases. Because of the typical alterations at the bronchioli, these lungs are also designated below as lungs with (chronic) bronchiolitis.

The patients of both groups had died suddenly. Lungs with preterminal alterations, e.g., diffuse edema, aspiration, or pneumonia, were excluded. The most frequent causes of death in the two groups were acute heart failure, acute hemorrhages (esophageal varices, gastrointestinal ulcers, traumas), multiple trauma, and death from acute failure of central nervous regulation.

III. Methods

The parameters studied, their abbreviations and their units of measurement are listed in Table 1. The measurements were generally performed about 24 h after death. For organizational reasons, a few lungs were first sealed in airtight containers and stored for up to 4 weeks at $-28°C$. In agreement with the investigations by *Pratt* and *Klugh* (1961) as well as by *Miller* et al. (1973), no significant difference in lung mechanics

Table 1. Parameters, abbreviations, and units. The symbol $\triangle$ is used to indicate a percentage change of measurement values

Abbreviation	Parameter	Unit
P	Pressure	
Pst	Static elastic recoil pressure	
Palv	Alveolar pressure	cm H_2O
Ppl	Pleural pressure	
Pbr	Lateral bronchiolar pressure	
Ptr	Tracheal pressure	
$\dot{V}$	Flow	liters/s
V	Volume	liters
Cst	Static lung compliance (always related to FRC)	liters/cm H_2O per liter
TLC	Total lung capacity	
VC	Vital capacity	
MV	Minimal lung volume	liters
RV	Residual lung volume	
FRC	Functional residual capacity	
TV	Tidal volume	
F	Frequency	breaths/min
Cdyn	Dynamic lung compliance	liters/cm H_2O
Rt	Total airways resistance	
Rc	Central airways resistance	cm H_2O/liter per second
Rp	Peripheral airways resistance	

could be demonstrated between numerous control measurements taken before and after deep freezing of the lungs. Usually the investigations were performed on the left lung, in some cases on both lungs.

Immediately before the measurements, and after ligation of the vessels and the bronchial stump in order to reduce autolytic changes of the pleura, the lungs were moistened for about 10 min on all sides with 10% formalin solution. Comparative measurements revealed that this procedure does not influence lung mechanics (*Wierich* 1974). During the studies, the pleura were continuously moistened with physiological saline solution. If necessary, mucus was sucked off from the bronchial system. Histological controls revealed that no mucous occlusions were left. Appropriate thin-walled cannulas were fixed in the main-stem bronchus of the lungs. The lungs were then placed with open pulmonary vessels and with the hilus downwards onto a water surface, and inflated and deflated several times up to a pressure of 25 cm H_2O to ventilate any area of atelectasis. During this process, a differing amount of blood flowed out of the pulmonary vessels. This amount of blood was established by weight controls, the average being 190 ± 12.8 ml. By immersing the inflated lungs under a water surface, pleural defects could be identified. Small pleural leaks not localized near the hilus were ligated and additionally coated with tissue glue (Histoakryl).

Direct measurements of Palv were performed at three sites at least. The chosen sites of measurement were consistently the mediastinal portions of the first, sixth, and tenth segments. The probes for measuring Palv were made from Teflon tubing with an internal diameter of 0.77 mm and a wall strength of 0.25 mm. Pieces of this tubing were pushed at one end onto a heated metal cone and dipped with the cone into cold water. After pulling the tubing from the cone, the end of the tubing was widened to an angle of about 120° in the form of a funnel. The diameter of the outer edge was about 1.5 mm.

At the places at which the Palv was to be measured, the pleura of an almost-collapsed lung was grasped in the center of a lobule with a forceps and pulled up. The pleura was cut off directly below the tip of the forceps, so that a small, roughly circular pleural defect arose. With a fine scissors, the pleura was then "undermined" over the entire circumference in the boundary area of the artificial defect. The edges of the pleural defects with the detached pleura reaching roughly to the boundary of the corresponding lobule were afterwards grasped with fine arterial clamps. The lungs were kept in the midinflatory position. After tightening the clamps and introducing the Palv probe tips, the pleura was ligated around the probe. In addition, the ligature was secured with tissue glue. The conical widening of the Palv probes was chosen in order to ensure a good fixation of the probes and to prevent the ends of the probes from pushing forward into the deeper pulmonary parenchyma.

Following *Macklem* and *Mead* (1967), Pbr was measured in order to be able to calculate Rc, Rp, and Rt. Pbr was measured consistently in the third and eighth pulmonary segments. In order to ensure exact localization and accurate fixation of the pressure probes at an angle of 90° to the longitudinal axis of the bronchiolus, the method of Macklem and Mead was substantially modified. These modifications ensured that the ends of the probes were in fact localized perpendicularly to the flow axis, and that they were not situated in an ostium, occluding the lumen. In contrast to the method of Macklem and Mead, the probes were pushed through the bronchial wall at right angles between branching points. These probes were also prepared from Teflon tubing. However, the edges of the free end of these probes were not widened only to 120°, but to 180°. The outer edges were treated in such a way that they were made circular, with a diameter of 0.8–0.9 mm. During insertion of the probes, the lungs were kept in the midinflation position. Before commencing the measurements, the positions of the probe tips were checked in intense transmitted light. The question of whether an erroneous measurement of Pbr occurs due to turbulences at the ends of the probe or by deformations of the corresponding bronchioli was investigated in detail. For this purpose, probes for measurement of Palv were applied in lung regions situated behind the Pbr probes. Pleural defects 2 mm in diameter were introduced directly beside the probes. The same procedure was followed in a neighboring subsegment. The primary bronchus was then connected to a valve with which a constant $\dot{V}$ could be adjusted. The air flowing into the lungs was able to escape only through the pleural defects beside the probes for the Palv measurement. The values of $\dot{V}$ and Palv were registered with varying $\dot{V}$ at the primary bronchus and with varying lung volumes. Identical values for Palv were measured at varying levels of $\dot{V}$ at the two measurement sites. Differences were found only with lung volumes of less than 15% of the defined VC. These repeatedly obtained results were taken as evidence that the tips of the probes for measurement of Pbr did not have any influence on the flow in the corresponding bronchioli, except at very low lung volumes.

For static measurements, the lungs were fractionally inflated and deflated. The individual volume fractions were about 5% of the TLC. The intrapulmonary pressure in the primary bronchus, the Palv, and the lateral bronchial pressures were registered simultaneously and transmitted to a computer. For the fractionated filling and emptying of the lungs, the individual volume changes were carried out at an interval of 60 s in order to ensure a complete intrapulmonary pressure equalization. During both the static and dynamic measurements, it proved absolutely necessary to close the stumps of the pulmonary arteries and veins. When this was not done, a volume loss of 3%–5% was very frequently observed at the end of a static measurement. This volume loss, which was also described by *Niewoehner* et al. (1974), must therefore take place via the pulmonary vessels. This is to be expected in the case of positive intrapulmonary pressure, because the parenchymal lesions caused by the probes can lead to small artificial links between the bronchial and vascular system. The static measurements were performed several times and P-V diagrams were constructed. Control measurements were performed after completion of the dynamic measurements. After complete deflation of the lungs, the cannula at the bronchial stump was closed and the MV was determined plethysmographically by measuring the volume displacement of the lungs, taking into account their weight.

Detailed information concerning the method of dynamic measurements has already been communicated (*Wierich* 1978). During these measurements, the lungs were ventilated indirectly in an artificial thorax, using a piston pump we have developed ourselves whose frequency and stroke volume can be adjusted continuously. The probes for the measurement of Palv, Pbr, Ptr, and Ppl were connected via Teflon tubes with differential pressure transducers (Gould-Statham, PM 5 ETC). The pressure differences were not measured directly against the pressure in the main-stem bronchus, because it has been shown that despite equal chamber volumes these transducers give erroneous measurement signals under dynamic conditions, especially at high pressure differences. According to the author's own investigations, this was due to the fact that the form of both chambers and their connection to the membrane are completely different. The problem of obtaining an exact measurement of the differential pressures was solved by continuous electronic subtraction of the absolute pressure signals. For measurement of $\dot{V}$, pneumotachographs (Fleisch) operating in the low, verified linear measuring rage were used. Because of their low values, the corresponding pressure differences could be measured directly with differential pressure transducers. The transducers were connected to extremely constant, self-balancing dc amplifiers (type DCB-4B, IFD Company). These amplifiers are especially suitable because the amplification factor can be varied either continuously or in constant steps from 1:1 to 1:10. The input signal can be filtered to different extents without phase shift in order to suppress, e.g., interfering high-frequency mechanical oscillations from the drive of the ventilation pump. Besides the on-line computing of the $\dot{V}$ signal, electronic integration was performed. The volume signal (V) obtained in this way, the signal for the flow rate, and all pressures were registered for control on a multichannel recorder (Hellige) and stored on magnetic tape (Philips EL 1020). For optical control, a storage oscillograph (Tektronix 565) was included in the measurement system. The entire measurement system was regularly tested under static and dynamic conditions, for accuracy, linearity, phase displacement, and frequency response, in accordance with the recommendations of *Fry* (1959). The absolute pressure signals and the $\dot{V}$ signal were digitalized and put on line in a data acquisition system with a process computer (model DAS 10/4, IFD Company) which has 16 analogous inputs with a resolution of 11 bits and polarity signs. The level of the digital conversion rate can be preselected according to the breathing rate in the experimental lung, and the respective measurement ranges of the amplifier and the pneumotachograph can be fed in via the program. During the static measurements, the P-V diagrams with the values of Cst and Pst are calculated by the computer and constructed graphically by the computer on a X-Y plotter (Gould). Furthermore, the measurement values of V, Cst, and Pst are printed out (Texas 810) for numerous diagram points. Cst was established as the slope of the inflatory limb of the diagrams over the TV range, because the P-V relation is almost linear here. For the Pst measurements, the more readily reproducible deflation branch of the diagrams was used. Details of the computer programs have already been published elsewhere (*Wierich* 1978). The measurements presented in this paper were calculated in analogy with clinical methods. Thus Cdyn was calculated from the quotient of $\triangle V/\triangle P$ at zero flow. The flow resistances were determined from the quotient of P and $\dot{V}$. Rt was calculated using the values of Palv measured at three points and averaged. Rc was calculated analogously using the mean values of Pbr. Rp was determined from the difference of Rt and Rc.

For the measurements performed in this investigation, various lung volumes had to be determined (Table 1). TLC was defined at a static intrapulmonary pressure of 25 cm H_2O. MV measured in collapse is designated as RV because of the good agreement with clinical values. VC was defined as the difference of TLC and MV. The volume of 50% of VC was established as the FRC. The lungs were ventilated with a TV of 10% of the TLC in the region of the FRC.

In order to achieve an approximate comparability of the measurement values with clinical values, the results measured in one lung were recalculated to include both lungs. A volume ratio of 55%/45% between the right and left lung was used as the conversion factor in accordance with the data of *Kluge* (1967) and *Whimster* and *Macfarlane* (1974). According to the author's own results, which were occacionally obtained from both lungs, a corresponding mean ratio of 53%/47% (SD ± 2.94%) was revealed. For a comparison of the postmortem resistance values with clinical values, it was furthermore to be considered that the resistance above the bifurcation is not registered in the postmortem measurements on isolated lungs. According to the results of various investigations, this percentage of the airway resistance has been reported, with variations, to be between 25% and 50% of the total resistance (*Hyatt* and *Wilcox* 1961; *Ferris* et al. 1964; *Jaeger* and *Matthys* 1968). According to the results of some of our own postmortem measurements, a mean percentage of 42% (SD ± 12.5%) was revealed for the proportion of the flow resistance between the bifurcation and the mouth. For correction of the resistance, this mean value was used in the present paper.

In the statistical processing of the measurement values, linear correlations could be formed for the life span investigated. The statistical calculations, including the correlation coefficient r, SD, SEE, and Student's test were performed according to the specifications of *Sachs* (1973). Probability levels of $P < 0.05$ for differences between means and for correlations coefficients were considered significant.

On completion of the studies, the lungs were fixed with formalin solution (8%). Before this fixation, a small amount of dye was injected via the Pbr probes, in order to facilitate later checking of the exact localization of the tips of the probes. The results from lungs in which the probes had not been placed correctly have been omitted. In order to preserve the epithelium and not flush away any accumulations of mucus, the lungs were not fixed via the bronchial system but were perfused with the fixation solution via the trunk of the pulmonary artery. In general, there was passage of formalin into the airways and alveoli. The fixation was performed for 2 days, during which time the lungs were inflated constantly to a pressure of 25 cm H_2O via the primary bronchus. Central, middle, and peripheral sections from all segments were investigated histologically. Furthermore, paper-mounted whole lung sections were prepared according to the technique of *Gough* and *Wentworth* (1958).

IV. Results

The lung volume measured at a pressure of 25 cm H_2O was defined as TLC, and MV measured in collapse was defined as RV. For comparison of these postmortem volumes with normal clinical values, the following formulas specified by *Cara* (1958, quoted by *Ulmer* et al. 1976) and *Islam* and *Ulmer* (1977) were used:

$$TLC = Bl^3 \times 1.33$$
$$RV = (0.2 + 0.003 \times age) \times Bl^3 \qquad [Bl, \text{ body length (m)}]$$

In Fig. 2a, the percentage deviation of the values measured for TLC and RV from the normal clinical values are shown in relation to age. There is a slight positive correlation with age, deviating from the normal clinical values both for the group of normal lungs (N group) and for the lungs with bronchiolitis (B group). These age-dependent differ-

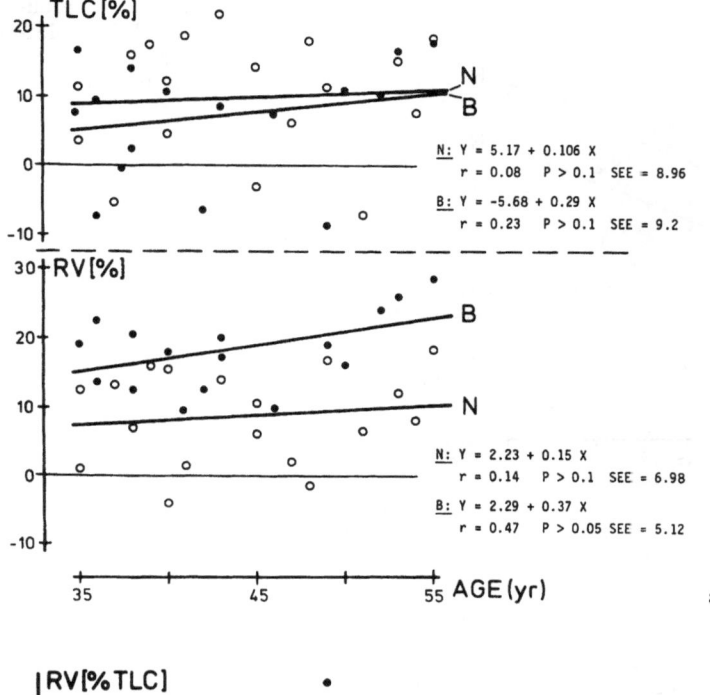

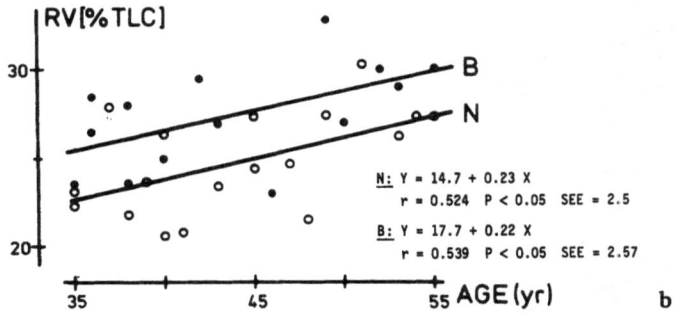

Fig. 2a. The percentage variations of *TLC* and *RV* from normal clinical values plotted against age. Clinical values according to the formulas given by *Cara* (1958) and *Islam and Ulmer* (1977). ○, values of normal lungs *(N)*; ●, values of lungs with bronchiolitis *(B)*. **b** Relations of percentage of *RV* in the volume of *TLC* and age. Symbols as in a

ences between clinical values and the author's own values are not statistically significant, however. There was a statistically significant difference (t = 4.44, $P < 0.001$) for the percentage deviation of RV between the mean values of the N group (+ 8.72% ± 6.8%) and the B group (+ 18.7 ± 5.57%). On the other hand, there were no statistically significant differences (t = 0.807, $P > 0.2$) between the two groups for the mean values of TLC. The mean absolute values of TLC were 7.84 ± 1.05 liters in the N group and 7.72 ± 0.81 liters in the B group. The mean absolute values of RV were 1.94 ± 0.27 liters and 2.13 ± 0.21 liters, respectively. In Fig. 2b, the percentage proportion of RV

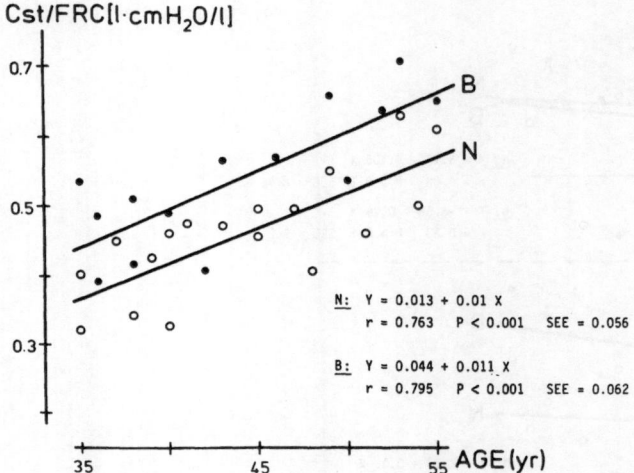

Fig. 3. Static compliance *(Cst/FRC)* plotted against age. Symbols as in Fig. 2a

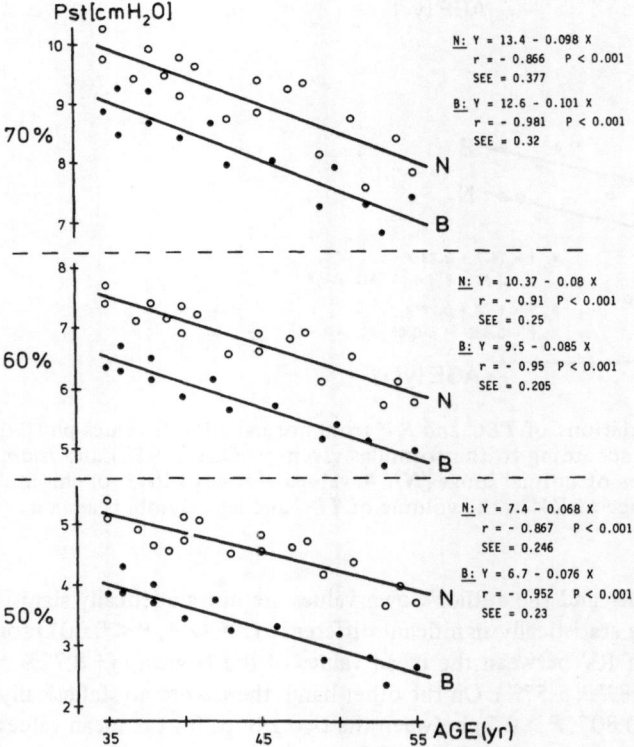

Fig. 4. Static elastic recoil pressure *(Pst)* at different lung volumes (%TLC) related to age. Symbols as in Fig. 2a

in TLC in relation to age is shown. The two groups had an almost identical positive correlation with age. The difference of the mean values is significant, with 27.4% ± 2.9% in the N group and 24.8% ± 2.8% in the B group (t = 2.5, $P < 0.02$).

The elastic properties of the lungs were investigated by measurement of Cst and Pst. The determinations of Cst were performed on the inflation limb of the P-V curves because there was a lineare P-V relation over the TV range. The values were specified because of the dependence between pulmonary volume and Cst. The FRC was chosen as

Table 2. Equations of regression lines, correlation coefficients, and standard errors at volumes of 80% and 90% TLC in normal lungs (N) and lungs with bronchiolitis (B)

	Regression	r	SEE
90% TLC	N: Y = 26.68 − 0.196 X	− 0.830	0.884
	B: Y = 27.02 − 0.200 X	− 0.878	0.823
80% TLC	N: Y = 18.72 − 0.140 X	− 0.840	0.606
	B: Y = 17.94 − 0.140 X	− 0.920	0.482

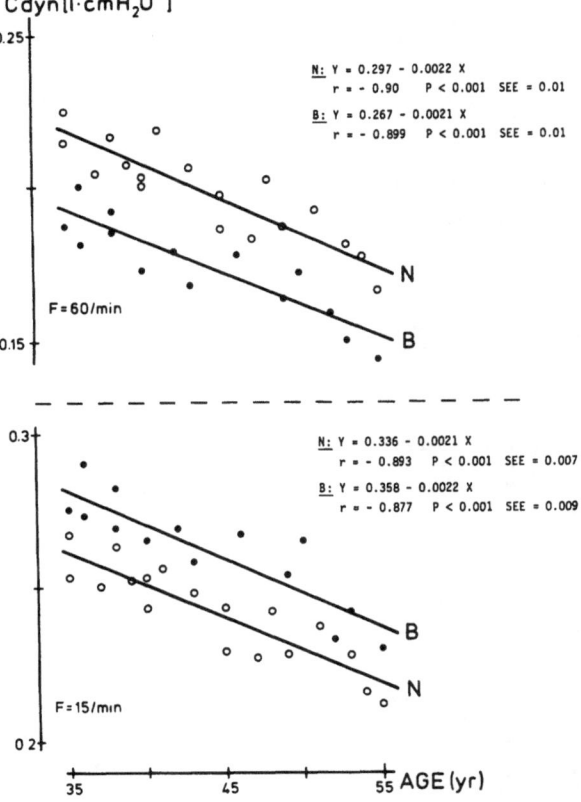

Fig. 5. Correlations between dynamic compliance *(Cdyn)* and age in forced breathing *(upper panel)* and in quiet breathing *(lower panel)*. Symbols as in Fig. 2a

reference volume in agreement with clinical data. As shown in Fig. 3, there were significant positive correlations between age and Cst in both the N group and the B group. The mean value of the B group is 0.439 ± 0.1, significantly above the mean value of 0.367 ± 0.08 measured in the N group ($t = 2.42, P < 0.05$). The measurements of Pst on the deflation limb of the P-V diagrams at different lung volumes (% TLC) were far more reproducible than the measurements of Cst. At all volumes measured, there was a significant negative correlation between age and Pst for both groups. The mean values of Pst were significantly below the values of the group of normal lungs at 50% ($t = 6.5$, $P < 0.0001$), 60% ($t = 4.32, P < 0.001$), and 70% ($t = 3.37, P < 0.01$) of TLC (Fig. 4). These significant differences were no longer observed at the higher inflation volumes of 80% ($t = 1.73$, $P > 0.05$) and 90% ($t = 0.63$, $P > 0.5$); regression equations and further statistical parameters are compiled in Table 2.

According to the results of the static measurements, the best separation for delimitation of the B group from the N group was provided by the measurements of Pst at volumes of 50% and 60% of TLC. It can clearly be seen from the results of Pst measurements that elasticity decreases with age and that there is a loss of ealsticity in the midinflation state in lungs with bronchiolitis.

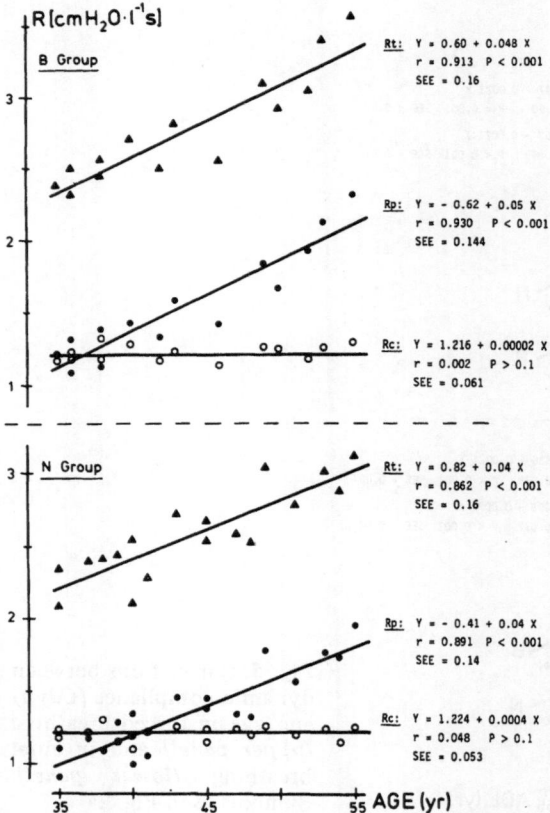

Fig. 6a. Airways resistances plotted against age in quiet breathing ($F = 15/\text{min}$). *Upper panel,* values of lungs with bronchiolitis *(B); lower panel,* values of normal lungs *(N).* ▲, Rt; ●, Rp; ○, Rc

The results of the dynamic measurements are restricted to presentation of the values in quiet breathing (F = 15/min) and forced breathing (F = 60/min). The individual values and the regression lines are shown in Fig. 5. There was a negative correlation between age and Cdyn for both groups. During quiet breathing, the mean value of the N group (0.241 ± 0.016), was significantly below the value of the B group (0.62 ± 0.017) (t = 3.57, $P < 0.002$). In forced breathing, a decrease of the measurement values was found in both groups; this was especially pronounced in the B group. The mean value of the B group at this frequency (0.173 ± 0.02) was significantly below the value of 0.199 ± 0.016 which was measured for the N group (t = 4.37, $P < 0.001$). With increase in frequency, the mean percentage decrease of Cdyn (ΔCdyn) in the B group (−52% ± 5.1%) was very significantly below the value of the N group (−21.7% ± 2.9%) (t = 21.25, $P < 0.001$).

The Rt, Rp, and Rc values were calculated from the quotients of the pressure differences and the flow rate. The mean values of Rt, Rp, and Rc, the mean percentage of Rp in Rt, and the mean percentage increase of the resistances with increase in frequency (ΔR) are displayed in Table 3 with the significant statisitcal parameters. In Fig. 6a, the individual values of Rt, Rp, and Rc measured in quiet breathing are shown in relation to age with the regression lines. There is a significant positive correlation between age and Rt, as well as Rp, for both groups, but there was no correlation with age for Rc.

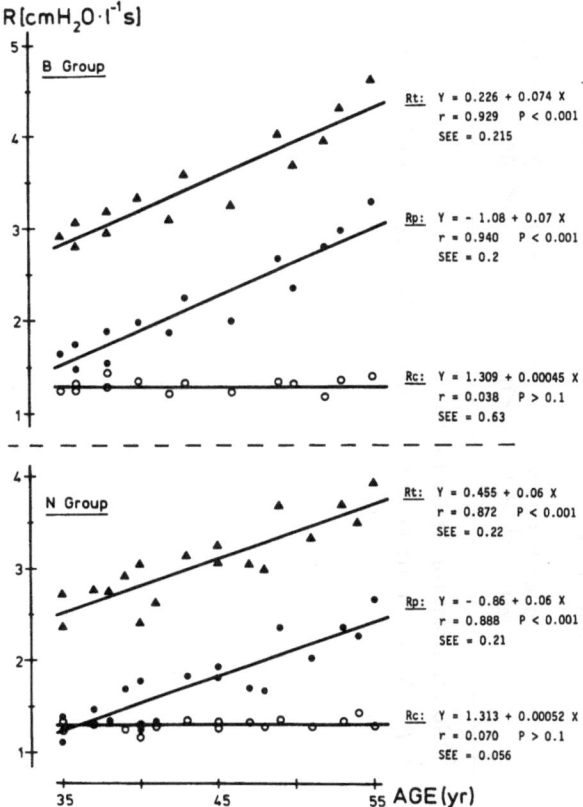

Fig. 6b. Airways resistances and age in forced brathing ($F = 60$/min). Representation and symbols as in a. Scale of the Y-axis is different from a

Table 3. Statistical parameters for airways resistances (Rt, Rp, Rc), the percentages of Rp in Rt at different breathing frequencies (F), and the frequency-dependent increase (ΔR)

	Rt (F = 15/min)	Rp (F = 15/min)	Rc	Rt (F = 60/min)	Rp (F = 60/min)	Rc	Rp (%Rt) F=15/min	Rp (%Rt) F=60/min	ΔRt (%)	ΔRp (%)	ΔRc(%)
Normal Mean	2.58	1.37	1.208	3.06	1.78	1.28	52.66	57.21	18.34	28.56	6.51
Slope	0.04	0.04	0.0004	0.06	0.06	0.00052	0.792	0.81	0.44	0.54	0.012
Correlation Coefficient (r)	0.862	0.891	0.048 [a]	0.872	0.888	0.056 [a]	0.890	0.883	0.810	0.772	0.085 [a]
Bronchio-litis Mean	2.77	1.55	1.216	3.47	2.18	1.295	55.38	61.86	25.03	39.79	6.59
Slope	0.048	0.05	0.00002	0.074	0.07	0.00045	0.73	0.78	0.431	0.47	0.032
Correlation Coefficient (r)	0.913	0.930	0.061[a]	0.929	0.940	0.038[a]	0.913	0.927	0.860	0.724	0.203[a]
Student's t test t	1.580	2.131	0.4118	2.327	2.284	0.396	1.386	2.189	5.340	7.740	0.216
P [b]	>0.05	<0.05	>0.5	<0.05	<0.05	>0.5	>0.1	<0.05	<0.001	<0.0001	>0.5

[a] No significant correlation to age

[b] $P < 0.05$, statistical significance of the difference between the group of normal lungs and the group with bronchiolitis. See text for explanation

The age-dependent increase of Rt and Rp is roughly the same in both groups. As can be seen from Table 3, the only significant difference between the N group and the B group (t = 2.13, $P < 0.05$), is for the mean value of Rp. Although the mean percentage of Rp in Rt is markedly raised in the B group, the difference from the value of the N group is not significant (t = 1.38, $P > 0.1$). In forced breathing, the values of resistances given in Fig. 6b were measured. There are significant correlations with age also at this frequency for Rt and Rp, but not for Rc. Statistical comparison of the mean values shows that there are significant differences between the two groups for Rp and Rt. There are also now significant differences between the two groups for the percentage share of Rp in Rt (Table 3). The percentage increase observed with rise in frequency is very marked for Rp and also for Rt in both groups. The mean values of the percentage increases of Rp and Rt in the B group are significantly above the values in the N group, but for Rc only a relatively slight percentage difference could be demonstrated between the two groups, not attaining statistical significance (see Table 3).

The percentage of Rp in Rt is regarded as very low, and according to the results of some recent experimental studies on normal lungs and on lungs with slight pathological alterations it is independent of age. However, the results of the measurements with a mean Rp of over 50% show that the percentage of Rp is by no means low. In Fig. 7, the individual values of the percentage share of Rp are given. A roughly similar significant correlation with age is found in both groups. As can be seen from Table 3, the mean value of the B group is significantly above that of the N group in forced breathing.

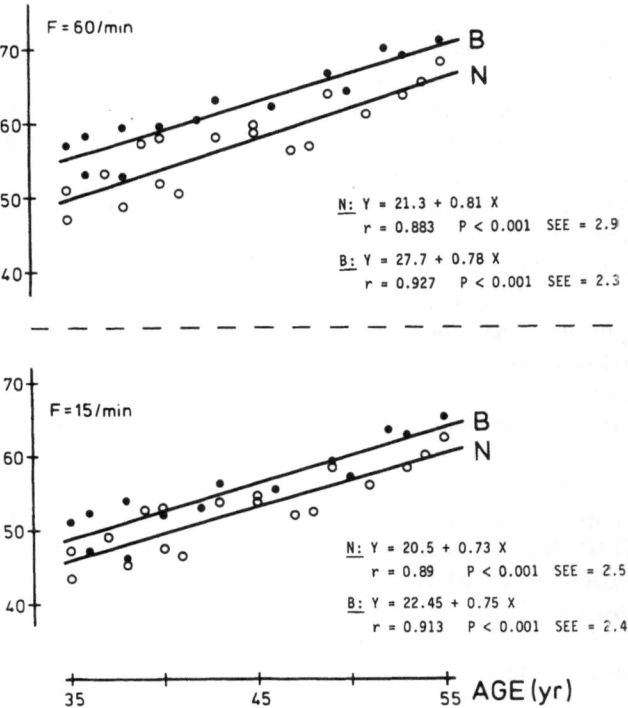

Fig. 7. Percentages of *Rp* in *Rt* (*Rt* = 100%) plotted against age. *Upper panel,* values in forced breathing; *lower panel,* values in quiet breathing. Symbols as in Fig. 2a

It can be seen from the graphical representation of the resistances (Fig. 6a, b), that the variations and the age dependent of Rt must be caused by alterations in the Rp. This assumption was checked by calculations of the correlations between individual values of Rp and Rt. For the N group, the correlation coeffecient in quiet breathing is $r = 0.880$ and in forced breathing, $r = 0.896$ ($P < 0.001$). The values from the B group were $r = 0.886$ and $r = 0.893$ ($P < 0.001$). On the other hand, in neither group were significant correlations found between the measurement values of Rc and Rt. It follows from the results of the resistance measurement that Rt is very substantially dependent on Rp in normal lungs and in lungs with chronic bronchiolitis. According to the results of the dynamic measurements, the best separation between the B group and N group is provided by measurement of the decrease in Cdyn with increasing frequency.

V. Discussion

Measurements of airway dynamics in isolated lungs are meaningful only when it can be assumed that significant alterations of the parameters of airway dynamics do not occur postmortem in the time period of these investigations.

The fact that pulmonary perfusion is lacking in such investigations might lead to effects on airway dynamics. As could be demonstrated by *Frank* (1959), *Frank* et al. (1959), *Gianelli* et al. (1967) and *Stemmler* and *DuBois* (1968), the lack of blood flow in the lungs does not appear to lead to significant repercussions on airway dynamics. According to the investigations by *McFadden* et al. (1970) and *Colebatch* and *Mitchell* (1971), and according to the results of investigations presented here, which in some cases commenced as soon as 30 min after death and were continued at regular intervals over 36 h, no alterations of airway dynamics are to be expected in this period of time. If autolytic processes were to lead to functionally significant repercussions on the properties of the fibrous tissue or the surfactant, then progressive and readily discernible alterations of parameters of airway dynamics would result.

For a standardized measurement of the parameters of airway dynamics of healthy and pathologically altered lungs, certain lung volumes and equivalent ventilation conditions would have to be established (Table 1). To establish lung volumes such as RV and TLC, it was desirable for practical and methodological reasons to define these volumes via a certain static pressure. The problems of satisfactorily defining lung volumes in accordance with vital conditions in postmortem investigations of airway dynamics have been emphasized by numerous authors (*Hartung* 1959; *Petty* et al. 1965; *Park* et al. 1969; *Stigol* et al. 1972; *Niewoehner* and *Kleinerman* 1974; *Pare* et al. 1978; *Thurlbeck* 1979).

In contrast to the author's own investigations, in comparable studies the TLC was mostly defined at a static intrapulmonary pressure of less than 25 cm H_2O. In general, this pressure was 20 cm H_2O (*Pratt* and *Klugh* 1961; *Hartung* and *Büttinghaus* 1967; *Silvers* et al. 1972, 1974; *Stigol* et al. 1972). In the investigations on isolated human lungs performed by *Niewoehner* and *Kleinerman* (1974), the TLC was defined at a static intrapulmonary pressure of 25 cm H_2O. In investigations on human autopsy lungs, *Thurlbeck* (1979) also defined the TLC at a static intrapulmonary pressure of 25 cm H_2O.

Most authors state that the minimum volume after deflation of the lungs is the most accurate reference parameter in determination of postmortem lung volumes, because this volume revealed good correlations with the clinical values of RV (*Pratt* et al. 1965; *Wohl* et al. 1968; *Pare* et al. 1978). The author's own measurements revealed a good agreement with normal clinical values for RV in the N group; the average difference was + 8.7% ± 6.8%. In the B group, the percentage deviation of normal clinical values (+ 18.7% ± 5.6%) was very much higher; the difference from the mean value of the N group was highly significant (t = 4.44, $P < 0.001$). On the other hand, the mean percentage deviation of TLC from the normal clinical values in the N group (+ 4.85% ± 8.7%), was somewhat higher than the value of the N group (+ 7.3% ± 9.1%). The difference between these mean values was not significant (t = 0.82, $P > 0.2$). The good correlation between the volumes of TLC and the normal clinical values defined postmortem in our investigations is in agreement with the recent experimental results of *Thurlbeck* (1979).

It was shown in an earlier study that surfactant damage in adult lungs leads to significant decreases in RV, but not to repercussions on TLC (*Wierich* 1980). The significant increase in RV demonstrated here in slight chronic bronchiolitis makes it evident that this parameter can be regarded as a subtle indicator for the presence of slight pathological changes in the lungs. It is also shown that TLC defined at a static pressure of 25 cm H_2O for normal lungs and for lungs with slight pathological changes constitutes the safest reference volume for postmortem investigations.

A mean value of 25% ± 2.8% was revealed in the N group for the percentage of RV in TLC. This value agrees astonishingly well with the corresponding mean clinical value of 24% specified by *Ulmer* et al. (1976) for the 35th to 55th years of life. The positive correlation between age and these values also corresponds to the clinical data. In the B group, this value (27.4% ± 8.5%) was significantly above the value in the N group (t = 2.5, $P < 0.02$). The significant increase in RV in chronic bronchiolitis can be explained by an increased tendency of the bronchioli to collapse. In analogy to clinical measurements of the closing volume, this results in an increase in RV in lungs with chronic bronchiolitis.

The measurement of Pst at different lung volumes (% TLC) revealed measurement values which were significantly higher than the values of normal lungs at volumes of 50%, 60%, and 70% TLC. The values of Cst related to the volume of FRC also showed a mean value in the bronchiolitis group which was significantly higher than the mean value of normal lungs. It was noticeable that the significance level between the two groups was far higher for Pst (especially at low TLC) than for Cst. The correlations with age were also far more rigid for Pst than for Cst (cf. Figs. 3, 4).

By measuring the static parameters Pst and Cst, information can be obtained both in vivo and in vitro on the elastic recoil pressure of the lungs. It has been shown that the results of Pst measurements have far better reproducibility and lead to more accurate results than is possible from determinations of Cst.

The recoil pressure of the lung results from a complex interaction between various elements. The fiber system of the lung has an overwhelming importance for the elasticity, and the surface tension at the alveolar interface also has a significant effect. As could be shown by static measurements on isolated lungs, roughly 30%–40% of Pst is attributable to surface tension forces even in adults (*Kluge* 1967; *Wierich* 1980). A corresponding effect of the surface tension forces on the dynamic process of breathing cannot be inferred from this result, however. On the contrary, it is probable that the surface tension forces have less importance in adults under dynamic conditions than in newborns (*Saibene* and *Mead* 1969; *Wierich* 1980).

Of the morphological structures, it is the elastic fibers which have essential importance for elasticity and elastic recoil of the lungs at physiological lung volumes (*Linser* 1900; *Dubreuil* et al. 1936; *Boyden* 1953; *Krahl* 1959; *Collet* and *Des Biens* 1974). Moreover, the elasticity of the lungs is determined not only by the individual properties of the elastic fibers, but also by their arrangement and interaction (*Carton* et al. 1962; *Hoppin* et al. 1975).

In the lower and midinflation state, the only slightly extensible collagen fibers have a subordinate importance for the elasticity of the lungs. These fibers are mainly regarded as limiting elements in high-inflation states of the lungs, in which the static P-V diagram flattens towards the pressure axis (*Hartung* 1960; *Giese* 1961; *Mead* 1961; *Pierce* et al. 1961a, b; *Radford* 1964; *Milic-Emili* 1974). In the inflation of normal lungs and lungs with bronchiolitis, a corresponding kink in the static P-V curve could be demonstrated in every case when the TLC was reached. It follows from this observation and from the fact that no significant differences were found for TLC that damage to the collagen fibers in the lungs cannot be present in bronchiolitis.

The greatly lowered Pst values at midlung volumes as well as the (less significantly) raised Cst values clearly indicate that damage to elastic fibers must be present in the lungs with bronchiolitis. This cannot be demonstrated morphologically, as is the case, for example, in emphysematous lungs. From the observation that the differences of Pst were most marked at midlung volume and became less with increasing volume, it can be inferred that elastic fibers are functionally damaged at moderate stretching in the cases with bronchiolitis.

The value of 0.2 was specified by *Ulmer* et al. (1976) as the normal value for Cst in clinical investigations. The mean value which was obtained in normal autopsy lungs, 0.459, is more than 100% above this normal clinical value. This discrepancy is likely to be essentially attributable to the fact that static measurement conditions can only be approximately realized in clinical studies. This is because it takes a certain time for the intrapulmonary pressure to equalize, especially in the periphery, even in healthy lungs. In the normal isolated human lung, a constant intrapulmonary and alveolar pressure is established during fractionated deflation after about 15 s in each case. In obstructive pulmonary diseases, this time interval is very much larger. Even when no pressure equilibration has yet taken place in the lung periphery, flow resistances are also included in the Cst value. Furthermore, it is known that in the clinical measurement of Pst, an unsystematic error of at least ± 20% is to be expected because of the different positions of the esophageal catheter and due to the muscular tonus of the esophagus. It is therefore understandable that clinical measurements of Cst become comparatively inaccurate and the values obtained are lower than is the case in solated lungs. Furthermore, it is to be expected that in clinical measurements of Pst in comparable lung volumes, the corresponding pressure values must be above the values measured post mortem.

Turner et al. (1968) reported on clinical measurements of Pst carried out in 44 healthy test subjects. In contrast to other studies, a compilation of the measured Pst

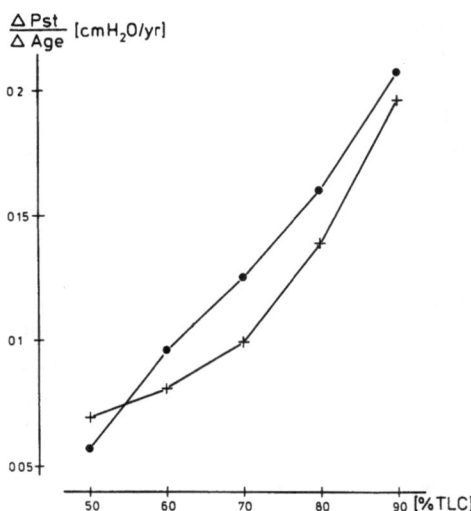

$\frac{\Delta \, Pst}{\Delta \, Age}$ [cmH₂O/yr]

Fig. 8. Slopes of the regression lines of *Pst* at different lung volumes (*%TLC*). Comparison of the author's own results obtained in normal lungs (+) with the clinical values (●) of *Turner* et al. (1968). Reproduced with permission of the American Physiological Society. See text for explanation

values in table form was presented. A comparison of these values with the author's own values shows that the values measured postmortem are lower throughout than those determined clinically. Moreover, the scatter of the individual values is appreciably wider. A comparison of the slopes of the regression lines for Pst at different lung volumes with the corresponding measurement values in normal lungs is given in Fig. 8. It is shown that these values agree relatively well. In contrast to the author's own results, which revealed an exponential relation between volume and pressure gradient, this relation is approximately linear according to the result of the clinical measurements. A nonlinear relationship between the volume and pressure difference was also demonstrated experimentally by *Salazar* and *Knowles* (1964) and *Niewoehner* et al. (1975).

In agreement with the clinical investigations by *Turner* et al. (1968), it can also be stated that there is an inverse relationship between age and elasticity of the lungs. The fact that the measurement values showed correlations with age in the group with bronchiolitis which were almost identical to the values of normal lungs proves that a uniform damage to the elastic fibers must be present in these lungs which summates to the normal age-dependent loss in elasticity. A decrease in pulmonary elasticity with increasing age was also demonstrated by numerous other authors (*Frank* et al. 1957; *Hartung* 1957; *Pierce* and *Ebert* 1958).

A morphologically demonstrable change in normal lungs due to age was described by *Hieronymi* (1961), *Ryan* et al. (1965), *Wagner* (1965), and *Otto* (1970). The diameter of the alveolar ducts increases with aging, and the alveoli become wider and shallower. This can readily be checked by experienced investigators using whole-lung sections after standardized fixation of the lungs. However, no functional interferences can be made from this observation because the above authors have performed their measurements on lungs fixed in the inspiration position. A "static observation" was thus involved. This does not allow a decision as to whether the results are the consequence of fibers which were already elongated in collapse, or whether they are the consequence of disturbed fiber elasticity.

In an extensive investigation on the dry weight of normal lungs, *Hieronymi* (1961) did not find any differences between the 20th and 70th year of life. Chemical analyses by *Pierce* et al. (1961a, b), *Pierce* and *Ebert* (1965), and *John* and *Thomas* (1972) did not reveal any alterations in the proportion of collagen or elastin or of the fiber protein in the lung tissue with age. Thus it can be assumed from the measurements of the dry weight and the result of these chemical analyses that the mass of the lung tissue does not increase with age. The increase in volume with age at a given recoil pressure must therefore be attributed to an alteration of the elastic properties of the fiber system, in the sense of a slackening.

There are only scanty descriptions in the literature of morphologically detectable alterations in the elastic and collagen fibers of the aging lung. *Wright* (1961) using light microscopy, found degenerative alterations to the elastic fibers of the lungs of aged subjects, but according to the result of the electron-microscopic investigations by *Adamson* (1968), the fibrous tissue of young people does not differ from the fibrous tissue of lungs of the elderly.

It remains to be noted that the cause of the loss in elasticity of the lungs with increasing age has not been sufficiently verified. Nevertheless, it is possible that an aging mechanism affecting the individual fibers or the interaction of the fibers, which cannot be demonstrated morphologically, is present here.

The dynamic investigations were performed at various frequencies. Of the parameters measured, the values of dynamic compliance as well as the results of the resistance measurements were presented. Only values which had been measured under comparable standardized conditions were presented.

Under dynamic conditions, the compliance Cdyn as a quotient of the pressure and volume change at the time of the flow reversal ($\dot{V} = 0$) cannot give exact information on pulmonary elasticity, because compliance is by definition bound to a static system. It was already indicated that in clinical measurements an incomplete pressure equilibration in the peripheral airways can lead to inclusion of flow resistances in the compliance value. Under dynamic conditions, this influence is naturally very much more manifest. Although the parameter of the dynamic P-V quotient is a functional parameter, the misleading term Cdyn introduced by *Comroe* et al. (1962) has gained general acceptance. However, according to the results of numerous investigations, this parameter can give approximate information on the elastic properties of the lungs only under certain conditions (*Paine* 1940; *Dean* and *Visscher* 1941; *Otis* et al. 1950; *Mount* 1955; *Mead* 1961; *Staub* 1963; *Ulmer* et al. 1976).

This observation is confirmed by an analysis of the results reported in the present paper. For normal lungs, there was a rigid correlation between the values of Cst and values of Cdyn in quiet breathing ($r = 0.842, P < 0.001$). The corresponding correlation was very much poorer ($r = 0.553, P < 0.05$) in lungs with bronchiolitis. It follows from this that the values of Cdyn still contain adequately accurate information concerning the elasticity of normal lungs in quiet breathing. In cases with bronchiolitis, this information is less, and other parameters of influence become evident. For the values of Cdyn measured during forced breathing, no correlations with static functional parameters could be demonstrated.

Numerous investigations on the parameters of influence contained in Cdyn have revealed that measurement of Cdyn and in particular its relation to the breathing rate, enables judgment of the distribution of the ventilation volume in the lungs (*Fowler* et al. 1952; *Otis* et al. 1956; *Mead* 1961; *Gomez* 1965; *Woolcock* et al. 1969; *Bobbaers* et al. 1975; *Ulmer* et al. 1976).

The ventilation volume can be distributed evenly or unevenly in the airspaces of the lungs. In this context, the terms ventilatory homogeneity and ventilatory inhomogeneity were coined (*Mead* et al. 1955; *Otis* et al. 1956; *Gomez* 1965). According to the results of the model concepts and investigations of *Otis* et al. (1956), *Hogg* et al. (1968), and *Woolcock* et al. (1969), it is assumed that normally there is an equal and frequency-independent product of R and C components in peripheral lung units (R x C = time constant t). The authors further concluded that regional differences in the elastic components and diseases of the *peripheral* airways lead to a frequency-dependent fall in Cdyn, i.e., to ventilatory inhomogeneity.

However, the author's own studies have already revealed a significant decrease in Cdyn with elevation of the frequency in normal lungs. In the group of normal lungs, there was a 21.7% mean decrease in Cdyn. It is therefore to be assumed that the ideal case of equal peripheral R-C products assumed by *Otis* et al. (1956) is not present even in the normal lung. The statement that a decrease in Cdyn with rising frequency is a manifestation of a disturbance of ventilatory distribution is not thereby restricted.

In the group of lungs with bronchiolitis, a 52% decrease in Cdyn was revealed with a rise in frequency. The difference between the mean values of the two groups is highly significant. This result confirms the assumption that alterations at the bronchioli lead to ventilatory and mechanical inhomogeneities with a strong effect of the frequency on Cdyn. An adequate morphological substrate, such as is found in emphysema with histologically recognizable loss of radial traction of the bronchioli, cannot be demonstrated for the minimal wall changes in chronic bronchiolitis, however. The fact, demonstrated by means of static measurements, that in the case with bronchiolitis the elastic fibers in the walls and in the adjacent tissue of the bronchioli must be functionally damaged, allows the conclusion that in these lungs, the stability of the bronchioli is severely damaged and must be reduced.

A statistically significant correlation between age and Cdyn in quiet breathing was found for both normal lungs and lungs with bronchiolitis. This correlation was to be expected, since a significant correlation was found between the values of Cst and Cdyn.

Numerous clinical investigations are unsuitable for comparison with the values presented here, because Cdyn is not given as an absolute value, but rather as a percentage deviation of the values of Cst, which differ from each other clinically and postmortem. The usable data concerning normal clinical values from comparable age groups display a relatively large variation. This is attributable to differences between the individual investigations, the methods, and the equipment used. *Comroe* (1968) and *Ulmer* et al. (1976) specified the normal value of Cdyn as 0.2. Other authors specified values of 0.15, 0.12, 0.19, 0.23, and 0.204 (*Frank* et al. 1957; *Hamm* et al. 1962; *Macklem* and *Becklage* 1963; *Bachofen* 1967; *Forkert* et al. 1975). The mean of these normal clinical values of Cdyn in normal breathing is 0.2. The mean value measured post mortem in normal lungs was 0.242. With a difference of less than 20%, there is thus very good agreement between the mean normal clinical values and the values of normal lungs determined post mortem. In agreement with the author's own results, it is also known that according to the results of clinical investigations, there is a negative correlation between age and Cdyn (*Frank* et al. 1956; *Pierce* and *Ebert* 1958; *Albright* and *Bondurant* 1965; *Woolcock* et al. 1969; *Seaton* et al. 1972; *Begin* et al. 1975).

The flow resistances were measured separately at the various frequencies as Rt, Rp, and Rc. A correlation of Rc with age was found neither in normal lungs nor in the group with bronchiolitis. Significant differences could not be demonstrated for the mean values of the two groups. The increase in Rc was only slight and roughly equal in the two groups even with increase in frequency (cf. Table 3).

Statistically significant positive correlations between age and Rt, as well as Rp, were found both for normal lungs and for the group with bronchiolitis. Only a few indications of a clinically determined correlation between age and Rt are found in the literature. *Pierce* et al. (1958), *Amrein* et al. (1969), and *Dosman* et al. (1975) did not find any positive correlation between age and Rt. On the other hand, positive correlations between age and Rt were demonstrated by *Dubois* et al. (1956), *Frank* et al. (1957), *Allen* and *Sabin* (1971), *Ulmer* et al. (1976), and *Islam* et al. (1978). The possible cause of the increase in Rt with increasing age is exclusively alterations in the lung periphery due to age, both in normal lungs and in lungs with bronchiolitis. This is because the same kind of age dependence could also be demonstrated for Rp, but not for Rc. A physiological ectasia of the alveolar ducts is not an explanation for this, since it only becomes evident in old age and would then be more likely to lead to a decrease in Rp. The reason for the positive correlations between age and Rt, as well as Rp, is doubtless revealed in part by the observation that the elastic recoil pressure decreases with age in the normal case and in bronchiolitis, and that the elastic recoil pressure in lungs with bronchiolitis was markedly lowered. The decrease in elastic recoil with increasing age was proved by the results of the static measurements as well as by the functional damage to the elastic fibers assumed in lungs with bronchiolitis. It leads to an increased radial traction with a declining wall stability of the membranous bronchioli. In consequence, there is an increase in the respiratory deformability of these airways with a corresponding rise in Rp (*Wierich* 1977). With age and in bronchiolitis, a functional alteration of the airway geometry of peripheral airways would thus be present which cannot be demonstrated morphologically.

Niewoehner et al. (1974) were able to demonstrate a further cause for the age-dependent increase of Rp according to the result of morphometric investigations on normal lungs. According to the result of this investigation, beyond the third decade of life there is a statistically significant negative correlation between age and mean bronchiolar diameter. This decrease of mean bronchiolar diameter likewise explains an inevitable increase in Rp (cf. Fig. 1b).

According to the results of static measurements, it was postulated that in bronchiolitis the significantly higher values of RV are attributable to weakness of the bronchioli, with increased tendency to collapse due to damage to elastic fibers. A dependence between RV and Rp would thus be expected. As can be seen from Fig. 9, there is such a significant correlation between the percentage deviations of RV from the predicted clinical values and the Rp measured in breathing. It follows from this that there must be a defective stability of the bronchioli in bronchiolitis. This causes raised Rp values and leads to a rise in RV via a raised tendency to collapse. This observation agrees with theoretical reflections and clinical investigations on the closing volume,

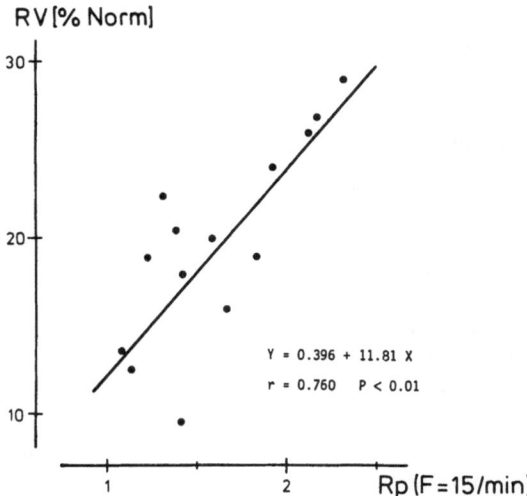

RV [% Norm]

30

20

10

Y = 0.396 + 11.81 X

r = 0.760   P < 0.01

1   2   Rp (F =15/min)

Fig. 9. Correlation between percentage deviations of *RV* from the clinical normal values and *Rp* during quiet breathing for lungs with bronchiolitis. See text for explanation

which is regarded as a sensitive parameter for diagnosis of pathological alterations in peripheral airways (*Begin* et al. 1975; *Buist* et al. 1973; *McCarthy* et al. 1972).

With increasing breathing frequency, a different percentage increase of Rt and Rp was observed (cf. Table 3). In quiet breathing, there was a significant difference only for Rp between normal lungs and lungs with bronchiolitis. In forced breathing, there was a significant difference between the two groups also for Rt, due to the large increase of Rp. There was a nonlinear correlation between $\dot{V}$ and Palv with increasing frequency in both groups. However, in the lungs with bronchiolitis the increase in Palv at the same $\dot{V}$ was steeper than in normal lungs. It follows from this observation that turbulent flow can also occur in peripheral airways in normal lungs, but in particular in bronchiolitis. According to the conventional model concepts, it is assumed that turbulences do not occur in the lung periphery, because the flow rates are low. However, the significance of the Hagen-Poiseoille law and the Reynold number, which is determined by numerous parameters of influence, is often not recognized. According to the results of numerous investigations, it is known that even at low frequencies the laminar flow described by the Hagen-Poiseoille law is not present in the bronchial system (*West* and *Hugh-Jones* 1959; *Long* et al. 1962; *Peslin* 1969; *Olson* et al. 1970; *Finucane* et al. 1975; *Drazen* et al. 1976). Besides the fact that this principle is basically only valid for stationary flow, and not for the periodic flow in breathing, it has been proved that turbulences can be induced in any region of the bronchial system by branching or other irregularities in the luminal shape of membranous bronchioli. This fact can readily be derived from the principles of engineering flow theories (*Bohl* 1975). It is to be assumed that the more severe turbulences in bronchiolitis are caused by respiratory-synchronous deformations of the more poorly stabilized bronchioli.

The first calculations on the distribution of the flow resistances in the bronchial tree were communicated by *Rohrer* (1915). According to the result of his own morphological investigations on collapsed unfixed lung tissue, *Rohrer* calculated that about 92% of Rp must be localized in bronchioles with a diameter of 2 mm. The result of this exceedingly thorough investigation was generally recognized.

The reflections of *Rohrer* on the distribution of flow resistance in the airways were called into question by the results of *Weibel* (1963) and *Horsefield* and *Cumming* (1968a, b), who performed morphometric investigations on human lungs fixed in the inspiratory state. The latter authors determined that *Rohrer* had underestimated the diameter of the peripheral airways. In contrast to *Weibel, Horsefield* and *Cumming* were able to demonstrate furthermore that the dichotomous branching of the bronchial tree is not symmetrical, but irregular. Theoretical reflections by *Kesic* and *Jaffrin* (1972), *Olson* et al. (1970), and *Pedley* et al. (1970) on the distribution of the flow rate in the bronchi and bronchioli, based on the morphometric measurements by *Weibel* (1963) and *Horsefield* and *Cumming* (1968a, b), revealed that the flow rate and the flow resistance in the membranous bronchioli must be very low, in contrast to the flow resistance in the cartilaginous bronchi. This analysis was supported and generally accepted after *Macklem* and *Mead* (1967) were able to demonstrate by the retrograde catheter technique in animal lungs and in two isolated human lungs that the flow resistance in the peripheral airways with a diameter of less than 2 mm only amounts to about 10% of Rp. Further investigations were performed by *Macklem* et al. (1968) and *Hogg* et al. (1970) on a total of ten isolated human lungs. These investigations revealed a similarly low percentage for Rp. Despite the relatively low size of the random sample, these authors came to the conclusion that the percentage of Rp can normally be ignored and is not age-dependent in the adult lung.

The measurements presented in this study are in clear contradiction to the results of the authors cited above. The mean proportion of Rp was 52% in the group of normal lungs during quiet breathing and 55% during forced breathing. In addition, there was an unequivocal positive correlation between age and Rp. The clinical investigations by *Silvers* et al. (1974), as well as the indirect Rp measurements performed by *Niewoehner* and *Kleinerman* (1974) on isolated human lungs, also revealed a high proportion for Rp and showed a correlation with age.

The question arises of whether there was a systematic error in the author's own measurements, leading to a substantial underestimation of Rc with an overestimation of Rp. On the other hand, both the results of the morphometric investigations by *Weibel* (1963) and the experimental results of *Macklem* and *Mead* (1967) and *Hogg* et al. (1970) should be considered critically.

An erroneous measurement of airway resistance could be attributable to too high a value for TV (defined as 10% of TLC) with too high a flow rate. However, this source of error appears improbable, because the values of TV defined in this way are clearly below the corresponding clinical values (*Ulmer* et al. 1976).

The calculation of Rt from the mean value of at least three Palvs directly measured in the author's own material can only be correct when these three pressures are representative of the Palv of the whole lung, indirectly determined clinically as an integral value. Single measurements with up to six Palv probes revealed a maximum difference between the individual Palvs of 22% in normal lungs and in lungs with bronchiolitis. This difference was on average only 11% in the measurement of the Palvs, which was performed in the usual way at three defined sites. That this difference is larger when many probes are used is attributable to several factors: the horizontal pressure gradient becomes effective because of the localization of such numerous probes and an isotropic volume change is not certain, especially in the dependent parts of the lung. However, the horizontal pressure gradient is far lower in the isolated lung (which is largely empty of blood) than is the case in vivo. This relatively lower pressure difference between the three measurement sites of the Palv did not have such a significant influence in the author's own studies on the determination of Rt and Rp performed via the mean value of Palv that it would explain the pronounced differences from the results of the other investigators. It is to be noted here that in the experiments of *Macklem* and *Mead* (1967) and *Hogg* et al. (1970) the Palv was not measured directly. For the values of lateral bronchiolar pressure measured at two sites in the bronchial system, no significant or systematic differences were found.

The localization of the lateral bronchial pressure probes proved to be correct in each of the evaluated cases when checked after fixation of the lungs. The technique by which the probes were introduced (cf. p. 5–6) is undoubtedly suitable to ensure a very much more exact and standardized localization of the probe tips from lung to lung than the method described by *Macklem* and *Mead* (1967). A further difference from the investigations cited above is that the probes were not inserted into collapsed lungs, but that the lungs were kept in the midinflatory position. It is conceivable that in the author's studies, the bronchial probe extended systematically further into the periphery than was the case in the investigations by *Macklem* and *Mead* (1967). If this was the case, however, a lower Rc with a higher percentage Rp would have resulted.

In contrast to the author's own studies, in the investigations by *Macklem* and *Mead* (1967) and *Hogg* et al. (1970) the necessary prerequisite of exact standardized measurement of lateral pressure was undoubtedly not met. This pressure measurement was performed on the human lungs by the above authors in such a way that a probe with an end widened in the form of a funnel to a diameter of about 2 mm must have been inserted into a bronchus with an internal diameter larger than 2 mm. According to the authors, the widened probe end is alleged to have fully closed the ostium of one bronchus (wedged position). The pressure which can be measured in this way corresponds to the pressure in the bronchus preceding the branch blocked at its exit point by the probe; the internal diameter of the bronchus would have to be larger than 2 mm. Because perpendicular bronchial branching is not found in healthy lungs, the pressure measurement could not be performed by measurement of the lateral pressure, which by definition has to be made perpendicularly to the flow axis. Instead, the pressure must be measured at a different angle to the flow axis, which depends on the FRC and alters synchronously during ventilation. In their original paper, *Macklem* and *Mead* (1967) also described the observation of a varying ventilation of the lung tissue distal to the bronchus blocked by the probe end. In the opinion of these authors, the ventilation took place via collateral airways. Thus the possibility does not appear to be excluded that besides a movement of the probe end synchronous with ventilation, the probe tip could also have been displaced into the lumen of the larger bronchus when the air which was trapped in the blocked lung tissue had developed an appropriate pressure. The investigations by *Macklem* and *Mead* (1967) differ from the author's own experimental design in one more important point: the lungs were ventilated directly and with unphysiologically high frequencies of a maximum of 600/min, produced by a loudspeaker. Even if the resonance frequency of the lungs was reached at such high frequencies, the possibility cannot be excluded that elastic components influenced the results even at this frequency because of the complex interrelationships of the R and C components. Because a normal ventilation was not performed in this high-frequency oscillation of the lungs, only minimal volumes have been moved during the measurements. These probably did not enable an exact registration of the flow resistances. In the measurement of the lateral bronchial pressure, local turbulences at the probe tip can likewise lead to an erroneous determination of Rp. In the studies by other authors, there is no information whether the respective probes with their widened tips were included in the dynamic calibrations. In the author's own investigations, turbulences at the narrow edges of the probe ends might likewise have led to an erroneous measurement of Rc. However, the slight influence of the frequency on Rc speaks against this. Furthermore, the possibility could not be excluded that the end of the probe fixed under slight traction may have strongly deformed the lumen or the course of the corresponding bronchiolus. As mentioned in the description of the method, this source of error could be excluded.

In conclusion, it is to be assumed that the methods used in this study provided exact measurement values and avoided serious systematic errors. Furthermore, for the reasons stated, a comparison of the author's own results, obtained from a relatively large number of lungs having high Rp values and definite correlation between age and Rp, with the measurements made by *Macklem* and *Mead* (1967) and *Hogg* et al. (1970) appears to have little value.

According to the results of the author's own direct measurements of resistance and the results of indirect resistance measurements from the detailed morphometric investigations by *Niewoehner* et al. (1974), the question also arises of whether the morphometric investigations by *Weibel* (1963) on five lungs from the 8th, 16th, 34th, 48th, and 74th year of life, as well as the investigations by *Horsefield* and *Cumming* (1968a, b), who merely studied the lung of a 35-year-old woman, were suitable in terms of the sample size to detect or exclude random morphological variance. Methodological errors are also not to be excluded in such investigations, since conclusions were drawn with regard to the dynamic process of breathing from a statically determined airway geometry which was measured by interpolation in lungs after fixation at the volume of the TLC. It appears to be entirely legitimate to reverse such inferences and to draw certain conclusions with regard to airway geometry on the basis of measurements of airway dynamic parameters at physiological lung volumes.

It has already been mentioned that a decrease in Cdyn with an increase in breathing rate is regarded as a sensitive parameter for pathological alterations in the bronchioli (*Otis* et al. 1956; *Mills* et al. 1963; *Woolcock* et al. 1969; *Ingram* and *O'Cain* 1971; *Seaton* et al. 1972; *McFadden* et al. 1974; *Ulmer* et al. 1976). As was shown, a frequency-dependent decrease in Cdyn could also be demonstrated in normal lungs. However, a much higher decrease was found in lungs with bronchiolitis. According to the results of reflections on the causes of the frequency dependence of Cdyn and according to the author's measurements with high Rp in normal lungs and in particular in lungs with bronchiolitis, it would be expected that a correlation exists between these parameters. As can be seen from Fig. 10, there is indeed a significant correlation between the frequency-dependent increase in Rp and the decrease in Cdyn. Therefore the bronchioli have a major functional significance even in the normal lung. This

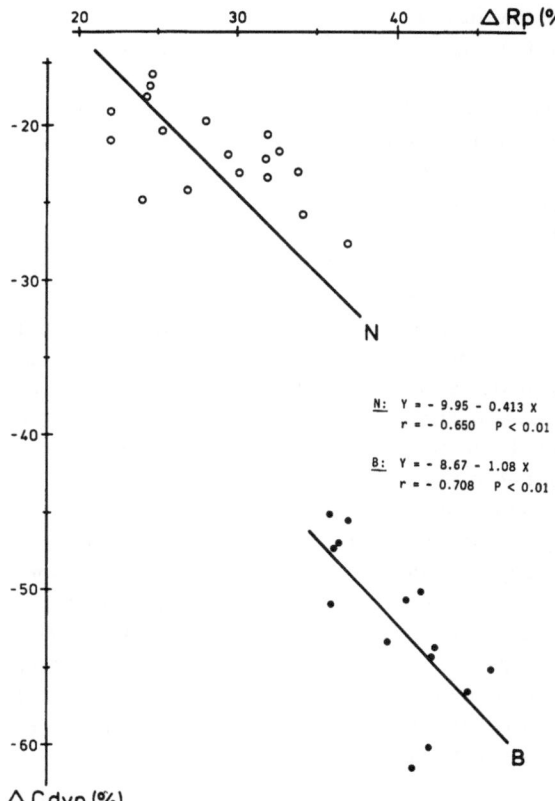

Fig. 10. Frequency-dependent increase in *Cdyn* (△ *Cdyn*) plotted against the corresponding values of *Rp* (△Rp) in the normal lungs (*N*) and in the lungs with bronchiolitis (*B*)

statement is consistent with the reflections by *Pardaens* et al. (1972) and *van de Woestijne* (1976), who found that no frequency dependence of Cdyn is to be expected with a small percentage of Rp.

The author's own results are in complete contradiction with the theoretical reflections of *Otis* et al. (1956) as well as with numerous other model concepts in which a decrease in C with an increase in R was not assumed in healthy lungs. This false conclusion results from ignorance of morphological structures and the use of overly simple models in which the extent of the complex linking of R and C components as well as their magnitude was inaccurately assessed.

According to the results of the author's own experimental investigations, it can be unequivocally stated that the bronchioli have a very important role in the normal lung and also in cases with minimal morphological alterations. The view held by *Mead* (1970) that this part of the bronchial system is the "quiet zone" of the lung undoubtedly requires correction. Such a "quiet zone" is more likely to be localized in the larger cartilaginous airways in normal lungs and in lungs with chronic bronchiolitis. It could be demonstrated by the static measurements that there is a loss of elasticity in lungs with chronic bronchiolitis. The parameters determined under dynamic conditions, especially the values of Rp (which are significantly higher than normal values), in combination with the strong frequency dependence of Cdyn, make it evident that the functionally important disturbances must be localized in the lung periphery. The possibility was discussed that elastic fibers in the walls of bronchioli and/or in their surrounding tissue must be functionally damaged, leading to a greater tendency toward bronchiolar collapse. However, no alterations were found histologically which might explain such damage to elastic fibers, nor was any cause found for the Rp values being significantly higher than those of normal lungs.

In lungs with bronchiolitis, on the whole comparable histological changes were evenly distributed in the terminal bronchioli and to a smaller extent also in respiratory bronchioli. With preserved texture, relatively dense infiltrates of lymphocytes and plasma cells as well as occasional neutrophilic granulocytes could be regularly demonstrated in the walls and in the adjacent tissue of the bronchioli. According to the histological appearance (morphometric investigations could not be carried out so far), there were no marked differences in the internal diameter of the bronchioli in the lungs with bronchiolitis compared with normal lungs.

In the group of normal lungs, such inflammatory changes were never found. However, in both groups goblet cell hyperplasia, chronic bronchitis, and epithelial metaplasia of varying intensity were very frequently demonstrable in all cartilaginous bronchial generations. Functional effects of these alterations could not be demonstrated.

In the lungs with bronchiolitis, with the exception of two cases, a remarkable additional histological finding could be demonstrated. Very numerous alveolar macrophages with fine granular brownish pigment in the cytoplasm were found in the alveoli, in the alveolar ducts, and occasionally also in the respiratory bronchioli (Fig. 11). By appropriate staining, it could be excluded that this pigment was hemosiderin. Although precise anamnestic data on the smoking habits were not always available in these cases, it is probable according to the result of numerous investigations that these patients had been cigarette smokers. *Niewoehner* et al. (1974), *Pratt* et al. (1969) and *Harris* et al. (1970) have demonstrated pigmented alveolar macrophages in smokers by endobronchial lavage.

The two test subjects in whom the same kind of inflammatory alterations were found in the peripheral airways, but which were not combined with a massive occurrence of pigmented alveolar macrophages, had worked in a rolling mill. More precise data on the working conditions, especially whether these subjects had been exposed to a particular inhalatory noxa, could not be obtained.

In smokers, discrete alterations of lung functional parameters have been observed in clinical studies. Thus *Ingram* and *O'Cain* (1971) found a significant increase in the closing volume in smokers. This finding is in agreement with the result of the author's own investigations in which the significant increase in RV can be compared with the increase in the closing volume. In the clinical investigations by *McCarthy* et al. (1972), a stronger frequency dependence of Cdyn was detected in a group of smokers. This finding is also in agreement with the author's own results.

As already emphasized, the cause of the marked loss of elasticity and the peripheral obstruction in the bronchiolitis group is by no means characterized by an adequate morphological correlate. According to results of investigations on the alveolar macrophages of smokers, there is the possibility that the elastic fibers in the bronchi-

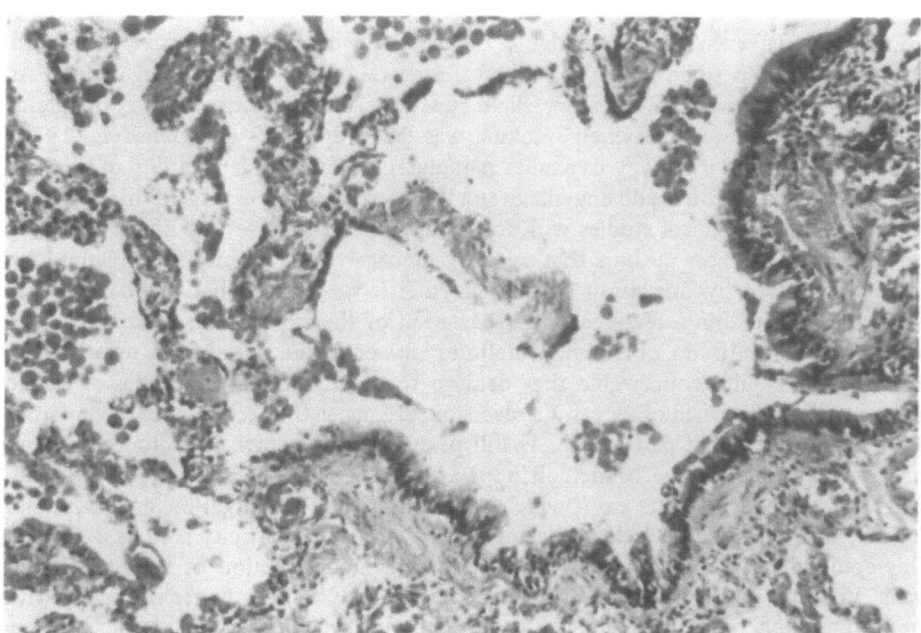

Fig. 11. Photomicrograph of a representative histological section from the group with bronchiolitis (smokers)

oles and in the surrounding tissue may be altered by an enzyme (protease) which is released by the macrophages. An additional factor, which likewise can only lead initially to a functional damage of the elastic fibers, is undoubtedly "smoker's cough". The probably irregularly distributed pressure peaks which occur in coughing might lead to sudden local overstretching of fibers, especially in the peripheral parts of the lung. Such a sudden inhomogeneous overstretching might damage the function of elastic fibers even though there is as yet no morphological demonstrable structural change. Some of the author's own studies in which lungs were ventilated at high frequencies against a central stenosis have shown that an irreversible loss of elasticity can occur without microscopically demonstrable morphological alterations.

The distinctly inhomogeneous ventilation with fall in Cdyn, which was demonstrated with increase of frequency, necessarily leads to inhomogeneous pulmonary circulation with local disturbances of diffusion. This results in a negative influence on the nutritive circulation of the lungs. Theoretically, this might result in a progressive damage to the lungs with disturbances of the regeneration capacity and decreasing resistance to infection.

In a few of the investigations previously mentioned concerning alveolar macrophages, but especially in a recent investigation by *Corrin* and *Soliman* (1978), it is assumed that surfactant synthesis can be disturbed in smokers. However, indications of an altered surfactant activity could not be found in lungs with bronchiolitis.

The question arises of whether functional damage to the elastic fibers and its repercussions on functional parameters, which is assumed in the group of lungs with bronchiolitis, is reversible or whether a manifest and possibly progressive damage to airway dynamics is to be expected even after removal of the corresponding irritant. As *Buist* et al. (1973) were able to show, slight functional disturbances of airway dynamics in smokers were reversible when smoking was given up. *Musk* and *Gandevia* (1976) reported alterations in airway dynamics parameters found in a large group of workers who had inhaled a proteolytic enzyme over a long period during detergent manufacture. The very detailed clinical studies with follow-up investigations left no doubt regarding the statement of these authors that selective damage to the elastic fibers in the lung tissue was caused by inhalation of this enzyme. It was shown that this damage was fully reversible within a few years after cessation of the exposure in most cases. The author's own results do not allow a definite answer to the question of reversibility. However, it is quite conceivable that damage to the functional properties of elastic fibers in chronic bronchiolitis can be reversible as long as the architecture of the bronchioli and the adjacent parenchyma is still preserved. In the case of prolonged inflammatory alterations to the bronchioli, especially when there are also leukocytic infiltrates, as is frequently the case, which according to the investigations by *Kuhn* and *Senior* (1978) can likewise release elastase, a further loss of elasticity is to be expected. This could finally lead to a morphologically evident destruction of the bronchiolar walls. Via a progressive deformation of the bronchiolar walls, a larger rise in Rp with severe functional bronchiolar stenosis can then occur, leading to the picture of irreversible obstructive pulmonary disease with poststenotic emphysema. The transition from (probably still reversible) inflammatory lesions to manifest chronic obstruction may take a very long time, and doubtless depends on the degree of severity of the injury and the duration of its action. According to the result of age-dependent physiological alterations in the lungs, it is to be assumed furthermore that the aging lung becomes increasingly vulnerable to minor degrees of bronchiolar narrowing and injury.

It has already been mentioned that according to a simple histological criterion no definite decrease in the internal diameter could be demonstrated in the bronchioli of lungs with bronchiolitis. An increase in the wall thickness with a decrease in the internal diameter, which can probably only be substantiated by morphometric methods, can be expected as an effect of the dense inflammatory wall infiltrates, however. Thus, besides the functional bronchiolar stenoses caused by raised deformability, a slight bronchiolar stenosis would also come into question as a cause of the increase in Rp. It is conceivable that a slight increase in the internal diameter is obscured by the fixation of the lungs at a pressure of 25 cm H_2O.

On the basis of the low Rp values determined experimentally in normal lungs, *Macklem* and *Mead* (1967) came to the conclusion that in chronic bronchiolitis, Rp must be roughly 40 times higher than normal before definite effects on Rt occur. Taking into account the morphometric data of *Niewoehner* and *Kleinerman* (1974) and assuming laminar flow, such an increase, which is already unrealistic according to the measurement results in normal lungs, would be expected when the diameter of all bronchioli decreases by more than half. Such a narrowing of the lumen was undoubtedly not present in the investigated lungs with bronchiolitis. These contradictory findings can be largely clarified by the results of the author's own investigations, which revealed high values for Rp even in healthy lungs, and by the morphometric investigations by *Niewoehner* and *Kleinerman* (1974). The high peripheral proportion of Rt demonstrated in healthy lungs shows, in combination with the results of the morphometric investigations, that the flow resistance localized in the peripheral airways is greater than was previously assumed. According to these results, an increase in Rp and in Rt is to be expected even with a relatively slight obstruction of the bronchioli, as was possibly the case in the bronchiolitic lungs. This is underscored by the findings of *Bignon* et al. (1969, 1970) as well as *Matsuba* and *Thurlbeck* (1972, 1973), who carried out morphometric investigations on lungs of patients in whom an increased Rt was known during life, and who mainly died of respiratory insufficiency. These authors found signs of chronic bronchiolitis in these lungs with locally different (but on the whole only very slight) decreases in the internal diameter of the bronchioli. An inhomogeneous ventilation and an increase in Rt with increasing breathing rate naturally results from this observation, especially at higher frequency.

According to the measurement results in normal isolated human lungs and in lungs with signs of slight chronic bronchiolitis and discrete airway obstruction, clinical methods should be found which can diagnose with certainty such functional alterations in the peripheral airways, because they possibly represent a reversible early form of "small airways disease".

The relatively simple static postmortem measurements revealed parameters allowing a definite demarkation between normal lungs and lungs with bronchiolitis. Such tests are not practicable for clinical investigations, because they merely allow measurements to be performed under quasi-static conditions, with relatively imprecise results.

The results of postmortem dynamic measurements showed that the frequency-dependent decrease in Cdyn ($\triangle$Cdyn) is by far the best parameter for distinguishing lungs with bronchiolitis from normal lungs ($t = 21.25, P < 0.0001$). As already mentioned, this parameter is also very suitable, even according to the results of clinical investigations, for diagnosis of peripheral airways diseases with slight obstruction. However, a routine use of this test cannot be realized because of its invasive nature and because of the elaborate method involved. A direct diagnostic measurement of Rp cannot be performed on live subjects.

According to the author's own investigations, one clinical diagnostic possibility involves routine use of a body plethysmograph. As was shown, there is a significant correlation between percentage changes in Rp and Cdyn with increase in frequency. In addition, a highly significant correlation was found between the values of Rp and Rt. It is thus to be expected that there is also a correlation between $\triangle$Rt and $\triangle$Cdyn. The calculation confirms this assumption: for normal lungs, the correlation coefficient is $r = 0.669$ ($P < 0.01$) and for the bronchiolitis group, $r = 0.810$ ($P < 0.001$). It follows from this that a clinical diagnosis of slight peripheral airways obstruction must also be possible from plethysmographic measurements of Rt. For this purpose it would be necessary to measure Rt at different breathing rates. The familar problem of an exact plethysmographic measurement of Rt at very dissimilar frequencies can already be solved satisfactorily by electronic compensations (*Smidt* 1980, personal communication). Important preconditions for exact clinical measurements are that the value of TV is defined as a percentage of another lung volume, e.g., TLC, and that both TV and FRC remain constant at different breathing frequencies. The values of Rt measured in this way should not be regarded as absolute values, because they depend greatly on the equipment of the respective laboratory. It would be better and more meaningful to analyze the correlation between frequency change and Rt. The degree of the percentage increase in Rt would have to be suitable in combination with appropriate normal values to diagnose with certainty a slight obstruction of the peripheral airways.

VI. Summary

Postmortem studies of airways dynamics were performed on isolated human lungs. Besides static measurements, dynamic measurements were performed in an artificial thorax. Eighteen normal lungs and 14 lungs with histological signs of slight chronic bronchiolitis from the 35th to the 55th year of life were investigated. The lungs with bronchiolitis differed from the normal lungs merely in somewhat irregularly distributed, but on the whole similar, slight infiltrates of lymphocytes, plasma cells, and occasional neutrophilic granulocytes in the walls and in the surrounding tissue of the bronchioli. Because numerous typically pigmented macrophages were found in the alveoli and alveolar ducts in 12 of these lungs, it was assumed that these individuals had been chronic cigarette smokers. The airway dynamics parameters of these lungs showed statistically significant variations from the values of normal lungs. In both groups, very distinct chronic inflammatory changes were found very frequently in large cartilaginous bronchi, in some cases with pronounced epithelial metaplasias without demonstrable functional repercussions. The measurement values from normal lungs showed a relatively good agreement with normal clinical values. Comparison of the postmortem lung volumes with predicted clinical values revealed that total lung capacity defined at a static pressure of 25 cm H_2O agrees best with clinical values. The values of the collapse volume (residual volume), which increase with age, and the static compliance, as well as the age-dependent decrease in the elastic recoil pressure measured in the midinflation position and the decrease in dynamic compliance, were interpreted as manifestations of an aging of the elastic fibers.

This fiber damage in the lung periphery also leads to loss of radial traction of the bronchioli with a marked rise in peripheral resistance. The mean values of the residual volume, but not the values of the total capacity, were significantly higher in the lungs with bronchiolitis than in normal lungs. From this observation and from the fact that the elastic recoil pressure was below normal values even only at midlung volumes, it was concluded that in chronic bronchiolitis the elastic fibers are damaged in moderate stretching, and that this damage is possibly reversible. In addition, it was shown that an aging process does not occur in the collagen fibers, and that these are not damaged in chronic bronchiolitis.

The mean values of the elastic recoil pressure at moderate lung volume have proved to be the best parameter for separating the two groups. In the dynamic measurements, the mean percentage decrease in dynamic compliance was the parameter with the highest significance level.

The proportion of peripheral resistance clearly increased with age: the mean value in the normal lungs was 52.7% in quiet breathing and 57.2% in forced breathing. In the lungs with bronchiolitis, the values were 55% and 61.9% respectively. These values are in clearly contradict to recent theoretical and experimental studies, according to the results of which this portion of airflow resistance should be so small that it could be neglected in normal lungs and lungs with slight chronic bronchiolitis. Wide variations of the measurement results, methodological inadequacies, and a very small number of investigated lungs compared with this author's own study render further comparisons of little value.

For clinical studies, measurement of the frequency-dependent increase in resistance affords the possibility of certain and relatively simple diagnosis of slight obstructive alterations in the peripheral airways.

References

Adamson JS Jr (1968) An electron microscopic comparison of the connective tissue from the lungs of young and elderly subjects. Am Rev Respir Dis 98:399–406

Albright CD, Bondurant S (1965) Some effects of respiratory frequency on pulmonary mechanics. J Clin Invest 44:1362–1370

Allen GW, Sabin S (1971) Comparison of direct and indirect measurement of airway resistance. Am Rev Respir Dis 104:61–71

Amrein R, Keller R, Joos H, Herzog H (1969) Neue Normalwerte für die Lungenfunktionsprüfung mit der Ganzkörperplethysmographie. Dtsch Med Wochenschr 94: 1785–1793

Avery ME, Fletcher BD (1974) The lung and its disorders in the newborn infant. Saunders, Philadelphia London Toronto

Bachofen H (1967) Physiologie und Pathophysiologie der Lungenmechanik. Beitr Klin Erforsch Tuberk Lungenkr 135:145–160

Begin R, Renzetti AD Jr, Bigler H, Watanabe S (1975) Flow and age dependence of airway closure and dynamic compliance. J Appl Physiol 38:199–207

Bignon J, Khoury F, Even P, Andre J, Brouet G (1969) Morphometric study in chronic obstructive bronchopulmonary disease. Am Rev Respir Dis 99:669–695

Bignon J, Andre J, Brouet G (1970) Parenchymal, bronchiolar and bronchial measurements in centrilobular emphysema. Thorax 75:556–567

Bobbaers H, Clement J, Pardaens J, van de Woestijne KP (1975) Simulation of frequency dependence of compliance and resistance in healthy man. J Appl Physiol 38:427–435

Bönninger M (1909) Zur Physiologie und Pathologie der Atmung. Z Exp Pathol Ther 5:409–427

Bohl W (1975) Technische Strömungslehre. Vogel, Würzburg

Boyden AE (1953) Observations on anatomy and development of the lungs. Lancet 73:509–512

Buist AS, van Fleet DL, Ross BB (1973) A comparison of conventional spirometric test and the test of closing volume in an emphysema screening center. Am Rev Respir Dis 107:735–746

Cara M (1958) Auswertung einer statistischen Untersuchung der ventilatorischen Funktionsgrößen bei normalen Personen. Europäische Gemeinschaft für Kohle und Stahl, Arbeitsdokument 6082/58d

Carson J (1820) On the elasticity of the lungs. Philos Trans R Soc 110:29–44

Carton RW, Clark JW, Dainauskas J (1962) Estimation of the tissue work of the lung (Abstr). Fed Proc 21:447

Cloetta M (1913) Untersuchungen über die Elastizität der Lunge und deren Bedeutung für die Zirkulation. Pflügers Arch 152:339–364

Colebatch HJH, Mitchell CA (1971) Constriction of isolated living liquid-filled dog and cat lungs with histamine. J Appl Physiol 30:691–702

34

Collet AJ, Des Biens G (1974) Fine structure of myogenesis and elastogenesis in the developing rat lung. Anat Rec 179:343–360

Comroe JH (1968) Physiologie der Atmung. Schattauer, Stuttgart

Comroe JH, DuBois AB, Briscoe WA, Carlsen E (1962) The lung. Year Book Medical Publishers, London, Lloyd-Luke Chicago

Corrin B, Soliman SS (1978) Cholesterol in the lungs of heavy cigarette smokers. Thorax 33:565–568

Dean RB, Visscher MB (1941) The kinetics of lung ventilation. Am J Physiol 134:450–468

Donders FC (1853) Beiträge zum Mechanismus der Respiration und Circulation in gesunden und kranken Zuständen. Z Ratio Med 3:287–302

Dosman J, Bode F, Urbanetti J, Antic R, Macklem PT (1975) Role of inertia in measurement of dynamic compliance. J Appl Physiol 38:64–69

Drazen JM, Loring SH, Ingram RH Jr (1976) Distribution of pulmonary resistance: effects of gas density, viscosity and flow rate. J Appl Physiol 41:388–395

DuBois AB, Botelho XY, Comroe JH (1956) A new method for measuring airway resistance in a man using a body plethysmograph: values in normal subjects and in patients with respiratory disease. J Clin Invest 35:327–335

Dubreuil G, Lacoste A, Raymond R (1936) Les étapes du development du poumon human et de son appareil élastique. C R Acad Sci (Paris) 121:244–246

Ferris BG Jr, Mead J, Opie LH (1964) Partitioning of respiratory flow resistance in man. J Appl Physiol 19:653–658

Finucane KE, Dawson SV, Phelan PD, Mead J (1975) Resistance of intrathoracic airway of healthy subjects during periodic flow. J Appl Physiol 38:517–530

Forkert L, Wood LDH, Cherniak RM (1975) Effect of gas density on dynamic pulmonary compliance. J Appl Physiol 39:906–910

Fowler WS, Cornish ER Jr, Kety SS (1952) Lung function studies: VIII. Analysis of alveolar ventilation by pulmonary N_2-clearance curves. J Clin Invest 31:40–50

Frank NR (1959) Influence of acute pulmonary vascular congestion on recoiling force of excised cats lungs. J Appl Physiol 14:905–908

Frank NR, Mead J, Siebens AA, Storey CF (1956) Measurements of pulmonary compliance in seventy healthy young adults. J Appl Physiol 9:38–42

Frank NR, Mead J, Ferris BG Jr (1957) The mechanical behavior of the lungs in healthy elderly persons. J Clin Invest 36:1680–1687

Frank NR, Radford EP Jr, Whittenberger JL (1959) Static volume pressure interrelationship of lungs and pulmonary vessels. J Appl Physiol 14:167–173

Fry DL (1959) Physiologic recording by modern instruments with particular reference to pressure recording. Physiol Rev 40:753–788

Gianelli JS, Ayres SM, Buehler ME (1967) Effects of pulmonary blood flow upon lung mechanics. J Clin Invest 46:1625–1642

Giese W (1961) Die allgemeine Pathologie der äußeren Atmung. In: Letterer E (Hrsg) Hilfsmechanismen des Stoffwechsels I. Springer, Berlin Göttingen Heidelberg. (Handbuch der allgemeinen Pathologie, Bd V/1, S 402–638)

Gomez DM (1965) A physico-mathematical study of lung function in normal subjects and in patients with obstructive pulmonary diseases. Med Thorac 22:275–294

Gough J, Wentworth JE (1958) Thin sections of entire organs mounted on paper. Harvey Lect 53:182–185

Gruenwald P (1958) The significance of pulmonary hyaline membranes in newborn infants. JAMA 166:621–623

Hamm J, Wettengel R, Fabel H (1962) Vergleichende Untersuchungen der Atemmechanik bei normaler Lungenfunktion, obstruktiven und restriktiven Ventilationsstörungen. Z Klin Med 157:133–155

Harris JO, Swenson EW, Johnson JE III (1970) Human alveolar macrophages: comparison of phagocytic ability, glucose utilisation, and ultrastructure in smokers and nonsmokers. J Clin Invest 49:2086–2096

Hartung W (1957) Die Altersveränderungen der Lungenelastizität nach Messung an isolierten Leichenlungen. Beitr Pathol Anat Allg Pathol 118:368–389

Hartung W (1959) Über Ausmaß und funktionelle Bedeutung des Elastizitätsverlustes bei verschiedenen Lungenerkrankungen. Beitr Pathol Anat Allg Pathol 120:178–213

Hartung W (1960) Histomechanik der Ventilationsstörungen. Verh Dtsch Ges Pathol 44:46–54

Hartung W, Büttinghaus K (1967) Messungen der dynamischen Volumendehnbarkeit isolierter normaler menschlicher Lungen. Med Thorac 24:348–370

Hieronymi G (1961) On the change in the morphology of the human lung due to age. Ergeb Allg Pathol 41:1–62

Hogg JC, Macklem PT, Thurlbeck WM (1968) Site and nature of airway obstruction in chronic obstructive lung disease. N Engl J Med 278:1355–1360

Hogg JC, Williams J, Richardson JB, Macklem PT, Thurlbeck WM (1970) Age as a factor in the distribution of lower-airway conductance and in the pathologic anatomy of obstructive lung disease. N Engl J Med 282:1283–1287

Hoppin FG Jr, Lee GC, Dawson SV (1975) Properties of lung parenchyma in distortion. J Appl Physiol 39:742–751

Horsefield K, Cumming C (1968a) Morphology of the bronchial tree in man. J Appl Physiol 24:373–383

Horsefield K, Cumming C (1968b) Functional consequences of airway morphology. J Appl Physiol 24:384–390

Hutchinson J (1846) On the capacity of the lungs and on the respiratory function. Med Chir Trans 29:127–148

Hyatt RE, Wilcox RE (1961) Extrathoracic airway resistance in man. J Appl Physiol 16:326–330

Ingram JR, O'Cain CF (1971) Frequency-dependence of compliance in apparently healthy smokers versus nonsmokers. Bull Physiol Patho Respir 7:195–210

Islam MS, Ulmer WT (1977) Der Strömungswiderstand in den Atemwegen und das Lungenvolumen. Dtsch Med Wochenschr 102:1187–1190

Islam MS, Buckup K, Ulmer WT (1978) Altersabhängigkeit der mechanischen Eigenschaften der Lunge. Dtsch Med Wochenschr 103:1482–1485

Jaeger MJ, Matthys H (1968) The pattern of flow in the upper human airways. Respir Physiol 6:113–127

Jaquet A (1908) Zur Mechanik der Atembewegungen. Arch Exp Pathol Pharmakol (Suppl) 309–322

John R, Thomas J (1972) Chemical compositions of elastins isolated from aortas and pulmonary tissues of humans of different ages. Biochem J 127:261–269

Kesci P, Jaffrin MY (1972) Predictions of pressure drop along the bronchial tree (Abstr). Proc Annu Conf Engin Med Biol 14:251

Kluge A (1967) Oberflächenspannung in der Lunge. Ergeb Gesamten Lungen Tuberkuloseforsch 16/10:69

Krahl VE (1959) Microscopic anatomy of the lung. Am Rev Respir Dis 80:24–44

Kuhn C, Senior RM (1978) The role of elastase in the development of emphysema. Lung 155:185–197

Liebermeister G (1907) Zur normalen und pathologischen Physiologie der Atmungsorgane. I. Über das Verhältnis zwischen Lungendehnung und Lungenvolumen. Zbl Allg Pathol 18:644–662

Linser P (1900) Über den Bau und die Entwicklung des elastischen Gewebes in der Lunge. Anat Hefte Arb Inst Wiesbaden 13:307–335

Long EC, Hull WE, Gebel EL (1962) Respiratory dynamic resistance. J Appl Physiol 17:609–612

Macklem PT, Becklage MR (1963) The relationship between the mechanical and diffusing properties of the lung in health and disease. Am Rev Respir Dis 87:47–56

Macklem PT, Mead J (1967) Resistance of central and peripheral airways measured by a retrograde catheter. J Appl Phyisol 22:395:401

Macklem PT, Hogg JC, Thurlbeck WM (1968) The flow resistance of central and peripheral airways in human lungs. In: Cumming G, Hunt LB (eds) Form and function in the human lung. Williams & Wilkins, Baltimore, pp 76—88

Matsuba M, Thurlbeck WM (1972) The number and dimensions of small airways in emphysematous lungs. Am J Pathol 67:265—276

Matsuba M, Thurlbeck WM (1973) Disease of the small airways in chronic bronchitis. Am Rev Respir Dis 107:552—558

McCarthy DS, Spencer R, Greene R, Milic-Emili J (1972) Measurement of closing volume as a simple and sensitive test for early detection of small airway disease. Am J Med 52:747—753

McFadden ER Jr, Newton-Howes J, Pride NB (1970) Acute effects of inhaled isoproterenol on the mechanical characteristics of the lungs in normal man. J Clin Invest 49:779—790

McFadden ER Jr, Kiker R, Holmes B, de Groot WJ (1974) Small airway disease. An assessment of the tests of peripehral airway function. Am J Med 57:171—182

Mead J (1961) Mechanical properties of lung. Physiol Rev 41:281—330

Mead J (1970) The lungs "quiet zone" (editorial). N Engl J Med 282:1318—1319

Mead J, Lindgren I, Gaensler EA (1955) The mechanical properties of the lungs in emphysema. J Clin Invest 34:1005—1016

Milic-Emili J (1974) Pulmonary statics. In: Guyton AC, Widdicombe J (eds) Respiratory physiology, ser 1, vol 2, pp 105—138. Butterworth, University Park Press, London Baltimore

Miller JA, Pratt PC, Capp MP (1973) Human bronchial and bronchiolar compressibility measured by postmortem bronchography. Lab Invest 29:465—477

Mills RJ, Cummings G, Harris P (1963) Frequency-dependent compliance at different levels of inspiration in normal adults. J Appl Physiol 18:1061—1064

Mount LE (1955) The ventilation flow-resistance and compliance of rat lungs. J Physiol (Lond) 127:157—167

Musk AW, Gandevia B (1976) Loss of pulmonary elastic recoil in workers formerly exposed to proteolytic enzyme (alcalase) in the detergent industry. Br J Ind Med 33:158—165

Neergard K von (1929) Neue Auffassungen über einen Grundbegriff der Atemmechanik. Die Retraktionskraft der Lunge, abhängig von der Oberflächenspannung in den Alveolen. Z Gesamt Exp Med 66:373—394

Niewoehner DE, Kleinerman J (1974) Morphologic basis of pulmonary resistance in the human lung and effects of aging. J Appl Physiol 36:412—418

Niewoehner DE, Kleinerman J, Rice DB (1974) Pathologic changes in the peripheral airways of young cigarette smokers. N Engl J Med 291:755—758

Niewoehner DE, Kleinerman J, Liotta L (1975) Ealstic behavior of postmortem human lungs: effects of aging and mild emphysema. J Appl Physiol 39:943—949

Niewoehner DE, Knoke JD, Kleinerman J (1977) Peripheral airways as a determinant of ventilatory function in the human lung. J Clin Invest 60:139—151

Olson DE, Dart GA, Filley GF (1970) Pressure drop and fluid flow regime of air inspired into the human lung. J Appl Physiol 28:482—494

Otis AB, Fenn WO, Rahn H (1950) Mechanics of breathing in man. J Appl Physiol 2:592—607

Otis AB, McKerrow CB, Bartlett RA, Mead J, McIlroy MB, Selverstone NJ, Radford EP Jr (1956) Mechanical factors in distribution of pulmonary ventilation. J Appl Physiol 8:427—443

Otto H (1970) Die Atmungsorgane. In: Meessen H, Roulet F (Hrsg) Die Organe. Springer, Berlin Heidelberg New York (Handbuch der allgemeinen Pathologie, Bd III/4, S 1—204)

Paine JR (1940) The clinical measurement of pulmonary elasticity. J Thorac Surg 9:550—567

Pardaens J, van de Woestijne KP, Clement J (1972) A physical model of expiration. J Appl Physiol 32:479—490

Pare PD, Boucher R, Michoud MC, Hogg JC (1978) Static lung mechanics of intact and excised rhesus monkey lungs and lobes. J Appl Physiol 44:547–552

Park SS, Yoo OH, Janis M, Williams MH Jr (1969) Postmortem evaluation of airflow limitation in obstructive disease. J Appl Physiol 27:308–312

Pattle RE (1955) Properties, function and origin of the alveolar lining layer. Nature 175:1125–1126

Pedley TJ, Schroter RC, Sudlow MF (1970) The prediction of pressure drop and variation of ressitance within the human bronchial airways. Respir Physiol 9:387–405

Peslin R (1969) Theoretical analysis of airway resistances on an inhomogenous lung. J Appl Physiol 24:761–767

Petty TL, Miercort R, Ryan S, Vincent T, Filley GF, Mitchell RS (1965) The functional and bronchographic evaluation of postmortem human lungs. Am Rev Respir Dis 92:450–458

Pierce JA, Ebert RV (1958) The elastic properties of the lungs in aged. J Lab Clin Med 51:63–71

Pierce JA, Ebert RV (1965) Fibrous network of the lung and its change with age. Thorax 20:469–476

Pierce JA, Hocott JB, Ebert RV (1961a) The collagen and elastic content of the lung in emphysema. Ann Intern Med 55:210–222

Pierce JA, Hocott JB, Hefley BF (1961b) Elastic properties and the geometry of the lung. J Clin Invest 40:1515–1524

Pratt PC, Klugh GA (1961) A technique for the study of ventilatory capacity, compliance, and residual volume of excised lungs and for fixation, drying, and serial sectioning in the inflated state. Am Rev Respir Dis 83:690–695

Pratt PC, Jutabha O, Klugh GA (1965) Quantitative relationship between structural extent of centrilobular emphysema and postmortem volume and flow characteristics of lungs. Med Thorac 22:197–208

Pratt SA, Finley TN, Smith MH (1969) A comparison of alveolar macrophages and pulmonary surfactant obtained from the lungs of human smokers and nonsmokers by endobronchial lavage. Anat Rec 163:497–508

Radford EP Jr (1964) Static mechanical properties of mammalian lungs. In: Fenn WO, Rahn H (eds) Respiration. Washington (Handbook of physiology, vol 1, pp 429–449)

Rahn H, Otis AB, Chadwick LE, Fenn WO (1946) The pressure-volume diagram of the thorax and the lung. Am J Physiol 146:161–169

Recklinghausen H von (1869) Über die Atemgröße des Neugeborenen. Pflügers Arch 62:451–493

Rohrer F (1915) Der Strömungswiderstand in den menschlichen Atemwegen und der Einfluß der unregelmäßigen Verzweigung des Bronchialsystems auf den Atmungsverlauf in verschiedenen Lungenbezirken. Pflügers Arch 162:226–229

Rohrer F (1925) Physiologie der Atembewegungen. In: Bethe, Bergman, Embden (Hrsg) Handbuch der normalen und pathologischen Physiologie. Springer, Berlin

Ryan SF, Vincent TN, Mitchell RS, Filley GF, Dart G (1965) Ductectasia; an asymptomatic pulmonary change related to age. Med Thorac 22:181–187

Sachs L (1973) Statistische Auswertungsmethoden. Springer, Berlin Heidelberg New York

Saibene F, Mead J (1969) Frequency dependence of pulmonary quasistatic hysteresis. J Appl Physiol 26:732–737

Salazar E, Knowles JH (1964) An analysis of pressure-volume characteristics of the lungs. J Appl Physiol 19:97–104

Scarpelli EM (1968) The surfactant system of the lung. Lead & Febiger, Philadelphia

Schoedel W (1971) Physikalische Grundlagen des Atemnotsyndroms. Verh Dtsch Ges Pathol 55:2–12

Seaton A, Lapp NL, Morgan WKC (1972) Lung mechanics and frequency dependence of compliance in coal miners. J Clin Invest 51:1203–1211

38

Silvers GW, Maisel JC, Petty TL, Mitchell RS, Filley GF (1972) Central airway resistance in excised emphysematous lungs. Chest 61:603–612

Silvers GW, Maisel JC, Petty TL, Filley GF, Mitchell RS (1974) Flow limitation during forced expiration in excised human lungs. J Appl Physiol 36:737–744

Staub NC (1963) Interdependency of pulmonary structure and function. Anesthesiology 24:831–854

Stemmler EJ, DuBois AB (1968) Pulmonary tissue and surface elastic forces at low lung volumes in rabbit. J Appl Physiol 25:473–478

Stigol LC, Vawter GE, Mead J (1972) Studies on elastic recoil of the lung in a pediatric population. Am Rev Respir Dis 105:552–561

Thurlbeck WM (1979) Post-mortem lung volumes. Thorax 34:735–739

Turner JM, Mead J, Wohl ME (1968) Elasticity of human lungs in relation to age. J Appl Physiol 25:664–671

Ulmer WT, Reichel G, Nolte D (1976) Die Lungenfunktion. Thieme, Stuttgart

van de Woestijne KP (1976) Spécificité des tests proposés pour le dépistage de la maladie des petites voies aériennes. Bull Eur Physiopathol Respir 12:477–486

Wagner W Jr (1965) Alveolar ductectasia as studied by microradiography. Med Thorac 22:188–195

Weibel ER (1963) Morphometry of the human lung. Academic Press, New York; Springer, Berlin Göttingen Heidelberg

Weibel ER, Gil J (1968) Electron microscopic demonstration of an extracellular duplex lining layer of alveoli. Respir Physiol 4:42–57

West JB, Hugh-Jones P (1959) Patterns of gas flow in the upper bronchial tree. J Appl Physiol 14:753–759

Whimster WF, Macfarlane AJ (1974) Normal lung weights in a white population. Am Rev Respir Dis 110:478–483

Wierich W (1974) Histomechanische Untersuchungen zum Atemnotsyndrom des Neugeborenen unter Berücksichtigung der Gesetze der Schwingungslehre. Medical dissertation, University of Münster

Wierich W (1977) Untersuchungen zur Atemmechanik von Früh- und Neugeborenen. II. Dynamische Messungen an isolierten Lungen. Respiration 34:21–30

Wierich W (1978) Erfassung und Auswertung atemmechanischer Größen an isolierten Lungen mit Hilfe eines Datenerfassungssystems. Atemwegs- und Lungenkrankh 4:201–204

Wierich W (1980) Atemmechanische Befunde an isolierten menschlichen Lungen mit Surfactantschaden. Prax Pneumol 34:348–355

Wierich W, Hartung W (1979) Measurements of total and intrabronchial resistances in normal and diseased isolated lungs. Bronchopneumologie 29/2:116–123

Wohl MEB, Turner J, Mead J (1968) Static volume-pressure curves of dog lungs in vivo and in vitro. J Appl Physiol 24:348–354

Woolcock AJ, Vincent NJ, Macklem PT (1969) Frequency-dependence of compliance as a test for obstruction in the small airways. J Clin Invest 48:1097–1106

Wright RR (1961) Elastic tissue of normal and emphysematous lungs. A tridimensional histologic study. Am J Pathol 39:355–367

Correlation Between Functional and Morphometrical Parameters in Chronic Obstructive Lung Disease

P. DALQUEN and M. OBERHOLZER

I. Introduction

Obstructive lung disease can be defined simply as an intermittent or permanent increase of bronchial resistance. Patients with this disease complain of dyspnea and a more or less productive cough. The underlying affection can be chronic bronchitis, destructive pulmonary emphysema, bronchial asthma, or bronchiectasis, all of which often occur in various combinations.

The airways obstruction has been attributed to emphysematous tissue destruction and to lesions of the bronchial system, which can be found in all these affections. However, until now detailed knowledge of how the morphological alterations act on pulmonary function has been lacking. Several attempts have been made to clarify this question, such as isolated interpretations of functional or morphological observations, correlations between roentgenological and functional findings, animal experiments, and clinicopathological correlation studies.

Isolated interpretations of functional or morphological findings have led to controversial theories: *Rohrer* (1915) concluded from the relief and the mode of ramification of the airways that 10% of airway resistance arises in nasal meatus and central bronchi, and 90% in peripheral bronchi with diameters of less than 3 mm. His opinion was accepted by most physiologists until recently when *Macklem* and *Mead* (1967) deduced from experimental findings in dogs that at least in healthy human subjects, the resistance arises mainly in central bronchi. Similarly, morphometrical findings (*Weibel* 1963) suggested that especially stenoses in central bronchi must influence airway resistance, because the "bottleneck" (narrowest part) of airways lies between the fourth and tenth bronchial generation (*Nolte* and *Ulmer* 1967). This suggestion is inconsistent with the experimental results of *Hogg* et al. (1968) who showed in isolated autopsy lungs that in obstructive lung disease the resistance is higher in bronchi with a diameter of less than 2 mm. For a long time, decrease in the forced expiratory volume within 1 s (FEV_1) was attributed to an early expiratory airway collapse. Loss of radial traction of bronchioli in destructive emphysema was regarded as a cause of this collapse (*Dayman* 1951). This interpretation, based on theoretical considerations and not on clinicopathological correlations, has been questioned by the morphological findings of others (*Park* et al. 1970).

Some authors have tried to establish the correlations between pulmonary emphysema and functional disorder by comparing X-ray findings with findings in lung-function tests (*Demedts* et al. 1978; *Martell* et al. 1974; *Simon* et al. 1973). However, this procedure cannot lead to conclusive results, because X-ray diagnosis of destructive emphysema often does not agree with the pathological findings (*Nicklaus* et al. 1966; *Otto* et al. 1969; *Thurlbeck* et al. 1978): moderate and severe emphysema are detected by X-ray examination in only 41% of cases (*Thurlbeck* et al. 1978). Grading and typing of emphysema is all the more difficult roentgenologically. Therefore, correlations between degree of emphysema and lung function cannot be studied in detail by this method.

The results of animal experiments cannot be assumed to be valid for man. Investigations in isolated canine lungs (*Hogg* et al. 1968) have certainly contributed much to our understanding of bronchial flow conditions, but the relations between pathological alterations and alterations of breathing mechanics cannot be imitated in animal experiments, since the structure of animal lungs is adapted to life conditions other than those of human lungs (*Horsfield* and *Cumming* 1968, 1976). Emphysema and chronic bronchitis are diseases typically found in man.

In laboratory animals they are rare and occur only in a modified or mitigated manner. Experimental induction of both emphysema and chronic bronchitis leads to inadequate alterations, and experimental emphysemas bear only a remote resemblance to human emphysemas. In most experiments an initial phase of highly acute inflammation, which has never been observed in man, precedes parenchymal destruction (*Frasca* et al. 1971; *Johanson* et al. 1971; *Marco* et al. 1971; *Pushpakom* et al. 1970; *Snider* et al. 1973). The experimental induction of chronic bronchitis (*Charkin* and *Saunders* 1974; *Wheeldon* and *Pirie* 1974) is difficult, because in laboratory animals nonphysiological irritants must be applied to overcome the nasal filter. In addition, animals are very sensitive to airway affections.

Therefore, findings in human autopsy lungs remain important for insight into respiratory mechanics. Measurements of functional parameters in isolated human lungs are of special interest (*Hartung* 1964; *Niewoehner* and *Kleinerman* 1977; *Park* et al. 1970; *Petty* et al. 1965; *Pratt* et al. 1962, 1965; *Silvers* et al. 1972; *Wierich* 1976; *Wierich* et al. 1978; *Wyatt* et al. 1964). These measurements showed that disturbances of lung recoil pressure, total lung capacity (TLC), and expiratory flow established in vivo can also be demonstrated post mortem (*Hartung* 1964; *Petty* et al. 1965; *Wierich* and *Hartung* 1978). They have given insight into the influence of extrapulmonary and skeletal alterations on pulmonary function (*Hartung* and *Kafarnik* 1966) and have already shed some light on the pathogenesis of airways obstruction. *Hartung* and *Kafarnik* (1966) showed that in autopsy lungs, intrabronchial mucus plugs increase the airway resistance considerably and impede pulmonary insufflation. They also demonstrated that in destructive emphysema, elasticity of the lung is actually diminished. Other investigations showed that in obstructive lung disease, airway resistance may largely arise in the small bronchi (*Hartung* and *Kissler* 1970; *Hogg* et al. 1968).

The results of all these investigations, however, have never been correlated with detailed morphometrical data. Only Reid's index and degree of emphysema were established in some studies (*Hartung* 1975; *Miller* et al. 1973).

Several authors compared functional data established in vivo with qualitative or quantitative postmortem findings (*Boushy* et al. 1968, 1971; *Burrows* et al. 1966; *Cullen* et al. 1970; *Dunnill* et al. 1969; *Gaensler* and *Lindgren* 1959; *Hossain* 1973; *Hossain* and *Heard* 1970; *Jenkins* et al. 1965; *Lyons* et al. 1972; *Martin* et al. 1970; *McKenzie* et al. 1969; *Mitchell* et al. 1976; *Otto* et al. 1967, 1969; *Park* et al. 1970; *Petty* et al. 1965; *Ryder* et al. 1970; *Sweet* et al. 1960, 1961; *Symonds* et al. 1974; *Takizawa* and *Thurlbeck* 1971; *Thurlbeck* 1963; *Thurlbeck* et al. 1970b; *Watanabe* et al. 1965; *Williams* and *Cane* 1965). The results of these studies have recently been summarized by *Thurlbeck* (1976): No clinical parameter allows the diagnosis of destructive emphysema. The degree of tissue destruction correlates best with carbon monoxide diffusing capacity (DCO) (*Boushy* et al. 1971; *Burrows* et al. 1966; *Hossain* 1973; *Park* et al. 1970; *Thurlbeck* et al. 1970b). There is also some concurrence of degree of emphysema and residual volume (RV) as well as TLC.

The correlations between bronchial lesions and pulmonary function have been studied less thoroughly. Only Reid's index has been compared with various functional parameters (*Bath* and *Yates* 1968; *Boushy* et al. 1970; *Lyons* et al. 1972; *Martin* et al. 1970; *Thurlbeck* et al. 1970b).

The aim of this study was to obtain more information about the correlations between morphological alterations and functional disorder. We therefore analyzed bronchi and lung parenchyma of autopsy cases by morphometrical methods and compared the results with those of lung-function tests carried out during life. The study comprised only cases with chronic obstructive lung disease caused by chronic bronchitis. Cases with bronchiectases or pure atopic bronchial asthma were excluded. The methodological problems are discussed in detail, because they may explain the contradictory results reported in the literature.

II. Material

Autopsy lungs of 188 patients (151 male, 37 female) were studied. All patients had lung-function tests during life. The tests were carried out because of the following diseases:

Chronic obstructive lung disease	42 cases	(22.3%)
Bronchial carcinoma	71 cases	(37.8%)
Pulmonary hypertension	6 cases	(3.2%)
Pneumoconiosis, tuberculosis	7 cases	(3.7%)
Pulmonary fibrosis	5 cases	(2.7%)
Preliminary surgical examination	25 cases	(13.3%)
Cardiovascular disease	19 cases	(10.1%)
Others	12 cases	(6.9%)

Preliminary surgical examination had been performed before operation of extra-pulmonary malignant tumors. The group "Others" comprises mainly cases of hematological or rheumatic disease.

The mean age at death was 64.4 ± 10.4 (SD) years. The mean period between lung-function test and death was 11.4 (0.1–53) months. It was less than 1 year in 64.5% of cases, less than 2 years in 84.4%, and less than 3 years in 93.5%.

The various problems were investigated in the following partially overlapping subgroups:

1. Subgroup E ($n = 138$): Correlations between destructive emphysema and lung function (Table 1).
2. Subgroup B ($n = 50$): Correlations between bronchial alterations and lung function (Table 2). In these patients lung function had been tested because of the following diseases:

Chronic obstructive lung disease	13 cases	(26%)
Bronchial carcinoma	16 cases	(32%)
Extrapulmonary carcinoma (preliminary surgical examination)	5 cases	(10%)
Hematological disease	3 cases	(6%)
Circulatory disease	1 case	(2%)
Malignant mediastinal lymphoma	8 cases	(16%)
Pulmonary fibrosis	1 case	(2%)
Laryngeal carcinoma	3 cases	(6%)

In this subgroup, 12 patients (10 men, 2 women) had a TLC of less than 90% of the predicted value. The decreased TLC suggests that these patients had restrictive pulmonary disease.
3. Subgroup F ($n = 8$): Examination of artificial shrinkage caused by fixation and embedding procedures (Table 3).

For further details of the subgroups see Tables 1–3.

Table 1. Survey of groups and subgroups in which correlations between destructive emphysema and clinical parameters were studied. E, degree of emphysema; CVPh, check-value phenomenon; RAW, resistance of airways at regular breathing

Group	n	Criterion for selection	Problem studied
E	138	Expiratory flow curve established	Interrelation between CVPh and degree of emphysema
E_1	128	Complete pulmonary function	Interrelation between bronchial obstruction and degree of emphysema
E_2	97	$E > 0.2\%$	Comparison of degree of emphysema with functional data
E_3	46	CVPh +	Connection between degree of emphysema and CVPh
$E_{3.1}$	44	CVPh +, RAW pathological	
E_4	92	CVPh −	
$E_{4.1}$	38	CVPh −, RAW pathological	
E_5	10	$E > 10\%$	Connection between degree of emphysema and FEV_1
E_6	10	$E = 0\%$ TLC $\geqslant$ 90 (% predicted	

Table 2. Survey of groups and subgroups on which correlations between morphological alterations of bronchi and pulmonary function parameters were studied. CVPh, check-value phenomenon; RAW, resistance of airways at regular breathing

Group	n	Criterion for selection	Problem studied
B	50	Morphometrical analysis of bronchi	Correlations of morphometrical parameters with each other, functional data, and age
B_1	5	Pulmonary function unchanged	Morphometrical normal data
B_2	9	CVPh + RAW equal,	Connection between bronchial structure and CVPh
B_3	10	CVPh − but increased	
B_4	38	TLC $\geqslant$ 90 (% predicted)	Correlations between FEV_1 and volume densities of bronchial glands and muscles

Table 3. Groups H and F, in which the influence of glutaraldehyde and formaldehyde on tissue shrinkage was compared

Group	n	Criterion for selection	Problem studied
H	32	Fixation by glutaraldehyde	Degree of pulmonary inflation
F	8	Random	Shrinkage of tissue

IV. Clinical Parameters

The following clinical parameters were available for clinicopathological correlations: TLC, vital capacity (VC), RV, FEV_1, resistance of airways at regular breathing (RAW), and the check-value phenomenon of the expiratory flow curve (CVPh). From these parameters the degree of disproportional decrease of FEV_1 (D_{FEV_1}) and obstructive ventilation disorder were estimated.

1. Degree of Disproportional Decrease of FEV_1

There is a close relation between RAW and FEV_1, the two main parameters of bronchial obstruction (Fig. 1). In some cases, however, especially if the expiratory flow curve shows the CVPh, FEV_1 is lower than expected on the basis of the RAW value. The degree of this disproportional decrease can be estimated as follows (*Herzog* et al. 1976): The values of RAW and FEV_1 are divided into five corresponding ranges referring to healthy persons whose airways resistance was artificially increased by progressive narrowing of the mouthpiece (*Herzog* et al. 1976). Ranges of RAW were given index numbers between 0 and IV, and those of FEV_1 index numbers between I and V (Table 4). When FEV_1 is disproportionally decreased, the measured FEV_1 value belongs to a higher range than the RAW value measured at the same time. The degree of disproportional decrease of FEV_1 corresponds to the difference between the FEV_1 range and the RAW range. This is illustrated in Table 5 by three examples.

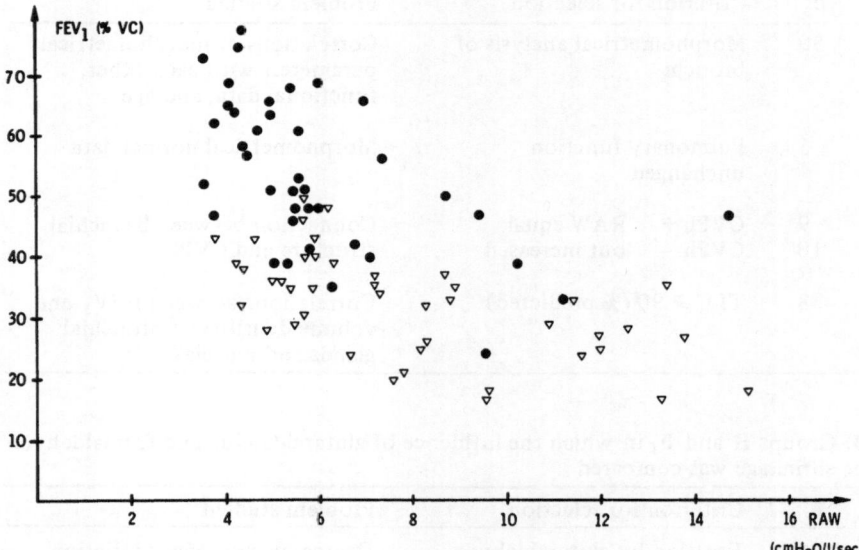

Fig. 1. Correlation between RAW and FEV_1. FEV_1 of cases with CVPh ($\triangle$) is disproportionately low. The graph contains only cases with increased bronchial resistance. $n = 82$, subgroups $E_{3.1}$ and $E_{4.1}$.

Table 4. Ranges of values of RAW and FEV$_1$ for establishment of degree of disproportional lowering of FEV$_1$

Range	RAW (cm H$_2$O/liter · s^{-1})	Range	FEV$_1$ (% VC)
0	<5.0		
I	5.1− 7.5	I	>55
II	7.6−10.0	II	46−55
III	10.1−15.0	III	36−45
IV	>15.0	IV	26−35
		V	<25

Table 5. Three examples of assessment of degree of disproportional lowering of FEV$_1$

	RAW (cm H$_2$O/liter · s^{-1})	Range	FEV$_1$ (% VC)	Range	Degree of disproportional decrease of FEV$_1$
Example 1	12	III	40	III	0
Example 2	12	III	40	IV	1
Example 3	12	III	20	V	2

2. Degree of Obstructive Ventilation Disorder

Increase of TLC, RV, and RAW, decrease of FEV$_1$ and VC, CHPh, and disproportional
decrease of FEV$_1$ are found in cases of obstructive lung disease. CVPh and D$_{FEV_1}$
point to particularly severe obstructive disease and are signs of unfavorable prognosis.
Generally, the functional parameters are more or less closely correlated (Table 6).
However, not only are FEV$_1$ and RAW not always equally changed, but there are also
considerable discrepancies between individual cases in the other parameters. Therefore,
all parameters have to be taken into account if the degree of obstructive ventilation
disorder is to be estimated. We did so by establishing five ranges for the values of RV
and FEV$_1$ and − to avoid overvaluing RV − two ranges for the values of TLC. The
ranges are indicated by numbers 0−IV. Thus, each measured value of TLC corresponds
to an index (I$_{TLC}$) of 0 or 1, and each measured value of RV and FEV$_1$ to an index
(I$_{RV}$, I$_{FEV_L}$) of 0−4. The total index I of obstructive ventilation disorder is the sum
of these indices plus D$_{FEV_1}$:

Table 6. Spearman coefficients of correlations between functional parameters

	RV (% TLC)	VC (% predicted)	FEV$_1$ (% VC)	FEV$_1$ (% predicted)	RAW
TLC (% predicted)	0.485[a]	0.169	−0.549[a]	−0.291[a]	0.437[a]
RV (% TLC)	−	−0.627[a]	−0.552[a]	−0.680[a]	0.693[a]
VC (% predicted)	−	−	0.120	0.500[a]	−0.381[a]
FEV$_1$ (% VC)	−	−	−	0.794[a]	−0.709[a]
FEV$_1$ (% predicted)	−	−	−	−	−0.725[a]

[a] 2 $P < 0.05$

$$I = I_{TLC} + I_{RV} + I_{FEV_1} + D_{FEV_1} \tag{1}$$

We distinguished three degrees of obstructive lung disease:

Mild	$I = 1-4$
Moderate	$I = 5-9$
Severe	$I \geqslant 10$

IV. Morphological Methods

1. Tissue Preparation

The following preparation techniques were used:

1. In each case the left lung was fixed in the inflated state by transbronchial instillation of 4% formol at filling pressures of 30–40 cm H_2O.
2. In 32 lungs the degree of inflation was estimated. For this purpose lung volume was measured immediately after formol instillation according to Archimedes' principle. The postmortem-estimated lung volume was then compared with intra vitam established TLC.
3. Fixed lungs were cut from the lateral side into 0.5- to 2.0-cm-thick sagittal slices. Only two-thirds of the lungs were sliced, so that central bronchi and arteries could be dissected as proposed by *Heard* (1969).
4. In 157 cases, paper-mounted macrosections of the slice with the largest circumference were prepared in the usual manner (*Gough* and *Wentworth* 1949; *Otto* and *Kemter* 1969).
5. From each lobe of the lung at least one piece of tissue was taken for paraffin sections.
6. For bronchus morphometry, rings were taken from three well-defined sites of the bronchial tree (Fig. 2). The bronchus rings were decalcified for 2 weeks in EDTA

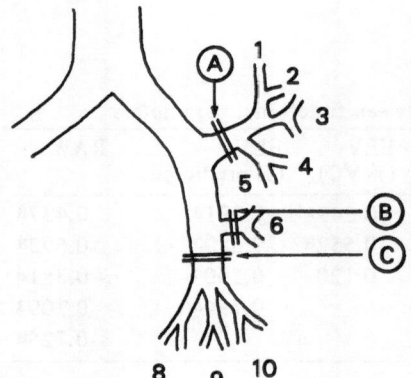

Fig. 2. Selection of three bronchus samples for histomorphometry. *A*, bronchus of upper lobe; *B*, bronchus of the upper segment of lower lobe; *C*, bronchus of lower lobe

(*Hunter* and *Nikiforok* 1954) and then embedded in paraplast. Sections (4–5 μ thick) were stained with H & E, van Gieson's elastica stain, and Goldner's trichrome method.

2. Morphometrical Models

a) Bronchus Morphometry

Morphometrical analysis of bronchi was carried out by point-counting. This method — first applied by *Dunnill* (1962) — was modified by introduction of new reference volumes and additional morphometrical parameters (*Oberholzer* et al. 1977). [For the stereological basis see *Weibel* (1973) and *Rohr* et al. (1976)]. Structures of bronchial walls whose volume density was determined are listed in Table 7. Additionally, the surface density of bronchial basement membrane was established. The structures underlined in Table 7 were chosen as reference volumes:

Reference volume B: 1 cm³ bronchus (bronchial lumen included)
Reference volume BWT: 1 cm³ bronchial wall tissue (cartilage included)
Reference volume BST: 1 cm³ bronchial wall tissue (cartilage excluded)

The symbol $V_{V(i/B)}$ means volume density of the bronchial structure (i) related to 1 cm³ bronchus including bronchial lumen.

Volume densities B and BWT are especially appropriate to correlation studies, whereas volume densities related to reference volume BST are recommended for comparisons of means (*Oberholzer* et al. 1977).

As test grid we used a double-square lattice with 64 and 1024 test points respectively [distance between test points (d), 13.0 and 3.3 mm respectively; total length of test lines (L_T), 832.0 mm (Fig. 3)]. Points were counted at 50-fold magnification using the projection microscope Visopan (Reichert). The whole bronchus section was covered

Table 7. Bronchial tissue compartments measured by bronchus morphometry. Reference volumes are framed

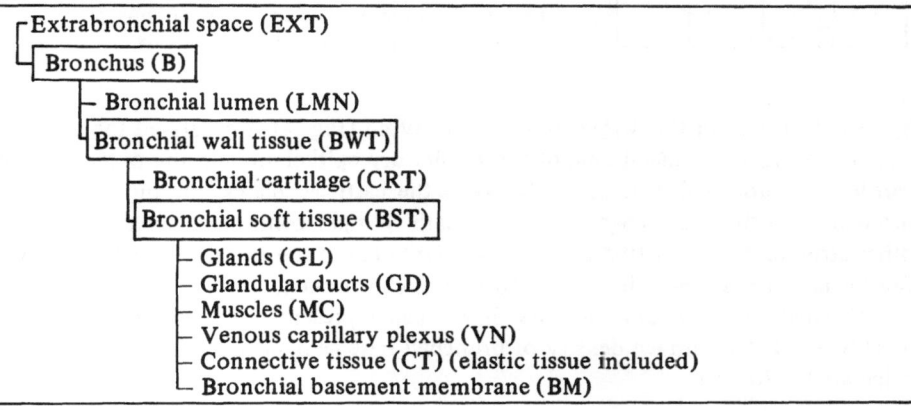

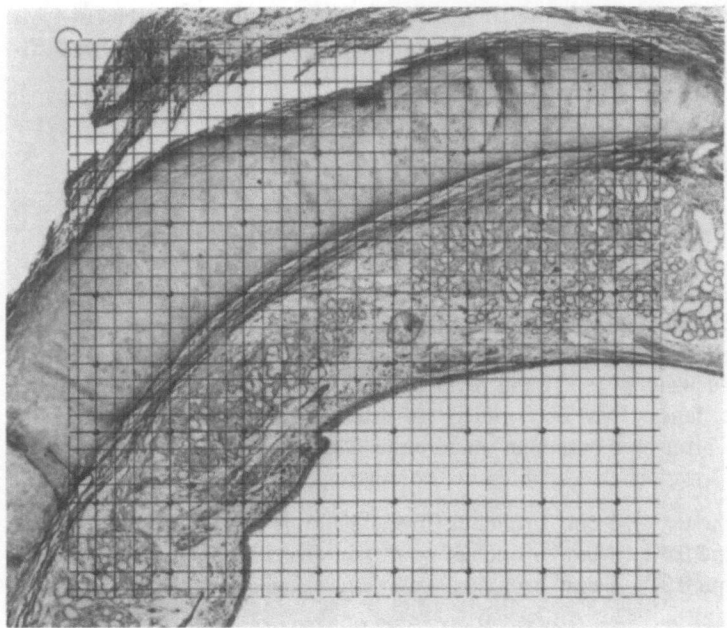

Fig. 3. Multipurpose test grid on a bronchial section. Total length of test lines is 832.0 mm. Distance between points: d_1, 13.0 mm; d_2, 3.3 mm

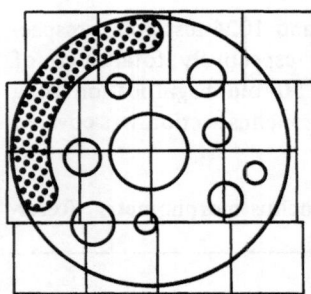

Fig. 4. Complete covering of bronchus sections by test fields for morphometrical analysis

by test fields and in this way completely analyzed (Fig. 4). We defined the tissue between the basement membrane of the respiratory epithelium and the outer limits of cartilage as bronchial wall tissue. Between the cartilage plates, the outer border of bronchi can often be recognized by a sheath of tight connective tissue. Glands and other structures beyond that sheath were attributed to the extrabronchial space. Artificial gaps of bronchial wall were added to bronchial lumen.

Calculations of volume densities have been represented in detail by *Oberholzer* et al. (1977). The surface density of bronchial basement membrane ($S_{V(BM/B)}$) was calculated as follows:

$$S_V(BM/B) = 2\,\frac{I_{BM}}{L_B}\ (cm^{-1}) \tag{2}$$

where I_{BM} is the number of intersections of test lines through bronchial basement membrane and L_B is the effective total length of test lines falling on bronchial tissue, which can be determined from the point distance (d) and the number of test points on bronchial tissue. Since only horizontal test lines are used, the following formula holds:

$$L_B = P_B \cdot d = P_B \cdot 2.59 \cdot 10^{-2}\ (cm) \tag{3}$$

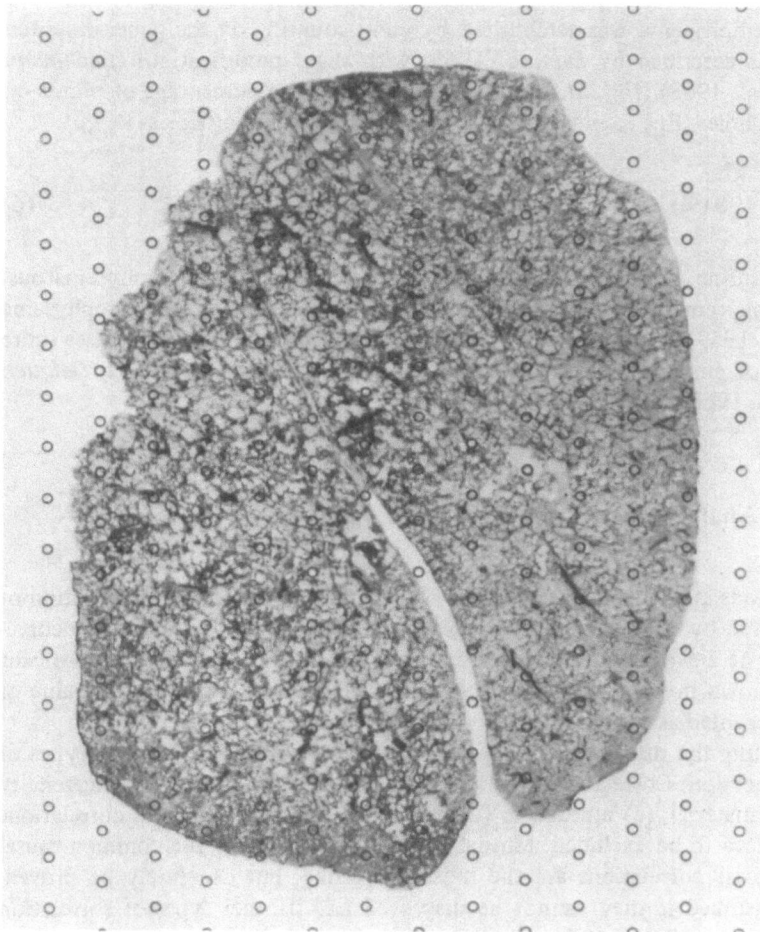

Fig. 5. Determination of degree of emphysema on paper-mounted macrosections of the lung. Section is covered by a test grid with small hollows. Distance between hollows was originally 1.5 cm

By analogy, the surface density of bronchial basement membrane related to bronchial wall tissue can be determined:

$$S_{V(MB/BWT)} = 2 \; \frac{I_{BM}}{P_{BWT} \cdot 2.59 \cdot 10^{-2}} \; (cm^{-1}) \tag{4}$$

Finally, volume and surface densities established separately for each of the three bronchi were averaged. For further details see *Oberholzer* et al. (1977).

b) Grading of Emphysema

The degree of emphysema was established by point-counting on the paper-mounted macrosections as described by *Dunnill* (1962) with slight modifications (*Bachmann* 1977; *Heath* et al. 1968) (Fig. 5). It has been defined as the percentage of points on emphysematous holes (P_E) to points on respiratory tissue including holes (P_{RSP}):

$$E = \frac{P_E}{P_{RSP}} \; 100 \; (\%) \tag{6}$$

Only holes measuring more than 1 mm in diameter were regarded as emphysematous. Typing of emphysema [aged lung, centroacinar, panacinar, perifocal emphysema (*Fletcher* et al. 1959)] was deliberately disregarded because in nearly all cases more than one type of emphysema occurs in the same lung (*Azcuy* et al. 1962; *Dalquen* 1974; *Otto* et al. 1968).

V. Statistical Analyses

Statistical methods applied in this study are listed in Table 8. Normal distribution of all data was tested by R/SD quotient. Regression analyses were carried out by curve-fitting. A value of $2P < 0.05$ (two-sided test) was accepted as statistically significant if it was not known in which direction the results would tend. Otherwise, a value of $P \leqslant 0.05$ was accepted as significant.

In interpreting the results of correlation analyses, we distinguished four types of correlative connection: Correlations may be (a) formal, (b) simulated by inhomogeneity of the original material, (c) mutual, or (d) causal. Formal and simulated correlations are futile and have to be excluded. Mutual correlations may hint at a common causal connection. Causal correlations are the most interesting, but can rarely be proved. They can be assumed if they cannot be disproved and if other types of correlation have been excluded (*Sachs* 1974). Partial correlation coefficients were used as an important tool in analyzing and interpreting correlative connections.

Table 8. Survey of statistical tests used

Proof of normal distribution	r/SD quotient
Correlation analyses	*Correlation coefficients*
Parametric	Pearson's
Nonparametric	Spearman's
	Partial
Curve-fitting analysis	*Mathematical models*
	Linear
	Logarithmic
	Exponential
	Parabolic
	Power
	Hyperbolic

VI. Discussion of Methods

Several sources of error have to be considered in clinicopathological correlation studies.

One source of error ist the *period between lung-function test and death.* In our patients this period was maximally 53 months, and on average as long as in similar studies (*Petty* et al. 1965; *Thurlbeck* et al. 1970b; *Watanabe* et al. 1965). It is not known how quickly morphological lesions, such as bronchial alterations and emphysema, which influence lung function, can change. Generally, pulmonary emphysema, for example, seems to develop over a long period, but quick formation in individual cases cannot be excluded. Therefore, some authors (*Boushy* et al. 1970; *Cosio* et al. 1978; *Gelb* et al. 1973) have used lungs from surgical pneumonectomies for clinico-pathological studies. So far we have refused these lungs because they obviously allow even less random sampling than autopsy lungs. It is not surprising that *Boushy* et al. (1970) found only 1 patient in 49 with lung resection who did not have cough, dyspnea, and airways obstruction; destructive emphysema; or enlargement of bronchial glands.

We examined the influence of the time between function test and death on the following correlations:

RAW	$= f(V_{V(MC/B)})$
RAW	$= f(V_{V(GL/B)})$
FEV_1 (% VC)	$= f(V_{V(MC/B)})$
FEV_1 (% VC)	$= f(V_{V(GL/B)})$

The results are shown in Table 9. There is a significant relation, regarding the whole group of 50 patients, between RAW and volume density of bronchial muscles. This correlation is also significant in the 21 cases in which the time between lung-function test and death did not exceed 1 year. In the 29 cases in which this interval was longer, the correlation was no longer significant. Furthermore, the dependence of this

Table 9. Dependence of some clinicopathological correlations on the period between lung-function tests and death. For details see text

| | Period between lung-function tests and death (years) | | | |
	< 0.5	< 1.0	< 2.0	All cases
RAW = f $(V_{V(MC/B)})$	$n = 15$ $r = 0.620^a$	$n = 21$ $r = 0.397$	$n = 32$ $r = 0.335$	$n = 50$ $r = 0.289^a$
RAW = f $(V_{V(GL/B)})$	$n = 15$ $r = 0.391$	$n = 21$ $r = 0.346$	$n = 32$ $r = 0.388^a$	$n = 50$ $r = 0.286^a$
FEV$_1$ = f $(V_{V(MC/B)})$	$n = 9$ $r = -0.689^a$	$n = 13$ $r = -0.333$	$n = 23$ $r = -0.241$	$n = 38$ $r = 0.304^a$
FEV$_1$ = f $(V_{V(GL/B)})$	$n = 9$ $r = -0.427$	$n = 13$ $r = -0.372$	$n = 23$ $r = -0.408$	$n = 38$ $r = -0.367^a$

[a] $2P < 0.05$

correlation on the time between function test and death is apparent, because correlation coefficients become less significant with increased time intervals. Only in the 38 cases without restrictive lung disease does FEV$_1$ show the same pattern of correlative connection with the two volume densities.

These findings suggest that at least the volume of bronchial muscle may change quickly. Nevertheless, we also include in this study cases with a time of more than 1 year between lung-function test and death, because clinical experience shows that obstructive lung disease develops over long periods of 10 or more years. Moreover we were encouraged by *Wierich*'s observations (*Wierich* and *Hartung* 1978), which suggest that FEV$_1$ values measured during life are reproducible up to 2 years post mortem.

Another error may arise if the real functional disturbance is obscured by *therapy effects*. Therefore we used only results of lung-function tests taken on or shortly after admission to hospital.

The reliability of clinical test results also depends on *accuracy of measurements* and on cooperation from patients. Cooperation is especially needed in measurements of FEV$_1$. TLC, RV, and RAW are measured by plethysmography and are therefore largely independent of cooperation.

Constancy of laboratory techniques over a long period is necessary, because it takes years to collect suitable cases for the clinicopathological studies. Therefore it is important to stress that in this study all lung-function tests were performed at the same laboratory.

Another point to be considered is that the validity of statistical results depends, among other things, on *selection and number of samples*. Samples should be selected at random. Our material, however, was obtained only from patients who had had lung-function tests. This implies preselection in a statistical sense, because the tests are only carried out on patients in whom respiratory disease is supposed. In fact, more than two-thirds of our patients had some kind of lung disease. Moreover, most patients of the Kantonsspital Basel come from a highly industrialized area, and thus the rural population is underrepresented in our material.

Thurlbeck (1976) regards differences in case selection as one of the main reasons for discrepancies among the results of various authors. Significant correlations between clinical and morphological data can be blurred if the group contains only cases with similar functional alterations. On the other hand, significant correlations are sometimes imitated by inhomogeneity of case groups and do not reflect causal relations. If one group, for example, contains a large number of patients with restrictive lung disease, correlations between TLC and morphometrical parameters or between age and any other data may be falsified. Finally, the composition of the cases may be inhomogeneous if in the same patient two or more diseases, e.g., restrictive and obstructive ventilation disorder, are superimposed.

Selection and number of samples are also important in morphometrical analyses. Valid results are obtained only if for measurement of volume densities a *minimal number of test points*, and for measurement of surface density a *minimal length of test lines*, are counted. This was guaranteed by pilot studies.

Artifacts introduced by *tissue preparation* are another source of error. *Ryan* (1969) reported emphysema-like alterations of lung tissue after fixation with formol steam. However, this kind of artifact occurs only in autolytic brittle lungs. We never saw such alterations after transbronchial instillation of a fluid fixative.

Fixation and embedding in paraffin leads to tissue shrinkage. The degree of shrinkage depends on the physiological density of the various tissue compounds, the embedding medium, and the fixative (*Bahr* et al. (1957). Cartilage shrinks less than other structures of the bronchial wall. Therefore variable-shrinking artifacts can change the volumetric relations between the tissue compounds (Fig. 6). Table 10 illustrates the different shrinkage effects on lung tissue after fixation with various fixatives. In con-

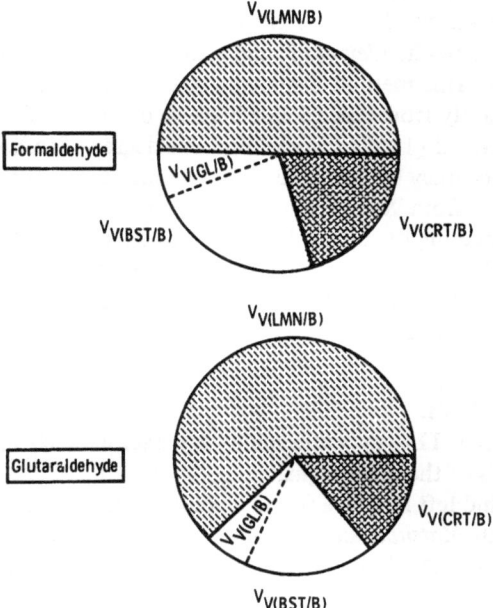

Fig. 6a, b. Relations of volume densities in reference volume B depending on different fixatives. Volume densities of lumen and cartilage differ significantly ($2P < 0.05$)

Table 10. Shift of volumetric relations between bronchial-wall compounds if different fixatives are used. Differences of volume densities are only listed if significant. The last column shows the mean deviation of volume densities as established in bronchi fixed with formaldehyde from those after fixation with glutaraldehyde. (Volume densities in the bronchus fixed with glutaraldehyde = 100%.)

	Formaldehyde 4% Mean ± SD ($n = 8$)	Glutaraldehyde 2.5% Mean ± SD ($n = 8$)	Deviation (%)
$V_V(LMN/B)^a$	0.499 ± 0.009	0.625 ± 0.025	79.8
$V_V(CRT/B)^b$	0.208 ± 0.019	0.146 ± 0.005	143.5
$V_V(BST/B)$	0.292 ± 0.013	0.260 ± 0.007	112.3
$V_V(GL/B)$	0.061 ± 0.005	0.049 ± 0.004	124.5
$V_V(MC/BWT)^c$	0.042 ± 0.003	0.063 ± 0.007	66.7
$V_V(MC/BST)^c$	0.072 ± 0.003	0.097 ± 0.010	74.2
$V_V(CT/BST)^c$	0.632 ± 0.011	0.584 ± 0.018	108.2

[a] $2P < 0.001$ [b] $2P < 0.01$ [c] $2P < 0.05$

trast to fixation and embedding, the usual staining methods do not influence morphometrical results.

Morphometrical measurements on lung tissue and bronchi can only be made if lungs are fixed at a constant, nearly physiological degree of inflation, because the geometrical structure of respiratory tissue remains unchanged only under this condition. The degree of inflation also influences the stretching of bronchi, and thereby the state of contraction, configuration, and volume density of bronchial muscles. To control inflation during fixation, various methods have been reported in the literature, some of which demand expensive equipment (*Blumenthal* and *Boren* 1959; *Hartung* 1963; *Heard* 1962; *Schubert* 1960; *Weibel* and *Vidone* 1961; *Wright* et al. 1974). Nevertheless, exact determination of inflation is difficult. *Weibel* (1963) estimated it from the weight and volume of the inflated lung. This method cannot be applied to diseased lungs, the weight of which varies significantly from case to case because of their different content of blood and edema fluid. *Heard* (1962) showed that the degree of inflation can be established with sufficient accuracy by comparing the volume of lungs expanded postmortem with TLC estimated from X-ray pictures taken during life. We established the degree of inflation by comparing the lung volume measured immediately after instillation of the fixative with TLC as measured intra vitam. We found that lungs fixed by transbronchial fluid instillation are inflated to 70%–80% of TLC (Fig. 7).

Discrepancies between lung volume estimated post mortem and that measured intra vitam may be caused by:

a) Different inflation effects of air and fluids.
b) Falsification of intra vitam measured TLC by extrapulmonary factors such as pleural effusions, tumors, or paralysis of the diaphragma.
c) Inequality of volume between right and left lung. We found a volume ratio between left and right lungs of 9:11, as did *Matsuba* and *Thurlbeck* (1972). However, individual deviations are very frequent. The left lung can even be bigger than the right one.

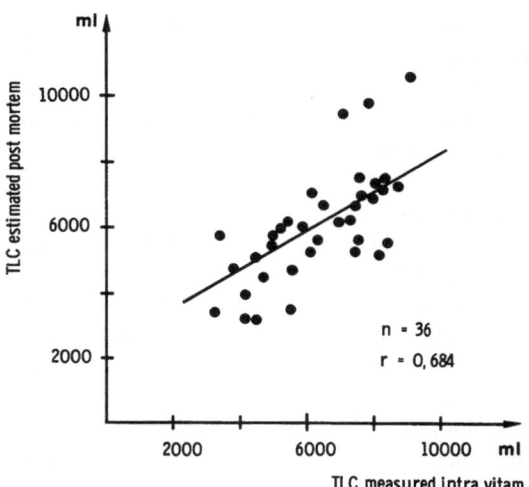

Fig. 7. Comparison between TLC as estimated post mortem and TLC as measured intra vitam for determination of the degree of inflation. $r_{SP} = 0.684$; $n = 36$; $P < 0.001$

Several methods have been described for *grading of emphysema* (*Dunnill* 1962, 1965; *Heard* 1969; *Jutabha* and *Lonngren* 1969; *Kory* et al. 1966; *Longfield* and *Hentel* 1969; *Prinsloo* 1966; *Ryder* et al. 1969; *Thurlbeck* and *Angus* 1967; *Thurlbeck* et al. 1970a). Point-counting (*Dunnill* 1962) has turned out to be the best for clinicopathological correlations because it discriminates minor differences of tissue destruction and delivers well-reproducible results (*Bachmann* 1977).

Anderson and *Dunnill* (1965) found in some cases considerable differences in degree of emphysema among the various slices of a lung. We share *Thurlbeck*'s opinion (1967) that such differences are avoided if the portion of destroyed tissue is related only to respiratory parenchyma and not to the whole lung, which also contains connective tissue, vessels, and bronchi. Errors in grading caused by different amounts of destroyed tissue in marginal and central parts of the lung can be minimized if the central slice, which is most representative of the whole lung, is taken for macrosection (*Bachmann* 1977). The degree of emphysema established in the left lung can be regarded as representative of the right lung, too (*Prinsloo* 1966). Finally, it could be demonstrated that the degree of emphysema established by macrosection corresponds well to the alveolar surface density as established by histomorphometry [r_{SP} (Spearman correlation coefficient) $= 0.828, n = 25$, see *Bachmann* (1977)]. Only minor degrees of tissue destruction are incorrectly established by the macrosection method. Nevertheless, we did not use a hand lens as suggested by others (*Jenkins* et al. 1965), because very low grade emphysema has no measurable influence on function (*Otto* and *Zeilhofer* 1969; *Pratt* and *Klugh* 1967; *Ryan* et al. 1965).

Some possible sources of error in bronchus morphometry and the *applicability of Reid's index* are discussed in detail elsewhere (*Oberholzer* et al. 1977, 1978). In addition, the inhomogeneous distribution of glands, muscles, capillaries, and so on within the bronchial system has to be considered if the number of bronchus samples is defined for the morphometrical study. Three samples seems to be a sufficient number, because we found that the variation coefficient of the volume densities of the various components of bronchial wall is smaller than 33%, the upper limit which is usually accepted (*Rohr* et al. 1976). Even if three samples meet this condition, the question has still to be answered whether all bronchi or at least all central ones are always affected in the same way so that the morphometrical results are representative. With few exceptions (*Niewoehner* et al. 1973), bronchial glands seem to react uniformly (*Reid* 1960; *Restrepo* and *Heard* 1963; *Sturgess* and *Reid* 1972). However, thickening of bronchial muscles seems to vary considerably from peripheral to central bronchi because the muscular compartment is smaller in the central ones (*Hale* et al. 1968; *Hayek* 1970). Therefore muscle hyperplasia manifests itself later in central bronchi and may easily be overlooked in early phases of obstructive disease. Atrophy of cartilage has been observed in bronchi beyond the segmental and subsegmental levels (*Maisel* et al. 1972; *Thurlbeck* et al. 1974; *Wright* and *Stuart* 1965). Therefore the chosen samples of central bronchi are probably not representative in regard to cartilage.

It will hardly be possible to estimate the influence on the development of bronchial lesions of such *concomitant affections* as bronchial carcinoma, pulmonary fibrosis, pneumonia, congestive lung disease, mechanical ventilation, and other factors which stress the pulmonary clearing system. Furthermore, we do not know within what time frame bronchial lesions change. In interpreting the results of a study, one has to consider these uncertainties as well.

VII. Baseline Data of Bronchus Morphometry

The baseline data of bronchus morphometry were established in five subjects with normal lung function. The mean volume densities of the most important tissue compounds are listed in Table 11 and are comparable to data available in the literature. For further details see *Oberholzer* et al. (1977).

Table 11. Baseline data in five cases displaying no functional disorder. (For further details see *Oberholzer* et al. 1977)

Reference volume Parameter	Unit	B Mean	SD	BWT Mean	SD	BST Mean	SD
V_V(LMN)	cm^3/cm^3	0.544	0.030				
V_V(CRT)	cm^3/cm^3	0.172	0.010	0.387	0.038		
V_V(BST)	cm^3/cm^3	0.284	0.034	0.613	0.041		
V_V(GL)	cm^3/cm^3	0.057	0.011	0.124	0.019	0.203	0.025
V_V(GD)	cm^3/cm^3	0.003	0.001	0.007	0.003	0.011	0.005
V_V(MC)	cm^3/cm^3	0.006	0.001	0.014	0.003	0.022	0.004
V_V(VN)	cm^3/cm^3	0.009	0.003	0.019	0.005	0.032	0.007
V_V(CT)	cm^3/cm^3	0.209	0.023	0.449	0.034	0.732	0.037
S_V(BM)	cm^2/cm^3	4.147	0.373	9.027	0.365		

VII. Correlations Between Morphometrical Parameters of Bronchial Wall

The correlations between morphometrical parameters of bronchial wall were examined in the 50 cases of group B (Tables 13–15).

Formal correlations exist between volume densities which are complementary within a reference volume. Such correlations are the more probable the larger the correlated volume densities. *Mutual correlations* occur because the obstructive disease manifest itself in various lesions, e.g., in thickening of smooth muscles, thickening of glands, and enlargement of glandular ducts. Therefore mutual correlations between morphometrical parameters are probably the basis of mutual correlations between functional parameters. It is a matter of *causal correlation* if the change in one bronchial compartment influences another. If, for instance, the volume of bronchial glands increases, the bronchial wall must become wider and thereby the bronchial lumen narrower. The mean volume densities are given in Table 12.

1. Formal Correlations

The following significant correlations are purely formal:

$$V_{V(LMN/B)} = f(V_{V(BST/BWT)}) \text{ (Table 13)}$$
$$V_{V(CRT/BWT)} = f(V_{V(BST/BWT)}) \text{ (Table 14)}$$
$$V_{V(GL/BST)} = f(V_{V(CT/BST)}) \text{ (Table 15)}$$

Other correlations seem to be partially formal, especially those between the volume density of bronchial lumen and the other volume densities in reference volume B. One must assume that in central bronchi, changes in bronchial wall volume lead only to changes in bronchial lumen, not to changes in the total bronchial diameter. (The reverse is only possible in bronchiectases, which were excluded from the study.) Accordingly,

Table 12. Mean values and standard deviation of the morphometrical parameters within the whole group B ($n = 50$)

Reference volume		B		BWT		BST	
Parameter	Unit	Mean	SD	Mean	SD	Mean	SD
$V_{V(LMN)}$[a]	cm³/cm³	0.434[a]	0.012				
$V_{V(BST)}$[a]	cm³/cm³	0.345[a]	0.010	0.600	0.010		
$V_{V(CRT)}$[a]	cm³/cm³	0.225[a]	0.008	0.403	0.012		
$V_{V(CT)}$	cm³/cm³	0.219	0.007	0.392	0.012	0.649	0.011
$V_{V(GL)}$[a]	cm³/cm³	0.083[a]	0.005	0.147[a]	0.007	0.245[a]	0.010
$V_{V(GD)}$[a]	cm³/cm³	0.009[a]	0.001	0.015[a]	0.002	0.025[a]	0.003
$V_{V(MC)}$[a]	cm³/cm³	0.014[a]	0.001	0.026[a]	0.001	0.043[a]	0.002
$V_{V(VN)}$[a]	cm³/cm³	0.012[a]	0.001	0.021[a]	0.002	0.035[a]	0.003
$S_{V(BM)}$[a]	cm²/cm³	4.006[a]	0.097	7.335[a]	0.260		

[a] Normal distribution

Table 13. Spearman rank correlation coefficients of correlations between morphometrical parameters in reference volume B

B	VV(BST)	VV(CRT)	VV(CT)	VV(GL)	VV(GD)	VV(MC)	VV(VN)	SV(BM)
VV(LMN)	-0.739[a]	-0.511[a]	-0.555[a]	-0.509[a]	-0.356[a]	-0.459[a]	-0.245	0.369[a]
VV(BST)	—	-0.067	0.753[a]	0.380[a]	0.294[a]	0.570[a]	0.307[a]	-0.098
VV(CRT)	—	—	-0.159	0.257	0.153	-0.059	-0.012	-0.346[a]
VV(CT)	—	—	—	-0.049	0.023	0.431[a]	0.160	-0.029
VV(GL)	—	—	—	—	0.370[a]	0.358[a]	-0.044	-0.276[a]
VV(GD)	—	—	—	—	—	0.124	0.030	-0.351[a]
VV(MC)	—	—	—	—	—	—	0.088	-0.181
VV(VN)	—	—	—	—	—	—	—	-0.046

[a] $2P < 0.05$

Table 14. Spearman rank correlation coefficients of correlations between morphometrical parameters in reference volume BWT

BWT	VV(CT)	VV(GL)	VV(GD)	VV(MC)	VV(VN)	SV(BM)
VV(BST)	0.687[a]	0.254	0.093	0.445[a]	0.023	0.111
VV(CT)	—	-0.399[a]	-0.239	0.139	-0.019	0.327[a]
VV(GL)	—	—	0.211	0.258	-0.150	-0.289[a]
VV(GD)	—	—	—	-0.008	-0.043	-0.389[a]
VV(MC)	—	—	—	—	0.022	-0.160
VV(VN)	—	—	—	—	—	-0.013

[a] $2P < 0.05$

changes in one tissue compartment must be balanced by an opposite change in bronchial lumen. Therefore the coefficients of correlations between volume density of lumen and the other compounds must be negative in reference volume B. This has been confirmed by our findings (Table 13). For the same reasons, similar correlations exist between volume density of bronchial wall tissue without cartilage ($V_{V(BST/B)}$) and the other tissue compartments in reference volume B (Table 13).

Reference volume BWT, however, is not constant, because the bronchial wall tissue can increase and decrease. Therefore only the volume densities of connective tissue and muscles are significantly correlated with that of bronchial tissue without cartilage (Table 14). The connective tissue is the largest compartment of the bronchial wall tissue without cartilage and therefore correlates closely with it.

The interpretation of the significant correlation between surface density of bronchial basement membrane and the volume density of connective tissue in the reference volume BWT is difficult. It suggests that the increase of bronchial surface is connected with decrease of connective tissue in the bronchial wall (Table 14), but is at variance with the correlation between surface density of basement membrane and volume density of bronchial lumen, which suggests that the bronchial surface related to the whole bronchus decreases with narrowing of the bronchial lumen. The correlation between basement membrane and connective tissue is probably formal, because the connective tissue behaves complementarily to the other tissue compounds. This explanation is supported by the negative correlation coefficients between surface density of bronchial basement membrane and volume density of glands and glandular ducts in the reference volume BWT (Table 14).

2. Mutual Correlations

Surface density of basement membrane and volume density of glandular ducts are significantly correlated in reference volumes B and BWT (Tables 12, 13). This means that the surface of bronchial mucosa decreases and the bronchial lumen gets narrower if glandular ducts are enlarged. This finding is surprising, because glandular ducts represent only 0.9% of the reference volume B and 1.5% of the reference volume BWT (Table 12). Even the maximum value amounts only to 3.0% in B and 5.2% in BWT, so

Table 15. Spearman rank correlation coefficients of correlations between morphometrical parameters in reference volume BST

BST	$V_{V(GL)}$	$V_{V(GD)}$	$V_{V(MC)}$	$V_{V(VN)}$	$S_{V(BM)}$
$V_{V(CT)}$	−0.920[a]	−0.454[a]	−0.211	−0.041	0.396[a]
$V_{V(GL)}$	−	0.268	0.143	−0.158	−0.301[a]
$V_{V(GD)}$	−	−	−0.004	−0.060	−0.271
$V_{V(MC)}$	−	−	−	−0.088	−0.212
$V_{V(VN)}$	−	−	−	−	−0.040

[a] $2P < 0.05$

that thickening of the bronchial wall as expressed by decreasing surface of bronchial mucosa cannot possibly be produced by increasing volume of glandular ducts. Therefore this correlation must be mutual, mediated by bronchial glands, the thickening of which is on the one hand significantly related to enlargement of glandular ducts (Table 14) and on the other hand leads to narrowing of bronchial lumen.

Since glands and glandular ducts represent a functional unit, the significant correlation between their volume densities can also be interpreted as mutual. The same is valid in regard to the relation between volume densities of glands and muscles in reference volumes B and BWT [in BWT, only after elimination of connective tissue as an influencing factor; r_{PART} (partial correlation coefficient) = 0.346], for glands and muscles are probably stimulated by the same mechanism in obstructive disease.

There is probably a mutual correlation between increase of muscles and bronchial wall tissue without cartilage, also mediated by glands (Tables 13, 14). This interrelation remains significant after elimination of the influence of connective tissue (r_{PART} = 0.312). The muscles themselves scarcely contribute to the width of bronchial wall tissue, because their volume comprise only 4.3% (2.1%–8.6%) of BST; in our cases, however, the glands comprise an average of 24.5% of BST (Table 12).

The significant connection between surface density of bronchial basement membrane and volume density of bronchial cartilage cannot be clarified. It may be that in chronic bronchitis, hypertrophy of cartilage leads to narrowing of bronchial lumen.

3. Causal Correlations

The following correlations must be causal:

$$S_{V(BM/B)} = f(V_{V(LMN/B)})$$
$$V_{V(GL/B)} = f(V_{V(LMN/B)})$$

The first of the two correlations suggests that the bronchial lumen is stenosed concentrically and not by protruding ridges of the mucosa, because lumen and bronchial surface change in the same sense. If ridges of mucosa had a stenosing effect on the lumen, the surface density of bronchial basement membrane would probably increase if the volume density of bronchial lumen decreased.

The concentric narrowing of lumen is produced by thickening of bronchial glands. This is shown by the second correlation, which remains highly significant even after elimination of cartilage and connective tissue as influencing factors (r_{PART} = −0.696). Moreover, the interrelation between surface density of basement membrane and bronchial lumen is weaker if the influence of bronchial glands is eliminated (r_{PART} = 0.276 instead of r_{SP} = 0.369). Conversely, the interrelation appears stronger if the influence of connective tissue is eliminated (r_{PART} = 0.424). This means that the bronchial lumen is influenced by thickening of the glands and not by the connective tissue. The correlations between surface density of bronchial basement membrane and volume densities of glands and glandular ducts must be interpreted in the same way (Tables 13, 14).

IX. Dependence of Clinical and Morphological Parameters on Age

Age dependence of lung function parameters is well known (*Amrein* et al. 1969; *Comroe* 1974; *Fletcher* et al. 1976; *Islam* et al. 1978). In the Basel lung-function laboratory, it was found that the predicted values of TLC (ml) and RV (% TLC) increase with age, whereas VC (% TLC) and FEV_1 (% VC) decrease (*Amrein* et al. 1969). These age-dependent changes of pulmonary function are equivalent to those of a slight obstructive ventilation disorder, which does not necessarily indicate the same morphological basis. If morphometrical parameters were to be correlated with age in the same way, the interrelations between them and lung-function parameters would have to be interpreted as mutual. Therefore, the age dependence of both clinical and morphometrical parameters was studied in the 50 cases of group B.

1. Age Dependence of Functional Parameters

Our findings are summarized in Table 16. The age dependence of RAW in our material is at variance with that reported by *Amrein* et al. (1969) but agrees with the findings of others (*Islam* et al. 1978; *Niewoehner* and *Kleinerman* 1974; *Wierich* and *Hartung* 1978). In our cases the correlation between age and RAW probably reflects the age dependence of obstructive disease, which, however, has not been confirmed by all investigators (*Penman* et al. 1970).

Other authors found a continuous decrease of FEV_1 in patients over the age of 20 (*Amrein* et al. 1969; *Anderhub* et al. 1974; *Fletcher* et al. 1976). Accordingly, there is a connection between age and FEV_1 (as % VC and % of predicted value) in our cases, too (Fig. 8). However, after elimination of RAW as an influencing factor, the correlation coefficient lies below the level of significance ($r_{PART} = -0.143$). The cause may be that the distribution of age is not random in our cases. We would expect that the relation between age and RV is also not as clearly demonstrable as in clinical studies; however, according to *Amrein* (1969) RV increases about 100% up to the age of 65. Within the same time, FEV_1 diminishes only 30%–40%. Age-dependent changes in FEV_1 are therefore less discernible than those in RV in a preselected group such as ours. The deviation of FEV_1 values with increasing age (Fig. 8) is in accordance with

Table 16. Dependence of functional parameters on age in the 50 cases with morphometrical analysis of bronchi

	r_{SP}
TLC (% predicted)	0.336[a]
RV (% TLC)	0.463[a]
VC (% predicted)	−0.252
FEV_1 (% VC)	−0.345[a]
FEV_1 (% predicted)	−0.323[a]
RAW (cm H_2O/liter $\cdot$ s^{-1})	0.353[a]

[a] $2P < 0.05$

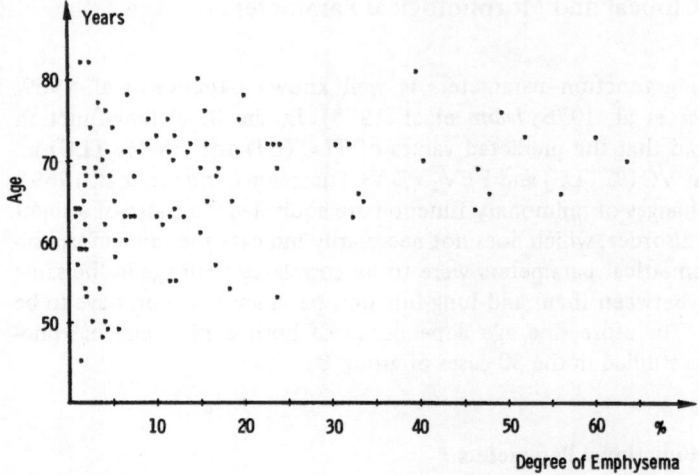

Fig. 8. Correlation between age and degree of emphysema. $r_{SP} = 0.311$; $n = 97$; $2P < 0.01$

the findings of *Fletcher* et al. (1976). It probably occurs because FEV_1 decreases faster the more severe the course of the obstructive diseases is.

The CVPh is not age-dependent.

2. Age Dependence of Morphometrical Parameters

No morphometrical compartment of the bronchial wall showed a correlation with age.

Within the group of 97 patients with emphysema (E_2, Table 1), a significant relation between degree of tissue destruction and age could be established ($r_{SP} = 0.311$; $2P < 0.01$). This correlation will be discussed later.

X. Influence of Emphysema on Pulmonary Function

The relations between degree of emphysema and pulmonary function were studied in the 97 cases in which a degree of tissue destruction of more than 2% had been established by point-counting on macrosections (group E_2, Table 1).

We found a significant interrelation between degree of emphysema and RAW (Table 17), but the deviation of RAW values was considerable at all degrees of emphysema. Therefore one must assume that tissue destruction scarcely influences the resistance at regular breathing. The findings suggest that RAW is the parameter of obstruction arising in bronchi. We took advantage of this in order to estimate the effect of emphysema alone on lung function by eliminating RAW as influencing factor in the calculation of partial correlation coefficients.

FEV$_1$ is more closely related to the degree of emphysema than is RAW (Table 17). The relation remains significant after elimination of RAW as an influencing factor (r_{PART} = −0.303, 2 P < 0.01). In cases with tissue destruction of more than 20%, FEV$_1$ is always below 50% VC (Fig. 9); however, there is a considerable deviation of FEV$_1$ values if tissue destruction amounts to less than 10%. From this it can be concluded that FEV$_1$ is not influenced only by emphysematous tissue destruction.

Finally, the question arises to what extent, even in cases with severe tissue destruction, is FEV$_1$ influenced by bronchial alterations, and not by emphysema itself. Therefore the behavior of FEV$_1$ in ten cases with emphysema over 10% (mean 22% ± 4%) and mean RAW of 2.4 ± 0.2 cm H$_2$O/liter per second was compared with that in ten cases without emphysema and a mean RAW of 2.3 ± 0.2 (groups E$_5$ and E$_6$). We found a significantly lower mean FEV$_1$ in the cases with emphysema ($\overline{FEV_1}$ = 51.0% ± 1.9% VC) compared with cases without emphysema ($\overline{FEV_1}$ = 66.0% ± 3.3% VC) (2 P < 0.005). However, the lowering of FEV$_1$ in cases with emphysema is only moderate and out of proportion to the severity of tissue destruction. We therefore presume that the influence of tissue destruction on FEV$_1$ cannot be very important.

The interrelations between CVPh and emphysema were studied in 138 cases of group E. In these cases the expiratory-flow curve was controlled: of the 138 patients,

Table 17. Spearman rank correlation coefficients between degree of emphysema and functional parameters (n = 97)

	r_{SP}
TLC (% predicted)	0.501a
RV (% TLC)	0.332a
FEV$_1$ (% VC)	−0.423a
RAW (cm H$_2$O/liter · s^{-1})	0.303a

a 2 P < 0.05

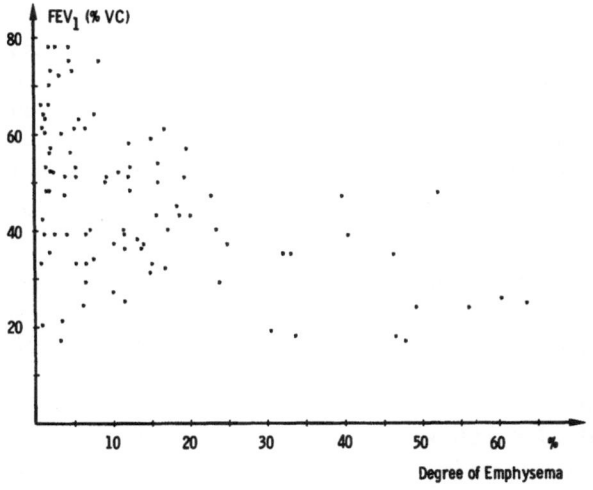

Fig. 9. Correlation between FEV$_1$ (% VC) and degree of emphysema. r_{SP} = −0.423, n = 97, 2 P < 0.001

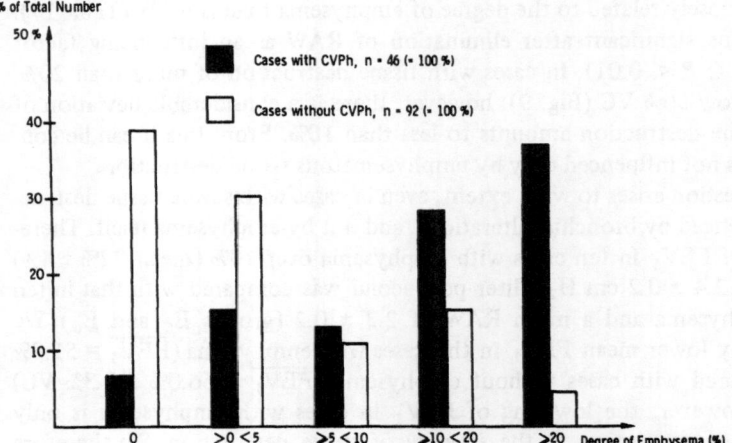

Fig. 10. CVPh related to degree of emphysema. Frequency of CVPh increases with increase of degree of emphysema, but CVPh occurs also in cases without emphysema

46 showed CVPh. Of these 46 patients, 44 had a raised RAW (group $E_{3.1}$.), but only 38 of 92 patients without CVPh showed an increased RAW (group $E_{4.1}$.).

From Fig. 10 it can be gathered that CVPh is more frequent in cases with a high degree of emphysema. However, on the one hand CVPh is missing in some cases with high-grade emphysema, whereas on the other hand it does occur in cases without a trace of tissue destruction. Therefore we believe that emphysema cannot possibly be the only cause of bronchial collapse as indicated by CVPh.

In 82 cases with raised RAW (groups $E_{3.1}$. and $E_{4.1}$.) the interrelations between CVPh, FEV_1, RAW, and emphysema were examined. The following conclusions were drawn:

1. The difference in RAW in cases with and without CVPh is independent of the degree of emphysema (Fig. 11).
2. As expected, FEV_1 is significantly lower in cases with CVPh, despite similar values of RAW. However, the difference decreases with degree of emphysema, which can be interpreted as the consequence of an additional effect of tissue destruction on FEV_1. The coefficient of correlation between FEV_1 and degree of emphysema in cases without CVPh is -0.429 ($2P < 0.01$). Presumably, severe emphysema can act on FEV_1 if central airways do not collapse, whereas collapse of central airways alone always leads to considerably lower FEV_1 (Fig. 12).

Among the 97 cases with emphysema (group E_2), a relatively close relation between degree of emphysema and TLC was found ($r_{SP} = 0.501$, $2P < 0.001$). However, there were some cases with low-grade emphysema and a TLC as high as 130%–160% of the predicted value.

The degree of emphysema does not correlate as well with RV ($r_{SP} = 0.332$, $2P < 0.01$) as with TLC ($r_{SP} = 0.501$, $2P < 0.001$). Nevertheless it is conspicuous that RV at parenchymal destruction of 20% or more lies routinely above 50% TLC. However, if

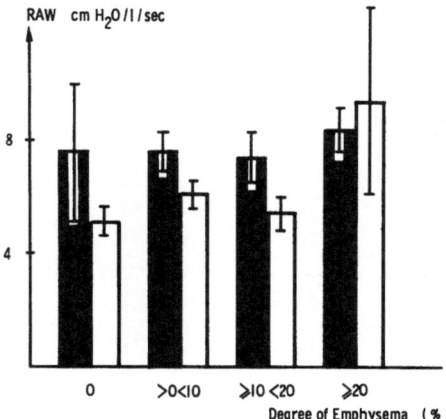

Fig. 11. CVPh related to bronchial resistance and degree of emphysema. RAW is usually higher in cases with CVPh *(black)* than in those without CVPh *(white)*, but is independent of degree of emphysema in either case

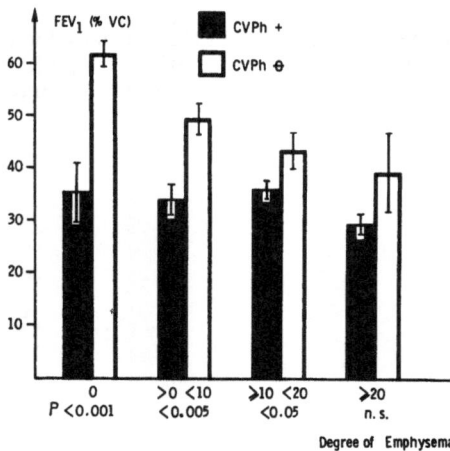

Fig. 12. CVPh related to FEV_1 and degree of emphysema. Independent of degree of emphysema, FEV_1 is disproportionally lowered in cases with CVPh *(black)*. There is a distinct correlation between FEV_1 and degree of emphysema only in cases without CVPh *(white)*. $r_{SP} = 0.429$; $n = 38$; $2P < 0.01$. *n.s.*, not significant

the degree of emphysema is lower than 20%, RV values deviate even more than TLC values. Also, the simultaneous increase of TLC and RV is not a sign of emphysema, as shown in Fig. 13.

If age is eliminated as an influencing factor, the correlation between emphysema and RV is still significant ($r_{PART} = 0.269$, $2P < 0.01$). this could be falsely interpreted as a pathogenetic connection. However, we could show a close interrelation between RV and RAW ($r_{SP} = 0.735$) in the 97 cases with emphysema (group E_2) as well as in the 50 cases of group B. Therefore it is more probable that increase in RV is caused by bronchial and/or bronchiolar lesions. Moreover, the correlation between emphysema and RV is no longer significant if the influence of the bronchial obstruction is eliminated ($r_{SP} = 0.132$). In summary, destructive emphysema cannot be clinically inferred from an increase of TLC and/or RV.

The integration of several clinical parameters also does not allow an unequivocal clinical diagnosis of destructive emphysema, as demonstrated in the 128 cases of group E_1. In all of these cases the severity of obstructive lung disease was established:

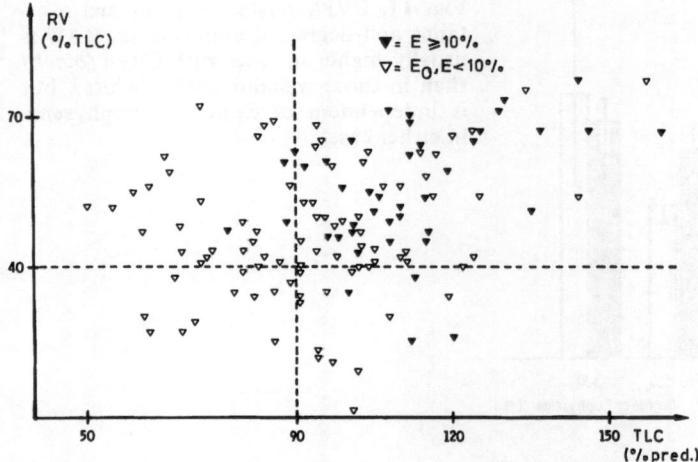

Fig. 13. RV and TLC related to degree of emphysema. RV and TLC are usually high in cases with degree of emphysema of more than 10% (▲). The combination of high RV and high TLC, however, can also be observed in many cases with low-grade emphysema (△)

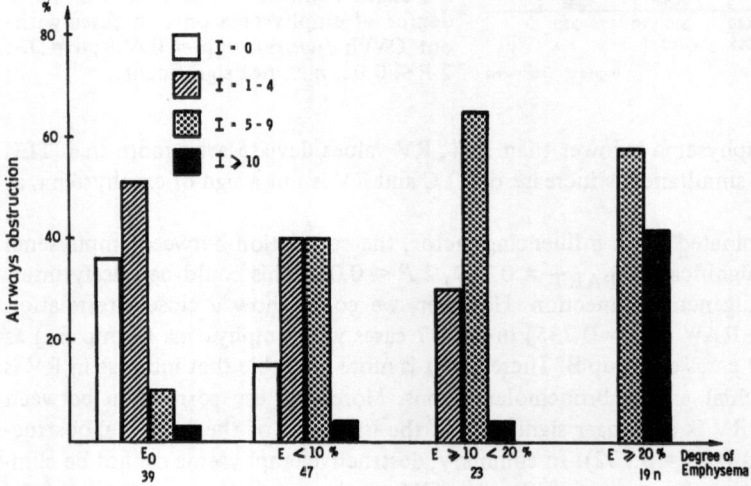

Fig. 14. Correlation between degree of airways obstruction and degree of emphysema. Cases with high-grade emphysema (E ⩾ 20%) always showed clinically moderate or severe functional disturbances, but similar functional disorder was also observed in cases without emphysema. *I*, degree of airways obstruction (Sect. C.II.)

46 (35.9%) showed slight, 49 (38.3%) moderate, and 12 (9.4%) severe obstructive ventilation disorder. We found severe functional disorder with all degrees of emphysema, even in patients without any trace of tissue destruction, but most cases of severe functional disorder showed advanced emphysema. All patients with 20% or more tissue destruction had moderate or severe functional disorder. Lung function was unchanged only in some cases in which the degree of emphysema was below 10% (Fig. 14).

Finally, we studied the relation between degree of emphysema and volume densities of bronchial glands and glandular ducts in 24 cases. There was a significant correlation to be noticed only in a subgroup of eight cases with CVPh ($r_{SP} = -0.909$, $n = 8$, $2P < 0.01$), which suggests that the glandular volume at a high level of hypertrophy decreases with increasing degree of emphysema.

XI. Correlations Between Clinical Parameters and Bronchial Alterations

The results given in the foregoing section suggest that the effect of tissue destruction is less important for function thatn the effect of bronchial and/or bronchiolar lesions. The bronchial lesions are the subject of the following analysis.

Coefficients of all relations studied are listed in Table 18. Significant interrelations were found between *volume density of bronchial lumen* and RAW as well as FEV_1 and VC (% predicted value). The findings show that narrowing of the bronchial lumen is paralleled by an increase in RAW and lowering of FEV_1 and VC. The relations between bronchial narrowing and RAW and FEV_1 are compatible with the usual pneumological conceptions. However, the connection between VC and bronchial width is not clear. It is probably based on a mutual correlation, because in obstructive disease VC is generally lowered by an increase in RV. Such an increase in RV and decrease in VC concur with an increase in bronchial resistance. Therefore the correlation between volume density of bronchial lumen and VC becomes insignificant after elimination of FEV_1 or RAW as influencing factors ($r_{PART} = 0.196$ and 0.214 respectively).

The *surface density of bronchial basement membrane* related to BWT correlates significantly with VC, FEV_1 (% predicted), and RAW, the same functional parameters with which the volume density of bronchial lumen related to B correlates. This supports our assumption that in central bronchi the surface of the basement membrane does not change without a change in the bronchial lumen.

The *volume density of bronchial wall without cartilage* correlated significantly with RV, VC, and RAW. Regression analysis showed nearly linear functions. The correlations correspond to those between volume density of bronchial lumen and clinical parameters, with the only difference being that the volume density of bronchial wall is also significantly related to RV in both reference volumes. This correlation, however, is lost if age and bronchial obstruction as influencing factors are eliminated ($r_{PART} = 0.030$). Thus changes in RV are probably caused by age-dependent and other morphological alterations. Since the increase in RV always takes place at the cost of VC, the statistical correlation between volume density of bronchial wall tissue without cartilage and VC must be regarded as mutual. Only the connection between bronchial lumen and RAW seems to be causal.

Table 18. Spearman rank correlation coefficients of correlations between functional and morphometric parameters in reference volume B

	VV(LMN/B)	VV(BST/B)	VV(GL/B)	VV(GD/B)	VV(MC/B)	VV(CT/B)	SV(BM/B)
TLC (% predicted)	−0.091	0.204	0.097	0.384[a]	−0.002	–	−0.001
RV (% TLC)	−0.263	0.319[a]	0.316[a]	0.304[a]	0.266	–	−0.108
VC (% predicted)	0.323[a]	−0.301[a]	−0.221	0.010	−0.244	–	0.212
FEV$_1$ (% VC)	0.246	−0.199	−0.301[a]	−0.471[a]	−0.255	0.021	0.152
FEV$_1$ (% predicted)	0.325[a]	−0.209	−0.401[a]	−0.403[a]	−0.264	0.044	0.287[a]
RAW (cm H$_2$O/ liter · s^{-1})	−0.364[a]	0.430[a]	0.283[a]	0.445[a]	0.284[a]	0.275	−0.176

[a] $2 P < 0.05$

The *volume density of bronchial glands* is significantly correlated in reference volume B with RV, FEV_1 (% VC), FEV_1 (% predicted), and RAW. The correlation between FEV_1 and volume density of bronchial glands is the only one which holds in all three reference volumes. Therefore we assume that changes in bronchial glands and secretions influence FEV_1 fundamentally.

The relation between gland volume and FEV_1 (% VC and % predicted) has already been established by others (*Boushy* et al. 1970; *Dunnill* 1974; *McKenzie* et al. 1969; *Thurlbeck* et al. 1970b). This relation means that FEV_1 decreases with increasing gland volume (Fig. 15). The correlation between gland volume and FEV_1 (% predicted) is closer than that between gland volume and FEV_1 (% VC) because of the greater accuracy of FEV_1 (% predicted) measurement (*Cullen* et al. 1970). With one exception (*McKenzie* et al. 1969), others reported lower correlation coefficients, probably because they compared gland thickness measured by Reid's index and not by pointcounting with functional parameters (*Oberholzer* et al. 1978).

The age-dependent decrease of FEV_1 (*Amrein* et al. 1969; *Fletcher* et al. 1976) was confirmed in our studies (Table 16). However, there is no relation between gland volume and age. This suggests a causal connection between gland thickening and loss of FEV_1 in obstructive disease.

The correlation between volume density of glands and RV does not seem to be age-dependent, because the correlation coefficient is even higher if age is eliminated as an influencing factor (in reference volume B: r_{PART} = 0.388, 2 P < 0.01). On the other hand, if the influence of bronchial obstruction in the form of FEV_1 or RAW is eliminated, the correlation disappears (r_{PART} = 0.065 and 0.176 respectively). These findings suggest that the correlation between gland volume and RV is mediated by airway obstruction and not by age.

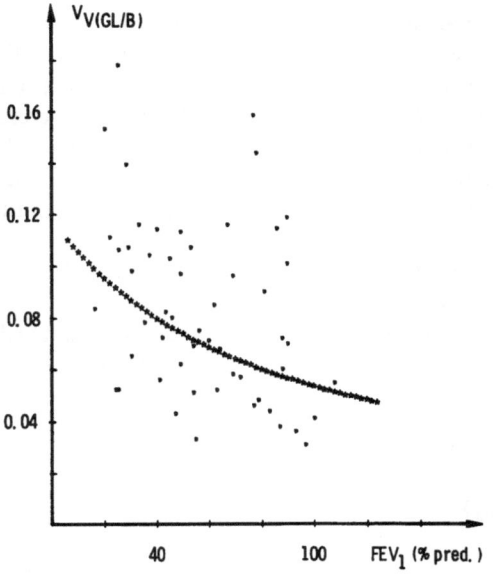

Fig. 15. Correlation between volume density of glands in reference volume B and FEV_1 (% predicted) r_{SP} = -0.401; n = 50; 2 P < 0.01)

There is a significant correlation in reference volume B only between volume density of bronchial glands and RAW (r_{SP} = 0.283, 2 P < 0.05). The correlation is weaker than that between volume density of glands and FEV_1 (% predicted) (r_{SP} = −0.401), though the accuracy of RAW measurements is generally better than that of FEV_1 measurements.

From these observations it may be concluded that resistances arising at regular breathing have other causes than those at forced expiration. Probably FEV_1 is more influenced than RAW by bronchial secretion.

Volume density of glandular ducts shows the best correlations of all morphometrical parameters with clinical data. It is also obvious that the correlations are closest if the volume density of glands is related to reference volume B (Table 18). The connection with RV, which is significant only in reference volume B, is probably mediated by mutual correlation with bronchial obstruction, since the correlation is no longer significant if RAW is eliminated as an influencing factor (r_{PART} = −0.007).

In the same way, the significant correlation between volume density of glandular ducts and TLC is probably a mutual one, because r_{PART} is only 0.235 (2 P < 0.1) or 0.160 after elimination of RAW and FEV_1 respectively. The significant correlation between volume density of glandular ducts and RAW as well as FEV_1 is not surprising, because enlargement of glandular ducts is also significantly related to thickening of the bronchial glands (Table 13).

The significant correlation between *volume density of bronchial muscles* and RAW in reference volume B depends on the period between lung-function test and death (Tabel 9), and is only significant within the whole group in cases in which this period was less than 1 year. The correlation suggests that muscular contraction mainly influences the resistance at regular breathing.

The *volume density of connective tissue* correlates significantly only in reference volume BST with FEV_1 (% VC and % predicted) (r_{SP} = 0.337, n = 50, 2 P < 0.05). The correlation coefficient is positive. Together with the fact that the correlation is closest in reference volume BST, and not in B, as expected, this suggests a formal correlation. Glands and connective tissue are large compartments in the bronchial wall. In BST, glands represent about 24.5%, and connective tissue about 64.9% of the total volume. Therefore, the correlations between connective tissue and clinical parameters mirror only those between gland thickness and clinical parameters. If the relative volume of glands increases, the relative volume of connective tissue must decrease. Thus correlation coefficients between clinical parameters and two volume densities must have opposite signs.

No significant correlations were found between *volume densities of cartilage* or *venous capillary plexus* and clinical parameters.

Special attention was given to the relations between volume density of bronchial wall structures and *CVPh*. These relations were studied in three specially selected groups of cases:

- Five patients with unchanged pulmonary function (group B_1)
- Nine patients with CVPh (group B_2)
- Ten patients without CVPh (group B_3).

Table 19. Comparison between the most important mean volume densities of bronchial-wall compounds in five cases without any airways obstruction, in nine cases with increased RAW and CVPh, and in ten cases with increased RAW but without CVPh

Group	V_V(GL/BST) (mean ± SD)	V_V(MC/BST) (mean ± SD)	V_V(LMN/B) (mean ± SD)	V_V(CRT/B) (mean ± SD)	V_V(BST/B) (mean ± SD)
B_1 Unchanged $n = 5$	0.203±0.025	0.022±0.004	0.544±0.030	0.172±0.010	0.284±0.034
B_2 Cases with obstruction and CVPh $n = 9$	c 0.337±0.025 c	0.047±0.005	0.402±0.021 b	0.228±0.015 a	0.373±0.026
B_3 Cases with obstruction, without CVPh $n = 10$	c 0.227±0.018	0.047±0.004	0.411±0.022 b	0.225±0.014 a	0.347±0.029

[a] $2P < 0.05$ [b] $2P < 0.005$ [c] $2P < 0.001$

Letters below numbers: Significance of differences between group B_1 and B_2
Letters above numbers: Significance of differences between groups B_2 and B_3

Groups B_2 and B_3 did not differ significantly in degree of emphysema or any clinical parameter except FEV_1. The mean resistance at regular breathing was nearly identical in both groups. The mean volume densities of various morphological structures within each group are given in Table 19. There were significant differences only between volume densities of bronchial glands and connective tissue related to bronchial wall without cartilage ($2P < 0.001$ and 0.01, respectively). The mean volume density of glands was higher in the nine cases with CVPh ($0.337 ± 0.25$) than in the cases without CVPh ($0.227 ± 0.018$). The mean volume density of connective tissue showed the reverse: it was lower in the cases with CVPh ($0.546 ± 0.027$) than in those without CVPh ($0.636 ± 0.030$). The volume densities of bronchial lumen, cartilage, and bronchial wall without cartilage related to reference volume B did not differ significantly.

Volume densities of glands, cartilage, and lumen were significantly different in both groups with raised RAW (B_2 and B_3) compared with the five patients without airways obstruction (Table 19). From these findings, it can be concluded that in cases with CVPh, glands in central bronchi are extremely hypertrophic. Thus bronchial wall atrophy cannot be the cause of airway collapse, because bronchial lumen is also smaller in cases without CVPh but with airways obstruction than in cases without any airways obstruction. The significantly lower volume density of connective tissue in cases with CVPh is the result of a formal correlative connection with gland volume in reference volume BST and not a sign of bronchial wall atrophy.

XII. General Discussion

In this study, both pulmonary emphysema and bronchial lesions were correlated with functional parameters of chronic airways obstruction. At first glance, the results seem to suggest that emphysema and bronchial lesions influence the airways conductance. Nevertheless we favor the hypothesis that the influence of bronchial lesions far outweighs that of emphysematous tissue destruction. This hypothesis is supported by many arguments gathered from our own findings and from the literature.

The *degree of emphysema* correlated significantly with FEV_1, and high-grade emphysema was usually connected with severe obstructive ventilation disorder, which is in agreement with the findings of others (*Boushy* et al. 1971; *Park* et al. 1970; *Watanabe* et al. 1965). However, some cases with and some without emphysema showed similar functional disorder. The significant correlation between degree of emphysema and RV, as shown in our study and others, seems to suggest that loss of pulmonary elasticity and radial traction on bronchioli are the main cause of increased RV in emphysema. Nevertheless very high RV is also observed in cases without emphysema. Similarly, TLC is increased in some cases without any trace of emphysema and it can even be transitorily augmented in asthmatic attacks (*Peress* et al. 1976). Other far-reaching discrepancies between pulmonary tissue destruction and clinical findings have been reported. About 10% of high-grade emphysemas are clinically silent (*Mitchell* et al. 1976; *Thurlbeck* and *Angus* 1963). *Jenkins* et al. (1965) did not find a significant correlation between FEV_1 and emphysema parameters despite FEV_1 being decreased in all cases with emphysema. *Gelb* et al. (1973) demonstrated that even in high-grade emphysema FEV_1 need not be decreased. *Pratt* and *Klugh* (1967) showed that 20%–30% of pulmonary parenchyma must be destroyed before airways obstruction occurs in each case. Even then the FEV_1 seems to be lowered only if the resistance at regular breathing is high (*Boushy* et al. 1971; *Levame* and *Brills* 1971).

Loss of pulmonary elasticity does not affect FEV_1 (*Leaver* et al. 1973; *Penman* et al. 1970). High-degree emphysema need not always be connected with irreversible obstruction. There are no functional differences among different types of emphysema (*Anderson* and *Foraker* 1973). It is not possible to discern an emphysematic and a bronchitic type of obstruction by clinical symptoms (*Burrows* et al. 1966). Furthermore, parenchymal destruction is hardly ever the functionally decisive factor. Only 20% of patients with relatively severe emphysema die of respiratory failure (*Otto* et al. 1967). In only 26% of cases of emphysema does pulmonary heart disease develop (*Otto* et al. 1967). *Thurlbeck* (1963) found right heart hypertrophy in only 40% of severe and 5% of moderate emphysema, but the weight of the right ventricle does not correlate with the degree of emphysema (*Bignon* et al. 1969; *Burrows* et al. 1966; *Hicken* et al. 1966; *Outhred* et al. 1970).

Finally, the various investigations have revealed a clear connection between emphysematous tissue destruction and function; however, this connection does not follow a distinct pattern. A possible explanation for the discrepancies is that alterations of the bronchial system, and not emphysematous tissue destructions, are the functionally decisive lesions. It is even reasonable to assume that high RV and TLC do not develop on the basis of "pulmonary relaxation" but on the basis of bronchiolar check-valve

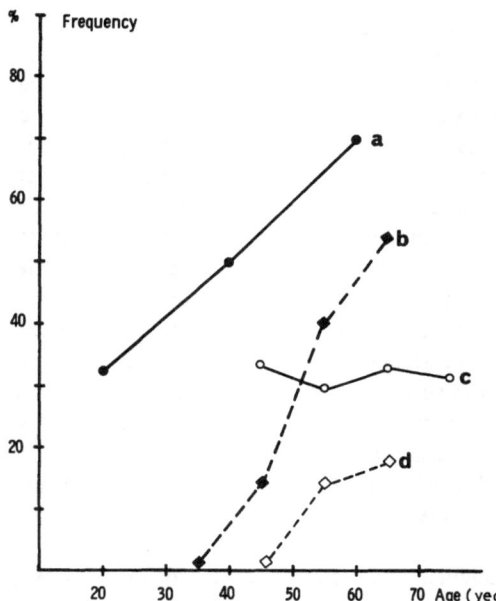

Fig. 16. Age dependence of a bronchial obstruction according to *Mueller* et al. 1971; b emphysema, all cases (*Dalquen* 1974); c high-grade emphysema (*Dalquen* 1974); d hypertrophy of bronchial glands according to *Scott* (1973)

mechanisms caused by inflammation, scars, or mucus plugs. These statements lead to the question how emphysema and bronchial alterations are connected.

Thurlbeck and *Angus* (1964) found *chronic bronchitis* in about 80% of cases with severe emphysema. In some cases deformation of bronchi can be seen on bronchograms (*Mueller* 1973a; *Stender* et al. 1969). Both emphysema and bronchitis occur mainly in males (*Auerbach* et al. 1972; *Dalquen* 1974; *Mueller* et al. 1971; *Otto* et al. 1968; and others). Some findings suggest that chronic bronchitis precedes destructive emphysema: chronic bronchitis frequently becomes apparent during the 3rd decade of life (*Ferris* et al. 1973; *Karon* et al. 1960; *Mork* 1970; *Mueller* et al. 1971; *Rufener* et al. 1972; *Ulmer* and *Reichel* 1970), whereas emphysema rarely occurs before the age of 40. Thereafter the frequency of chronic bronchitis increases up to a plateau between the ages of 60 and 70 (*Boushy* et al. 1968; *Breining* et al. 1971; *Dalquen* 1974; *Dieplinger* 1974; *Otto* et al. 1968). High-grade emphysema occurs only after a further lag phase beyond the age of 50 (*Dalquen* 1974; *Sutinen* et al. 1978) (Fig. 16).

The correlation between bronchial gland thickening, as the main morphological criterion of chronic bronchitis, and emphysema is not as clear as the relation between clinical symptoms and emphysema. Some authors found such a correlation (*Greenberg* et al. 1967; *Ryer* et al. 1971; *Thurlbeck* and *Angus* 1964); others did not (*Martin* et al. 1970; *Mitchell* et al. 1966). In high-grade emphysema lower gland volume has been established as expected (*Greenberg* et al. 1967; *Ryder* et al. 1971; *Thurlbeck* and *Angus* 1964). This was confirmed in our patients with high-grade emphysema and CVPh.

We believe that these deviating results can be explained by superimposition of hypertrophic and atrophic changes within the bronchial glands in long-standing chronic bronchitis. With increasing duration of chronic bronchitis, some acini of the bronchial glands grow larger and others become smaller. In the later stages of chronic bronchitis the atrophic changes can no longer be balanced by progressive hypertrophy of the remaining acini, so that the gland volume as a whole inevitably decreases. This process of combined hypertrophy and atrophy of bronchial glands may also be reflected in the positive, but not very close correlation between the volume densities of glands and glandular ducts: enlargement of the glandular ducts, which is an important criterion of bronchial wall atrophy, correlates well with duration of chronic bronchitis (*Stender* et al. 1969). Superimposition of hypertrophic and atrophic changes in chronic bronchitis may also explain the fact that hypertrophy of bronchial glands occurs in the 5th decade of life as frequently as it does in old age, though clinical observation suggests that the frequency of chronic bronchitis increases continuously with age (Fig. 16).

The concurrence of destructive emphysema and bronchial wall atrophy is suggested by *Wright* and *Stuart* (1965), who found an atrophy of glands and cartilage within intermediate bronchi of patients with destructive emphysema. The correlation between volume density of glandular ducts and TLC in our cases may even point to an atrophy of bronchiolar walls resulting in pathological airway collapsibility and air-trapping. Thus the incongruency between morphological chronic bronchitis and emphysema does not disprove the suggested connection between bronchial lesions and airways obstruction in emphysema.

Bronchial lesions may affect the bronchial conductance in two different ways, that is by narrowing the lumen and by changing the surface structure of the bronchial mucosa. Narrowing of the lumen is effective at regular breathing and at forced respiration. At regular breathing the bronchial resistance responds mainly according to Hagen-Poisseyle's law and is inversely proportional to the fourth power of the total bronchial radius, which increases with airways generations. If this is true, the main portion of airway resistance must arise in central bronchi (*Nolte* and *Ulmer* 1967), in which, according to morphometrical findings (*Weibel* 1963), the "bottleneck" of airways is situated.

At forced respiration turbulences arising within the bronchi become a more decisive factor for the airflow resistance. With a speeding up of the airflow, and under pathological conditions, turbulences may develop at wrinkles in the bronchial mucosa, at muscular bulges, and at mucus plugs. The resistance can then be estimated according to Fanning's equation (*Arnott* et al. 1971), which states that under conditions of turbulent flow, the resistance is proportional to the square of velocity of flow and inversely proportional to the fifth power of the radius. We therefore suggest that the different constellations of functional alterations reflect different patterns of bronchial and/or pulmonary lesions.

We attempted to demonstrate this by studying the airway resistance arising at low and high flow velocity. The main measure of resistance at low flow velocity is RAW, and that at high flow velocity is FEV_1, because RAW is determined at regular breathing, and FEV_1 at forced expiration. In discussing our findings, we had to consider that the morphological alterations as such cannot simply be taken as the cause of functional disturbances. They also imply pathophysiological processes. Hypertrophy of bronchial glands, for example, may not only lead to bronchial narrowing, but also implies increasing viscosity of bronchial secretions. Hypertrophy of bronchial muscles as such can never significantly narrow the bronchial lumen, since the muscles comprise too small a portion of the bronchial wall. However, their hypertrophy indicates recurrent and strong bronchoconstriction.

In agreement with *Martin* et al. (1970) and *McKenzie* et al. (1969), we observed *narrowing of central bronchi* amounting to 26% (Table 19) on average in cases with airways obstruction. It remains open whether this narrowing contributes to resistance. Possibly it does, because the volume densities of bronchial lumen and glands correlate significantly with RAW (Table 18). Nevertheless, mutual correlations among the three parameters cannot be excluded. The loss of lumen results in a reduction of only 14% of the bronchial radius. According to *Nolte* and *Ulmer* (1967), this reduction of the radius would hardly affect the resistance even in segmental and subsegmental bronchi which belong to the narrowest part of the bronchial system. Possible causes of bronchial narrowing in chronic obstructive lung disease are: hypertrophy of bronchial cartilage, congestion of venous capillary plexus, bronchial wall edema, thickening of smooth muscles and bronchoconstriction, scarred stenoses, hypertrophy of bronchial glands, mucus plugging, and bronchial collapse.

Hypertrophy of bronchial cartilage in chronic bronchitis has already been described by *Hart* and *Meyer* (1928) and is interpreted as the sequel to chronic inflammatory irritation. We showed a statistical relation between volume density of cartilage in reference volume B and the surface density of bronchial basement membrane (Table 13). This signifies that the surface density of bronchial basement membrane, and therefore the bronchial lumen, decreases with increasing volume of cartilage, but it remains unclear why FEV_1, and not RAW, correlates significantly with the volume density of cartilage.

Congestion of the bronchial capillary plexus may occur in left as well as in right heart failure. However, the enlargement of the capillary plexus can rarely reach such an extent that it narrows the bronchial lumen, because its volumetric portion in the central bronchi is extremely small (Table 12). Thus the lack of significant correlation between volume density of bronchial capillary plexus and functional parameters is not surprising.

Lumen-narrowing by scars, e.g., in deforming hilary silicosis, was rare in our material, so scars can hardly be a significant cause of bronchial obstruction. It remains unsettled whether bronchial distortion as shown by bronchograms (*Gregg* and *Trapnell* 1969; *Mueller* 1973a; *Reid* 1955; *Reid* and *Simon* 1959; *Scott* and *Steiner* 1975; *Simon* and *Galbraith* 1953) actually corresponds to scarred stenoses rather than to mucus plugs or muscular bulges.

Clinicians often regard allergic or inflammatory *bronchial wall edema* as the major cause of bronchial narrowing in obstructive lung disease (*Hayes* 1976). This edema must manifest itself by an increase of bronchial connective tissue. However, we showed that the bronchial lumen is probably not narrowed by edema, because there is no significant causal correlation between volume density of bronchial connective tissue and clinical parameters. Therefore we agree with *Dunnill* (1974), who does not believe that bronchial wall edema contributes much to obstruction. It is true that wall edema may play a role in acute bronchitic or asthmatic attacks, but as no patient in our study died in an acute attack, bronchial edema could not be observed.

Lumen-narrowing by bronchoconstriction is indicated by hypertrophy of bronchial muscles. Since bronchial obstruction increases with time, the muscular hypertrophy may reflect the duration as well as the dimension of bronchospasms. Hyperplasia of bronchial muscles is a frequent morphological finding in bronchial asthma and chronic bronchitis (*Fischer* 1889; *Fukushi* 1914; *Hossain* and *Heard* 1970; *Huber* and *Koessler* 1922; *Liebow* et al. 1953; *Sobonya* and *Kleinerman* 1972), but its significance is not quite clear. *Huber* and *Koessler* (1922) were the first to objectify hyperplasia in bronchial asthma by morphometry. With one exception, *Dunnill* et al. (1969) found thickening of bronchial muscles only in patients who had died in asthmatic crisis, the exception being a patient suffering from chronic bronchitis. *Hoassain* and *Heard* (1970) believe, however, that hyperplasia of bronchial muscles is characteristic in both chronic bronchitis and asthma. *Takizawa* and *Thurlbeck* (1971) found muscular hyperplasia in patients with wheezing, irrespective of the underlying disease. Our results concur with those of *Takizawa* and *Thurlbeck,* because we compared the volume density of bronchial muscles with functional parameters irrespective of other symptoms of obstructive lung diesease. We suppose that bronchial constriction influences the resistance most at regular breathing, because the volume density of bronchial muscles correlate significantly with RAW but not with FEV_1.

The narrowing of bronchial lumen, as established post mortem, is due to thickening of bronchial glands, as discussed earlier. Nevertheless, the hypertrophy of glands implies an additional narrowing effect on the lumen by mucus plugging (*Chen* and *Delfano* 1978). Mucus plugs are in fact a characteristic roentgenological feature in chronic bronchitis (*Bates* et al., quoted by *Thurlbeck* 1976; *Mueller* 1973a; *Reid* 1955; *Simon* 1959; *Stender* et al. 1969). They are regularly found in small bronchi of empyhsematous lungs (*Matsuba* and *Thurlbeck* 1972; *McLean* 1957) and can cause suffocation in status asthmaticus (*Gloor* 1954). Apart from death in status asthmaticus, however, their functional significance is difficult to assess in autopsy lungs, where they may merely reflect terminal failure of bronchial clearance (*Cullen* et al. 1970).

There is also clinical evidence that hypersecretion in chronic bronchitis leads to loss of bronchial conductance (*Cochrane* et al. 1977). This effect seems to be more pronounced at forced expiration than at regular breathing, as in our study the volume density of glands corresponds better with FEV_1 than with RAW (Table 18). Volume density of bronchial glands was usually increased in cases with low FEV_1 (Fig. 15), but in no case with FEV_1 over 60% was it higher than 0.075 (reference volume B). Therefore it seems reasonable to assume that *mucus plugs* change the surface relief of bronchial mucosa and intensify airflow turbulence. The lack of a relation between the amount of sputum and FEV_1 (*Fletcher* et al. 1976) does not speak against this connection, since *Clarke* et al. (1973) and *Keal* (1973) have shown a highly significant correlation between FEV_1 and sputum viscosity, and the amount of sputum is small at high viscosity (*Fletcher* et al. 1976).

In some cases the gland volume is not increased despite low FEV_1 (Fig. 15). This observation has also been made by other investigators (*Dunnill* et al. 1969; *Oberholzer* 1978; *Ryder* et al. 1971; *Thurlbeck* and *Agnus* 1967). The following methodological reasons have to be considered:

– The hypertrophy of glands may be distributed unevenly within the bronchial tree (*Karpick* et al. 1970; *Niewoehner* et al. 1973) so that it can be overlooked in the bronchus samples examined.
– Since hypertrophy of glands is established by measuring Reid's index, large errors must be taken into account.

In our opinion, however, focal atrophy of some bronchial glands may mask functionally important hypertrophy of others.

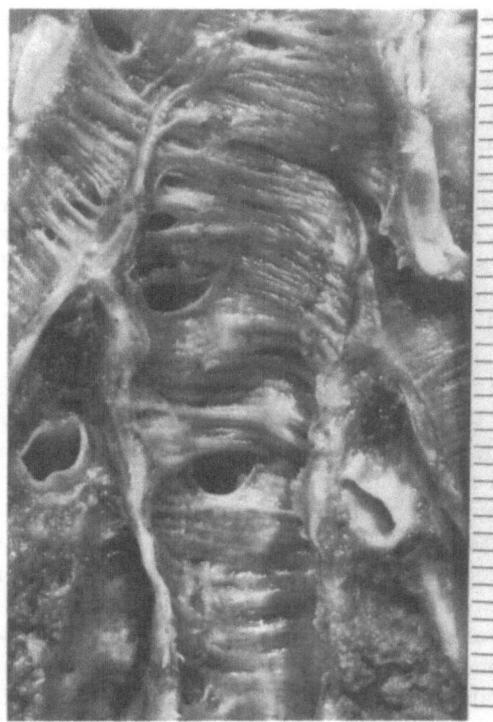

Fig. 17. Deforming chronic bronchitis. The bulges of bronchial mucosa correspond to thickened muscular bundles. Light spots represent squamous cell metaplasia of bronchial epithelium

Compared with mucus plugs, wrinkles of mucosa and muscular bulges seem to play a minor role in changing the bronchial surface relief. However, our morphometrical findings are not compatible with the *wrinkling of the mucosa* described by *Giese* (1960) and *Hart* and *Mayer* (1928). *Longitudinal folds* would result in an increase of bronchial surface density. Therefore we would have expected that in cases with chronic obstructive lung disease the narrowing of bronchial lumen would be accompanied by an increase in the bronchial surface density. On the contrary, we found that the surface density of bronchial basement membrane even decreases significantly with bronchial narrowing (Table 13). Furthermore, one would expect a lowering of FEV_1 to be connected with an increase of bronchial surface density, but the opposite is true: with decreasing FEV_1 the bronchial surface density also decreases (Table 18). Hence, at least in central bronchi, longitudinal foldings of the mucosa, which can be seen on cross-sections of bronchi, do not seem to play any role in the origin of resistance at forced expiration. *Transversal corrugations* of the mucosa become apparent with thickening of the smooth muscles within the bronchial wall (Fig. 17). They probably do not influence the resistance at high flow velocity, because FEV_1 and volume density of muscles do not correlate significantly (Table 18).

Finally, airways collapse has to be considered as an important cause of bronchial narrowing. In obstructive lung disease the collapse can be observed using bronchokinematograms (*Stender* et al. 1969) or endoscopy (*Jackson* 1950; *Lell* 1946). It often occurs in only a few bronchi, but occasionally in bronchial asthma the whole bronchial system collapses (*Gayrard* and *Charpin* 1967). This collapse develops by a shifting of the equal pressure point between intra- and extrabronchial pressure during expiration from the central to the peripheral bronchi (*Macklem* and *Mead* 1967). Pathological shifting of the equal pressure point occurs if the intrabronchial pressure decreases or if the wall of the central bronchi is destabilized. If the intrabronchial pressure is diminished, the peripheral bronchi collapse early during forced expiration or a coughing fit, whereas in healthy lungs they collapse only late, at the end of expiration. Under pathological conditions, the collapse may continue into the central bronchi. In healthy lungs the central bronchi, the walls of which are armored by a tunica elastica and cartilage, withstand even high extrabronchial pressures, as in coughing fits.

There are various causes of central tracheobronchial collapse under discussion, such as inborn malformation of trachea and large bronchi (*Johnston* and *Green* 1965), atrophy of bronchial walls (*Levame* and *Brille* 1971; *Maisel* et al. 1972; *Silvers* et al. 1972; *Wright* 1960; *Wright* and *Stuart* 1965), loss of radial traction of bronchi by emphysema (*Herzog* and *Keller* 1970), and decrease of intrabronchial expiration pressure by peripheral closure of bronchi and bronchioli, e.g., by mucus plugs.

Tracheobronchial collapse caused by malformation is called "primary" or "idiopathic." The other forms are termed "secondary." The symptoms are bascially the same in both: At forced expiration or coughing the pars membranacea of the trachea encroaches on the lumen and sometimes touches the front of the tracheal wall, producing a severe coughing attack which ends in apnea. The central expiratory airway collapse causes CVPh and disproportional lowering of FEV_1 (*Herzog* et al. 1968). There is often no airway obstruction in primary collapse at regular breathing (*Campbell* and *Faulks* 1965; *Frank* and *Menges* 1977; *Guest* and *Anderson* 1977; *Herzog* and *Nissen* 1954; *Hunter* et al. 1975; *Koblet* and *Wyss* 1953; *Lell* 1946).

Idiopathic tracheobronchial collapse is rare and occurs in children and young adults. Sixty-nine cases were described up to 1973 (*Himalstein* and *Gallagher* 1973).

The morphological basis is a tracheobronchomegaly, which is attributed to alteration of the tunica fibroelastica of the pars membranacea (*Herzog* and *Nissen* 1954), degeneration of cartilage (*Berant* et al. 1974; *Hermann* et al. 1977; *Meyenburg* 1936), or hereditary ectasia (*Johnston* and *Green* 1965). In our correlation study, such cases were not considered.

Secondary tracheobronchial collapse develops mostly in older people with obstructive lung disease, and is characterized by pronounced collapsibility of the whole airway system. It seems reasonable to assume that this collapsibility is due to alterations of the bronchial wall. One of these lesions may be atrophy of cartilage, which has been demonstrated in the intermediate bronchi of individuals with obstructive disease and pulmonary emphysema (*Maisel* et al. 1972; *Tandon* and *Campbell* 1969; *Thurlbeck* et al. 1974; *Wright* and *Stuart* 1965). The process of aging, inflammation, and frequent compression of bronchi by chronic coughing are under discussion as possible causes (*Miller* et al. 1973; *Tandon* and *Campbell* 1969; *Wright* and *Stuart* 1965). However, central tracheobronchial collapse cannot be explained by the loss of cartilage armoring. We found hypertrophy rather than atrophy of cartilage (Table 19) in the central bronchi in cases with CVPh. This is in agreement with the findings of *Restrepo* and *Heard* (1963), who also studied central bronchi. *Maisel* et al. (1972) demonstrated incongruity of collapse and cartilage atrophy: the collapse, for example, occurred in bronchi of the upper lobe, whereas atrophy of cartilage could be established only in bronchi of the lower lobe.

Destruction of fibroelastic tissue in segmental and subsegmental bronchi, as described by *Wright* and *Stuart* (1965) in cases of chronic bronchitis and emphysema, is difficult to prove. Nevertheless, *Wilson* et al. (1974) found no difference in bronchial compressibility between individuals with and without airways obstruction. *Tammeling* and *Sluiter* (1965) saw no tracheal lesion which could explain bronchial collapse in patients with bronchial obstruction; neither did *Bryant* et al. (1965).

As bronchial wall atrophy and emphysema frequently occur together (*Tammeling* and *Sluiter* 1965; *Thurlbeck* et al. 1974; *Wright* 1960; *Wright* and *Stuart* 1965), it is tempting to assume that emphysema contributes to airways collapse. *Dayman* (1951) was the first to suggest that loss of radial traction of bronchioli in emphysema leads to airway collapse and thus to a decrease of FEV_1. Other investigators had the idea that the collapse caused by emphysema begins in peripheral bronchi and continues even into the trachea (*Herzog* and *Keller* 1970; *Park* et al. 1969; *Rainer* et al. 1963). This assumption is supported by the good correlation between degree of emphysema and loss of lung recoil (*Park* et al. 1970; *Thurlbeck* et al. 1970b). Additionally, the equal pressure-point between intra- and extrabronchial pressure has shifted beyond segmental bronchi to the periphery (*Hartung* and *Kafarnik* 1966). The reason for this is said to be an increase of peripheral resistance, partially caused by loss of radial traction of bronchioli (*Hartung* and *Kafarnik* 1966). In fact, loss of radial traction has been proved (*Lamb* and *Reid* 1969); so has destruction of bronchioli in emphysema (*Anderson* and *Foraker* 1967; *Bignon* et al. 1969, 1975; *DePierre* et al. 1972; *Matsuba* and *Thurlbeck* 1972). Nevertheless, airways collapse in obstructive lung disease cannot be explained sufficiently by emphasematous tissue destruction, because CVPh does not correlate in each case with a high degree of emphysema. CVPh and disproportional lowering of FEV_1 occur in children (*Hofmann* and *Geubelle* 1974), who rarely have destructive emphysema (*Dalquen* 1974; *Otto* et al. 1968). *Maisel* et al. (1972) noticed that bronchial collapse correlates better with bronchial obstruction than with emphysema. In bronchograms of chronic bronchitis, *Gayrard* and *Charpin* (1967) observed alternating overinflated and collapsed bronchi, unevenly distributed over the bronchial tree. Similar to *Bryant* et al. (1965), they have interpreted the collapse as a result of a flow-check by scarring strictures, local muscle contraction, or mucus plugs.

All phenomena of bronchial collapse observed in chronic obstructive lung disease can be easily explained if one assumes that they are mainly caused by mucus plugs. This would explain their independence from emphysema (*Maisel* et al. 1972) and their disappearance after antibronchitic treatment (*Herzog* and *Dalquen* 1979; *Herzog* et al. 1971). Indeed, mucus plugs seem to be the main reason for bronchial collapse, because they are always accompanied by considerable bronchial hypersecretion (*Herzog* et al. 1968; *Stender* et al. 1969) and because CVPh and thickening of bronchial glands correlate significantly.

Obviously, bronchi narrowed by mucus plugs close completely at forced expiration by compression from outside. Thus the intrabronchial pressure diminishes downstream. Additionally, hypersecretion may lead to an increase in the surface tension within the peripheral bronchi (*Macklem* et al. 1970), which may promote their collapsibility. If in these ways many peripheral bronchi collapse, the intrabronchial pressure may also diminish in central bronchi and the collapse may spread into them.

XIII. Closing Remarks

We have endeavored to reconcile many divergent findings from our own investigations and those of others, and are aware of one weak point in our interpretation. For the argument to be conclusive it should be known what happens in airways between the central bronchi and the terminal airways. *Hogg* et al. (1968) suppose, and many others with them, that alterations in small bronchi are mainly responsible for airways obstruction, but so far there is little information (*Cosio* et al. 1978) about relations between morphological alterations of small bronchi and lung function. It is not clear to what extent "small bronchi" as understood by physiologists coincide with small bronchi or bronchioli as defined by anatomists. Does "small-airways disease" actually exist separate from disease of large airways or vice versa? What is the real morphological basis of the irreversibility of airways obstruction? Before these questions can be answered, new and even more sophisticated morphometrical models have to be developed. It is to be hoped that lungs whose function has been tested during life and by postmortem methods, as applied by *Wierich* (1976), will give further insight into the intriguing problems of clinicopathological correlations in obstructive lung disease.

XIV. Summary

Correlations between destructive emphysema, alterations in central bronchi, and obstructive lung disease were examined in various subgroups of 188 autopsy cases. All patients had been given lung-function tests a maximum of 53 months before death. The mean age of death was 64.4 ± 10.4 years. About 60% of the patients had been admitted to hospital because of bronchial carcinoma or chronic bronchitis.

Clinical parameters taken into account were total lung capacity (TLC), vital capacity (VC), residual volume (RV), forced expiratory volume within one second (FEV_1), and check-valve phenomenon (CVPh) of the forced expiratory flow curve. From these parameters, degree of disproportional lowering of FEV_1 and degree of obstructive ventilation disorder were derived.

All lungs were fixed in the inflated state by instillation of 4% formol or 2.5% glutaraldehyde into the bronchial tree and dissected into sagittal slices. Paper-mounted macrosections were prepared from the central slice. Samples of the bronchi of the upper lobe, lower lobe, and apical segment of the lower lobe were taken for bronchus morphometry.

The degree of pulmonary emphysema was established by point-counting on macrosections. Point-counting was also used in bronchus morphometry, which was carried out in a subgroup consisting of 50 cases. Volume densities of bronchial lumen, bronchial wall tissue with and without cartilage, glands, glandular ducts, connective tissue, muscles, and venous capillary plexus of bronchial mucosa were measured. Additionally, the surface density of bronchial basement membrane was established by the intersection method. The morphometrical parameters were related to three reference volumes — B, total bronchus section; BWT, bronchial wall tissue, cartilage included; BST, bronchial wall tissue, cartilage excluded. Morphometrical models and methodological problems of clinicopathological correlations are discussed in detail. Interrelations of functional and morphometrical parameters and correlations between functional and morphometrical parameters were tested.

Close correlations between those functional parameters (RAW, FEV_1 and RV) usually altered in obstructive lung diesease could be demonstrated ($2\ P < 0.001$, $|r| = 0.552-0.709$). These three parameters were correlated to a lesser degree with TLC ($|r| = 0.291-0.549$).

The functional parameters TLC, RV, FEV_1, and RAW were significantly related to age ($|r| = 0.323-0.463$, $2\ P < 0.05-<0.01$), whereas the morphometrical parameters were not. The age dependence of the functional parameters probably reflects the age dependence of obstructive lung disease.

In a subgroup consisting of 138 cases, relations between degree of emphysema and functional parameters were studied. It is suggested that the statistical correlation between degree of emphysema and RAW ($r_{SP} = 0.303$) is probably not a causal one. FEV_1 is lowered, even in high-grade emphysema, only if at the same time RAW is high. CVPh does not occur in all cases with high-grade emphysema.

Analysis of interrelations among morphometrical parameters showed that causal relations exist between surface density of bronchial basement membrane and bronchial lumen ($r_{SP} = 0.369$) and between bronchial lumen and glands ($r_{SP} = -0.509$). It seems obvious that the inner surface of bronchi decreases if the bronchus lumen is narrowed by thickening of glands. In cases with obstrutive lung disease, the sectional area of the lumen is about 26% less than in cases with normal lung function. Narrowing of the bronchial lumen is correlated with an increase of RAW ($r_{SP} = -0.364$), and a lowering of FEV_1 (% predicted) ($r_{SP} = 0.325$) and VC ($r_{SP} = 0.323$). Thicking of bronchial glands is more closely related to a lowering of FEV_1 ($r_{SP} = -0.401$) than to an increase of RAW. These relations can hardly be explained by the narrowing of the bronchial lumen. Thickening of glands probably signifies secretion of a more viscous mucus and intrabronchial mucus plugging, which influences the bronchial resistance mainly at forced expiration. CVPh is found in cases displaying the highest volume density of bronchial glands (0.337 ± 0.025); cases without CVPh but with similar resistance at regular breathing show a volume density of 0.227 ± 0.018. It is therefore suggested that mucus plugs cause a diminution of the intraluminal pressure in the downstream bronchi. Therefore these bronchi are compressed by the extramural pressure at forced expiration. The bronchial collapse causes the CVPh.

The volume density of bronchial muscles correlates significantly only with RAW ($r_{SP} = 0.284$), indicating that muscular contraction influences the airway resistance mainly at regular breathing.

Acknowledgments. Above all we would like to thank Prof. H. Herzog, for the functional data established in his laboratory at the Kantonsspital Basel and for stimulating discussion. We are obliged to Prof. H.P. Rohr and Dr. P. Sandoz for methodological and statistical advice. H. Wyss, M. Huber, W. Bachmann, M. Wyss and L.V. Segesser helped in the point-counting. B. Amsler, M. Richner, M. Suter, H.R. Zysset and M. Nebiker rendered technical assistance.

References

Amrein R, Keller R, Joos H, Herzog H (1969) Neue Normalwerte für die Lungen-funktionsprüfung mit der Ganzkörperplethysmographie. Dtsch Med Wochenschr 94:1785–1793

Anderhub HP, Keller P, Herzog H (1974) Spirometrische Untersuchungen der forcier-ten Vitalkapazität, Sekundenkapazität und maximalen Atemstromstärke bei 13.798 Personen. Dtsch Med Wochenschr 99:33–38

Anderson AE, Foraker AG (1967) Populations of nonrespiratory bronchioles in pul-monary emphysema. Arch Pathol 83:286–292

Anderson AE Jr, Foraker AG (1973) Centrilobular emphysema and panlobular emphy-sema: two different diseases. Thorax 28:547–550

Anderson JA, Dunnill MS (1965) Observations on the estimation of the quantity of emphysema in the lungs by the point sampling method. Thorax 20:462–466

Arnott WM, Clarke SW, Jones JG (1971) Mass movement of gas in respiratory tubes. Prog Respir Res 6:2–14

Auerbach O, Hammond EC, Garfinkel L, Benante C (1972) Relation of smoking and age to emphysema. Whole lung section study. N Engl J Med 286:853–857

Azcuy A, Anderson AE, Foraker AG (1962) The morphological spectrum of aging and emphysematous lungs. Ann Intern Med 57:1–17

Bachmann W (1977) Zum Problem der morphologischen Emphysemgraduierung. Medical dissertation, University of Basel

Bahr GF, Bloom G, Friberg U (1957) Volume changes of tissues in physiological fluids during fixation in osmium tetroxide or formaldehyde and during subsequent treat-ment. Exp Cell Res 12:342–355

Bath JC, Yates PA (1968) Clinical and pathological correlations in chronic airways obstruction – observation on patients with pulmonary resection. In: Current research in chronic airways obstruction. 9th Aspen Emphysema Conference. Public Health Publication 1717, pp 293–308

Bernant M, Varsano I, Duparc A, Liban E (1974) Congenital bronchomalacia. An unusual cause of expiratory stridor. Helv Paediatr Acta 29:181–184

Bignon J, Khury F, Even P, Andre J, Brouet G (1969) Morphometric study in chronic obstructive bronchopulmonary disease. Am Rev Respir Dis 99:669–695

Bignon J, Hem B, Molinier B (1975) Morphometric and angiographic studies in diffuse interstitial pulmonary fibrosis. Prog Respir Res 8:141–160

Blumenthal BJ, Boren HG (1959) Lung structure in three dimensions after inflation and fume fixation. Am Rev Respir Dis 79:764–772

Boushy SF, Greenberg SD, Jenkins DE (1968) The prevalence of emphysema in 67 unselected male necropsies. Dis Chest 53:497–501

Boushy SF, Helgason AH, Billig DM, Gyorky FG (1970) Clinical, physiologic and morphologic examination of the lung in patients with bronchogenic carcinoma and the relation of the findings to postoperative deaths. Am Rev Respir Dis 101:685–695

Boushy SF, Aboumrad MH, North LB, Helgason AH (1971) Lung recoil pressure, air-way resistance and forced flows related to morphologic emphysema. Am Rev Respir Dis 104:551–561

Breining H, Hinüber GV, Otto H (1971) Zur Epidemioloige des Lungenemphysems am Beispiel von Aachen, Erlangen, Cardiff und Stockholm. Prax Pneumol 25:323–328

Bryant LR, Eiseman B, Gan HK (1965) The significance of tracheobronchial collapse in obstructive emphysema. Med Thorac 22:244–257

Burrows B, Fletcher CM, Heard BE, Jones NL, Wootliff JS (1966) The emphysematous and bronchial types of chronic airway obstruction: A clinicopathological study of patients in London and Chicago. Lancet I:830–835

Campbell AH, Faulks LW (1965) Expiratory air-flow pattern in tracheobronchial collapse. Am Rev Respir Dis 92:781–791

Charkin LW, Saunders LZ (1974) Experimental chronic bronchitis. Pathology in the dog. Lab Invest 30:145–154

Chen TM, Dulfano MJ (2978) Mucus viscoelasticity and mucociliary transport rate. J Lab Clin Med 91:423–431

Clarke SW, Cochrane GM, Webber B (1973) Effects of sputum on pulmonary function (Abstr). Thorax 28:262

Cochrane GM, Webber BA, Clarke SW (1977) Effects of sputum on pulmonary function. Br Med J II:1181–1183

Comroe JH (1974) Physiology of respiration. An introductory text, 2nd edn. Year Book Medical Publishers, Chicago

Cosio M, Ghezzo H, Hogg JC, Corbin R, Loveland M, Dosman J, Macklem PT (1978) The relations between structural changes in small airways and pulmonary-function tests. N Engl J Med 298:1277–1281

Cullen JH, Kaemmerlen JT, Daoud A, Katz HL (1970) A prospective clinical-pathologic study of the lungs and heart in chronic obstructive lung disease. Am Rev Respir Dis 102:190–204

Dalquen P (1974) Incidence of pulmonary emphysema, a study of 467 randomized autopsy cases. Beitr Pathol 153:330–338

Dayman H (1951) Mechanics of airflow in health and in emphysema. J Clin Invest 30:1175–1190

Demedts M, Cosemans J, deRoo M, Billiet L, van de Woestijne KP (1978) Emphysema with minor airway obstruction and abnormal tests of small airway disease. Respiration 35:148–157

Depierre A, Bignon J, Lebeau A, Brouet G (1972) Quantitative study of parenchyma and small conductive airways in chronic non-specific lung disease. Use of histologic stereology and bronchial casts. Chest 62:699–708

Dieplinger P (1974) Vergleichende Untersuchungen zur Pathologie des Lungenemphysems. Prax Pneumol 28:299–322

Dunnill MS (1962) Quantitative methods in the study of pulmonary pathology. Thorax 17:320–328

Dunnill MS (1965) Quantitative observations on the anatomy of chronic nonspecific lung disease. Med Thorac 22:261–274

Dunnill MS (1974) The contribution of morphology to the study of chronic obstructive lung disease. Am J Med 57:506–519

Dunnill MS, Massarella GR, Anderson JA (1969) A comparison of the quantitative anatomy of the bronchi in normal subjects, in status asthmaticus, in chronic bronchitis and in emphysema. Thorax 24:176–179

Ferris BG Jr, Higgins ITT, Higgins MW, Peters JM (1973) Chronic nonspecific respiratory disease in Berlin, New Hampshire, 1961 to 1967. A follow-up study. Am Rev Respir Dis 107:110–122

Fischer W (1889) Über die feineren Veränderungen bei Bronchitis und Bronchiektasie. Beitr pathol Anat 5:453–468

Fletcher CM, Gilson JG, Hugh-Jones P, Scadding JG (1959) CIBA Guest Symposium 1958. Terminoloy, definitions and classification of chronic pulmonary emphysema and related conditions. Thorax 14:286–299

Fletcher C, Peto R, Tinker C, Speizer FE (1976) The natural history of chronic bronchitis and emphysema. Oxford University Press, Oxford New York Toronto

Frank P, Menges V (1977) Tracheobronchomegalie. ROEFO 127:599–601

Frasca JM, Auerbach O, Parks VR, Jamieson JD (1971) Electron microscopic observations on pulmonary fibrosis and emphysema in smoking dogs. Exp Mol Pathol 15:108–125

Fukushi M (1914) Über das Verhalten der Bronchialmuskulatur bei akuter und chronischer Bronchitis. Virchows Arch 217:16–55

Gaensler EA, Lindgren I (1959) Chronic bronchitis as an etiologic factor in obstructive emphysema. Am Rev Respir Dis (Suppl 2/2) 80:185–193

Gayrard P, Charpin J (1967) Evaluation of the role of the large bronchi in the genesis of air obstruction in normal subjects and in various diseases. Am Rev Respir Dis 97:1076–1088

Gelb AF, Gold WM, Wright RR, Bruch HR, Nadel JA (1973) Physiologic diagnosis of subclinical emphysema. Am Rev Respir Dis 107:50–63

Giese W (1960) Die Atmungsorgane. (Lehrbuch der speziellen pathologischen Anatomie). de Gruyter, Berlin

Gloor F (1954) Zur Pathologie des Asthma bronchiale. Virchows Arch 325:189–210

Gouch J, Wentworth JE (1949) The use of thin sections of entire organs in morbid anatomical studies. J R Microsc Soc 3:231–235

Greenberg SD, Boushy SF, Jenkins DE (1967) Chronic bronchitis and emphysema: correlation of pathologic findings. Am Rev Respir Dis 96:918–928

Gregg I, Trapnell DH (1969) The bronchographic appearances of chronic bronchitis. Br J Radiol 42:132–139

Guest JL, Anderson JN (1977) Tracheobronchomegaly (Mounier-Kuhn-syndrome). JAMA 238:1754–1755

Hale FC, Olsen CR, Mickey MR Jr (1968) The measurement of bronchial wall components. Am Rev Respir Dis 98:978–987

Hart C, Mayer E (1928) Kehlkopf, Luftröhre und Bronchien. In: Henke O, Lubarsch F (Hrsg) Atmungswege und Lungen. Springer, Berlin (Handbuch der speziellen pathologischen Anatomie und Histologie, Bd 3, S 288)

Hartung W (1963) Untersuchungsmethoden an Lungen und Thorax zur postmortalen Analyse der Atmungsfunktion. Ergeb Allg Pathol 43:121–160

Hartung W (1964) Lungenemphysem. Morphologie, Pathogenese und funktionelle Bedeutung. Springer, Berlin Heidelberg New York

Hartung W (1975) Mechanical effects of structural lesions within the lungs on ventilation and pulmonary circulation. In: Schüren KP, Hüttemann U, Schröder R (eds) Chronisch obstruktive Lungenkrankheiten und Cor pulmonale. Symposium in Berlin, Oktober 1974. Schattauer, Stuttgart New York, pp 17–27

Hartung W, Kafarnik D (1966) Zur Statik des Thorax-Lungen-Systems an der Leiche. II. Einfluß krankhafter Veränderungen und experimenteller Variation der Versuchsbedingungen auf die Volumendehnbarkeit. Med Thorac 23:77–94

Hartung W, Kissler W (1970) Distribution of resistances in artificially ventilated human autopsy lungs. Respiration 27:176–199

Hayek H von (1970) Die menschliche Lunge. Springer, Berlin Heidelberg New York

Hayes JA (1976) The pathology of bronchial asthma. In: Weiss EB, Segal S (eds) Bronchial asthma, mechanisms and therapeutics. Little Brown, Boston, p 347

Heard BE (1962) Fixation of the lung with respect to lung volumes and air space size. In: de Reuck AVS, O'Connor M (eds) CIBA Foundation Symposium on Pulmonary Structure and Function. Churchill, London, pp 291–296

Heard BE (1969) Pathology of chronic bronchitis and emphysema. Churchill, London

Heath D, Brewer D, Hicken P (1968) Cor pulmonale in emphysema. Mechanisms and pathology. Thomas, Springfield

Herrmann R, Zillesen E, Büchele U, Kühn H (1977) Die rezidivierende Polychondritis. Eine Fallbeobachtung mit letaler Tracheobronchomalazie. Med Klin 72:893–898

Herzog H, Dalquen P (1979) Base morphologique pour le collapsus des voies aériennes dans les maladies obstructives du poumon. XXVII. Congrès de l'Association Internationale du Broncho-Pneumologie, Toulouse, 4–6.5.1978. Bronchopneumologie 29:134–152

Herzog H, Keller R (1970) Correlation between forced expiration and airways resistance during quiet breathing in obstructive lung disease. In: Bronchitis III. Proceedings of the third international symposium on bronchitis at Groningen. van Gorcum, Assen, pp 219–226

Herzog H, Nissen R (1954) Erschlaffung und exspiratorische Invagination des membranösen Teils der intrathorakalen Luftröhre und der Hauptbronchien als Ursache der asphyktischen Anfälle beim Asthma bronchiale und bei der chronischen Bronchitis des Lungenemphysems. Schweiz Med Wochenschr 84:217–221

Herzog H, Keller R, Baumann HR, Joos H (1968) Folgen chronisch-obstruktiver Atemwegserkrankungen aus klinischer Sicht. In: Bopp KP, Hertle FH, Heymer A (Hrsg) Chronische Bronchitis. Schattauer, Stuttgart, S 301–320

Herzog H, Knuchel R, Nosbaum J, Baumann HR, Keller R (1971) Funktionelle Erfolge in der Behandlung der chronischen Bronchitis. Progr Respir Res 6:181–200

Herzog H, Dalquen P, Specht H (1976) Grading of pulmonary emphysema. Comparison of functional to morphological data in 134 patients. Prog Respir Res 10:81–99

Hicken P, Heath D, Brewer D (1966) The relation between the weight of the right ventricle and the percentage of abnormal air space in the lung in emphysema. J Pathol Bacteriol 9:519–528

Himalstein MR, Gallagher JC (1973) Tracheobronchomegaly. Ann Otol Rhinol Laryngol 82:223–227

Hofmann D, Geubelle F (1974) Die Sekundenkapazität und der Lungengesamtwiderstand bei Kindern mit Asthmasyndrom. Helv Paediat Acta 29:269–280

Hogg JC, Macklem PT, Thurlbeck WM (1968) Site and nature of airway obstruction in chronic obstructive lung disease. N Engl J Med 278:1355–1360

Horsfield K, Cumming G (1968) Morphology of the bronchial tree in man. J Appl Physiol 24:373–383

Horsfield K, Cumming G (1976) Morphology of the bronchial tree in the dog. Respir Physiol 26:173–182

Hossain S (1973) Quantitative measurement of bronchial muscle in men with asthma. Am Rev Respir Dis 107:99–109

Hossain S, Heard BE (1970) Hyperplasia of bronchial muscle in chronic bronchitis. J Pathol 101:171–184

Huber HL, Koessler KK (1922) The pathology of bronchial asthma. Arch Intern Med 30:689–760

Hunter HA, Nikiforuk G (1954) Staining reaction following demineralization of hard tissues by chelating and other decalcifying agents. J Dent Res 33:136

Hunter TB, Kuhns LR, Roloff MA, Holt JF (1975) Tracheobronchiomegaly in an 18-months-old child. AJR 123:687–690

Islam MS, Buckup K, Ulmer WT (1978) Altersabhängigkeit der mechanischen Eigenschaften der Lunge. Dtsch Med Wochenschr 103:1482–1485

Jackson C (1950) Bronchial obstruction. Dis Chest 17:125–150

Jenkins DE, Greenberg SD, Boushy SF, Schweppe HI, O'Neal RM (1965) Correlation of morphologic emphysema with pulmonary function parameters. Trans Assoc Am Physicians 78:218–230

Johanson WG Jr, Pierce AK, Reynolds RC (1971) The evolution of papain emphysema in the rat. J Lab Clin Med 78:599–607

Johnston RF, Green RA (1965) Tracheobronchiomegaly. Report of five cases and demonstration of familial occurrence. Am Rev Respir Dis 91:35–50

Jutabha O, Lonngren KE (1969) Measurement of pulmonary emphysema using a microwave technique. A feasibility study. Am Rev Respir Dis 99:101–103

Karon EH, Koelsche GA, Fowler WS (1960) Chronic obstructive pulmonary disease in young adults. Mayo Clin Proc 35:307–316

Karpick RJ, Pratt PC, Asmundsson T, Kilburn KH (1970) Pathological findings in respiratory failure. Goblet cell metaplasia, alveolar damage, and myocardial infarction. Ann Intern Med 72:189–197

Keal EE (1973) Relationship between sputum rheology and pulmonary function (Abstr). Thorax 28:262

Koblet H, Wyss F (1956) Das klinische und funktionelle Bild des genuinen Bronchialkollapses mit Lungenemphysem. Helv Med Acta 23:553–560

Kory RC, Rauterkus LT, Korthy AL, Coté RA (1966) Quantitative estimation of pulmonary emphysema in lung macrosections by photoelectric measurement of transmitted light. Am Rev Respir Dis 93:758–768

Lamb D, Reid L (1969) Histochemical types of acidic glycoprotein produced by mucous cells of the tracheobronchial glands in man. J Pathol 98:213–229

Leaver DG, Tattersfield AE, Pride NB (1973) Contributions of loss of lung recoil and of enhanced airways collapsibility to the airflow obstruction of chronic bronchitis and emphysema. J Clin Invest 52:2117–2128

Lell WA (1946) Bronchoscopy as an aid in the diagnosis and treatment of allergic pulmonary disease. Arch Otolaryngol 43:49–58

Levame M, Brille D (1971) Les lésions anatomiques de l'arbre bronchique dans les bronchopneumopathies obstructives sans emphysème. Aspects histologiques, siège et distribution. Prog Respir Res 6:223–231

Liebow AA, Loring WE, Felton WL (1953) The musculature of the lungs in chronic pulmonary disease. Am J Pathol 29:885–911

Longfield AN, Hentel W (1969) Quantitation of pulmonary emphysema. Am J Med Sci 257:171–176

Lyons JP, Ryder R, Campbell H, Gough J (1972) Pulmonary disability in coal worker's pneumoconiosis. Br Med J I:713–716

Macklem PT, Mead J (1967) Resistance of central and peripheral airways measured by a retrograde catheter. J Appl Physiol 22:395–401

Macklem PT, Proctor DF, Hogg JC (1970) The stability of peripheral airways. Respir Physiol 8:191–203

Maisel JC, Silvers GW, Gerge MS, Dart GA, Petty TL, Mitchell RS (1972) The significance of bronchial atrophy. Am J Pathol 67:371–383

Marco V, Mass B, Meranze DR, Weinbaum G, Kimbel P (1971) Induction of experimental emphysema in dogs using leucocyte homogenates. Am Rev Respir Dis 104:595–598

Martelli NA, Hutchison DCS, Barter CE (1974) Radiological distribution of pulmonary emphysema. Clinical and physiological features of patients with emphysema of upper or lower zones of lungs. Thorax 29:81–89

Martin CJ, Katsura S, Cochran TH (1970) The relationship of chronic bronchitis to the diffuse obstructive pulmonary syndrome. Am Rev Respir Dis 102:362–369

Matsuba K, Thurlbeck WM (1972) The number and dimensions of small airways in emphysematous lungs. Am J Pathol 67:265–275

McKenzie HI, Glick M, Outhred KG (1969) Chronic bronchitis in coal miners: ante-mortem-post-mortem comparisons. Thorax 24:527–535

McLean KH (1957) The pathogenesis of pulmonary emphysema. Am J Med 25:62–74

Meyenburg R von (1936) Über Chondromalazie. Schweiz Med Wochenschr 66:1239

Miller JA, Pratt PC, Capp MP (1973) Human bronchial and bronchiolar compressibility measured by postmortem bronchography. Lab Invest 29:465–477

Mitchell RS, Ryan SF, Petty TL, Filley GF (1966) The significance of morphologic chronic hyperplastic bronchitis. Am Rev Respir Dis 93:720–729

Mitchell RS, Stanford RE, Johnson JM, Silvers GW, Dart G, George MS (1976) The morphologic features of the bronchi, bronchioles and alveoli in chronic airway obstruction: a clinicopathological study. Am Rev Respir Dis 114:137–145

Mork T (1970) Bronchitis in the United Kingdom and the United States of America. J Chronic Dis 23:345–350

Mueller KM (1973a) Chronische Bronchitis und Emphysem. Eine vergleichende röntgenographische und morphologische Strukturanalyse. Fischer, Stuttgart

Mueller KM (1973b) Die Morphologie der sogenannten Bronchialwanddivertikel im Bronchogramm bei chronischer Bronchitis. ROEFO 118:136–145

Mueller RE, Keble DL, Plummer J, Walker SH (1971) The prevalence of chronic bronchitis, chronic airway obstruction and respiratory symptoms in a Colorado City. Am Rev Respir Dis 103:209–228

Nicklaus TM, Stowell DW, Christiansen WR, Renzetti AD Jr (1966) The accuracy of the radiological diagnosis of chronic pulmonary emphysema. Am Rev Respir Dis 93:889–899

Niewoehner DE, Kleinerman J (1974) Morphologic basis of pulmonary resistance in the human lung and effects of aging. J Appl Physiol 36:412–418

Niewoehner DE, Kleinerman J, Knoke JD (1973) Regional chronic bronchitis. Am Rev Respir Dis 105:586–593

Nolte D, Ulmer WT (1967) Die Strömungswiderstände im normalen Tracheobronchialbaum und bei obstruktiven Atemwegserkrankungen. Beitr Klin Tuberk 136:320–329

Oberholzer M, Dalquen P, Huber M, Rohr H-P (1977) Stereology, a complement to respiration research. Bronchus morphometry: methodology and baseline data. Microsc Acta 79:205–223

Oberholzer M, Dalquen P, Rohr HP (1978) The applicability of the gland/wall ratio (REID-Index) to clinicopathological correlation studies. Thorax 33:779–784

Otto H, Kemter I (1969) Die Technik der papiermontierten Großflächenschnitte. Med Lab 22:5–11

Otto H, Zelihofer R (1969) Lungenfunktion und Strukturbefund unter besonderer Berücksichtigung der obstruktiven Ventilationsstörung und des Lungenemphysems. Respiration 26:262–286

Otto H, Zelihofer R, Leutschaft R, Kulke H (1967) Vergleichende klinisch-morphologische Untersuchungen zur Symptomatik, Diagnostik und Dignität des chronischen Lungenemphysems. Klin Wochenschr 45:68–72

Otto H, Orell SR, Guettich R (1968) Vergleichende Untersuchungen zur Epidemiologie des Lungenemphysems. Prax Pneumol 22:481–487

Otto H, Zelihofer R, Reisinger O (1969) Vergleichende Untersuchungen zu Klinik und Symptomatik morphologisch gesicherter Emphysemfälle. Prax Pneumol 23:776–785

Outhred KG, McKenzie HI, White KH (1970) Some findings on the post-mortem association of right ventricular wall thickness and chronic obstructive bronchitis, pneumoconiosis, emphysema and tuberculosis. Med J Aust 57/2:950–954

Park SS, Yoo OH, Janis M, Williams MH (1969) Postmortem evaluation in obstructive lung disease. J Appl Physiol 27:308–312

Park SS, Janis M, Shim CS, Williams MH Jr (1970) Relationship of bronchitis and emphysema to altered pulmonary function. Am Rev Respir Dis 102:927–936

Penman RWB, O'Neill RP, Begley L (1970) Lung elastic recoil and airway resistance as factors limiting forced expiratory flow. Am Rev Respir Dis 101:528–535

Peress L, Sybrecht G, Macklem PT (1976) The mechanism of increase in total lung capacity. Am J Med 61:165–169

Petty TL, Meicort R, Ryan S, Vincent T, Filley GF, Mitchell RS (1965) The functional and bronchographic evaluation of postmortem human lungs: Clinical, physiologic, roentgenologic and pathologic correlations in normal subjects and patients with emphysema and chronic bronchitis. Am Rev Respir Dis 92:450–458

Pratt PC, Klugh GA (1967) Chronic expiratory air flow obstruction – cause or effect of centrilobular emphysema. Dis Chest 52:342–349

Pratt PC, Haque A, Klugh GA (1962) Correlation of postmortem function and structure in panlobular pulmonary emphysema. Lab Invest 11:177–187

Pratt PC, Jutabha O, Klugh GA (1965) Quantitative relationship between structural extent of centrilobular emphysema and postmortem volume and flow characteristics of lungs. Med Thorac 22:197–208

Prinsloo I (1966) The determination of the degree of emphysema on autopsy material. Lab Invest 15:947–961

Pushpakom R, Hoog JC, Woolcock AJ, Angus AE, Macklem PT, Thurlbeck WM (1970) Experimental papain-induced emphysema in dogs. Am Rev Respir Dis 102:778–789

Rainer WG, Hutchinson D, Newby JP, Hamstra R, Durrance J (1963) Major airway collapsibility in the pathogenesis of obstructive emphysema. J Thorac Cardiovasc Surg 46:559–566

Reid L (1955) Correlation of certain bronchographic abnormalities seen in chronic bronchitis with the pathological changes. Thorax 10:199–204

Reid L (1960) Measurement of the bronchial mucous gland layer: A diagnostic yardstick in chronic bronchitis. Thorax 15:132–141

Reid L, Simon G (1959) Pathological findings and radiological changes in chronic bronchitis and emphysema. Br J Radiol 32:291–305

Restrepo G, Heard BE (1963) The size of the bronchial glands in chronic bronchitis. J Pathol Bacteriol 85:305–310

Rohr HP, Oberholzer M, Bartsch G, Keller M (1976) Morphometry in experimental pathology: methods, baseline data and applications. Int Rev Exp Pathol 15:233–325

Rohrer F (1915) Der Strömungswiderstand in den menschlichen Atemwegen und der Einfluß der unregelmäßigen Verzweigung des Bronchialsystems auf den Atmungsverlauf in verschiedenen Lungenbezirken. Pfluegers Arch 162:225–299

Rufener C, Rey P, Press P (1972) Epidémiologie de la bronchite chronique à Genève. Schweiz Med Wochenschr 102:1461–1466

Ryan SF (1969) Artificial emphysema. Am Rev Respir Dis 99:801–803

Ryan SF, Vincent TN, Mitchell RS, Filley GF, Dart G (1965) Ductectasia; an asymptomatic pulmonary change related to age. Med Thorac 22:181–187

Ryder RC, Thurlbeck WM, Gough J (1969) A study of interobserver variation in the assessment of the amount of pulmonary emphysema in paper-mounted whole lung sections. Am Rev Respir Dis 99:354–364

Ryder R, Lyons JP, Campbell H, Gough J (1970) Emphysema in coal-worker's pneumoconiosis. Br Med J II:481–487

Ryder RC, Dunnill MS, Anderson JA (1971) A quantitative study of bronchial mucous gland volume, emphysema and smoking in a necropsy population. J Pathol 104:59–71

Sachs L (1974) Angewandte Statistik, 4. Aufl. Springer, Berlin Heidelberg New York

Schubert W (1960) Über die Wiederentfaltung der Lungen und Verdeutlichung von Emphysemen durch Unterdruckfixierung. Verh Dtsch Ges Pathol 44:172–178

Scott KWM (1973) An autopsy study of bronchial mucous gland hypertrophy in Glasgow. Am Rev Respir Dis 107:239–245

Scott KWM, Steiner GM (1975) Postmortem assessment of chronic airways obstruction by tantalum bronchography. Thorax 30:405–414

Silvers GW, Maisel JC, Petty TL, Mitchell R, Filley GF (1972) Central airway resistance in excised emphysematous lungs. Chest 61:603–612

Simon G (1959) Radiological changes in chronic bronchitis. Br J Radiol 32:299–305

Simon G, Galbraith HJB (1953) Radiology of chronic bronchitis. Lancet II:850–852

Simon G, Pride NB, Jones NL, Raimondi AC (1973) Relation between abnormalities in the chest radiograph and changes in pulmonary function in chronic bronchitis and emphysema. Thorax 28:15–23

Snider GL, Hayes JA, Korthy AL, Lewis GP (1973) Centrilobular emphysema experimentally induced by cadmium chloride aerosol. Am Rev Respir Dis 108:40–48

Sobonya RE, Kleinerman J (1972) Morphometric studies of bronchi in young smokers. Am Rev Respir Dis 105:768–775

Stendler HS, Wagner HH, Kahlstorf J (1969) Dynamische Bronchographie bei chronischer Bronchitis. ROEFO 111:763–769

Sturgess J, Reid L (1972) Secretory activity of the human bronchial mucous glands in vitro. Exp Mol Pathol 16:362–381

Sutinen S, Vaajalahti P, Pääkö P (1978) Prevalence, severity and types of pulmonary emphysema in a population of deaths in a Finnish city. Correlation with age, sex and smoking. Scand J Respir Dis 59:101–115

Sweet HC, Wyatt JP, Kinsella PW (1960) Correlation of lung macrosections with pulmonary function in emphysema. Am J Med 29:277–281

Sweet HC, Wyatt JP, Fritsch AJ, Kinsella PW (1961) Panlobular and centrilobular emphysema. Correlation of clinical findings with pathologic patterns. Ann Intern Med 55:565–581

Symonds G, Renzetti AD, Mitchell MM (1974) The diffusing capacity in pulmonary emphysema. Am Rev Respir Dis 109:391–394

Takizawa T, Thurlbeck WM (1971) Muscle and mucous gland size in the major bronchi of patients with chronic bronchitis, asthma and asthmatic bronchitis. Am Rev Respir Dis 104:331–336

Tammeling GJ, Sluiter HL (1965) The influence of lung volume, flow rate and eso-phageal pressure on the sagittal diameter of the trachea in patients with and without airway obstruction. Am Rev Respir Dis 92:919–931

Tandon MK, Campbell AH (1969) Bronchial cartilage in chronic bronchitis. Thorax 24:607–612

Thurlbeck WM (1963) A clinico-pathological study of emphysema in an American hospital. Thorax 18:59–67

Thurlbeck WM (1967) Measurement of pulmonary emphysema. Am Rev Respir Dis 95:752–764

Thurlbeck WM (1976) Chronic airflow obstruction in lung disease. Saunders, Philadelphia

Thurlbeck WM, Angus E (1963) The relationship between emphysema and chronic bronchitis as assessed morphologically. Am Rev Respir Dis 87:815–819

Thurlbeck WM, Angus GE (1964) A distribution curve for chronic bronchitis. Thorax 19:436–442

Thurlbeck WM, Angus GE (1967) The variation of Reid index measurements within the major bronchial tree. Am Rev Respir Dis 95:551–555

Thurlbeck WM, Simon G (1978) Radiographic appearance of the chest emphysema. AJR 130:429–440

Thurlbeck WM, Dunnill MS, Hartung W, Heard BE, Heppleston AG, Ryder RC (1970a) A comparison of three methods of measuring emphysema. Hum Pathol 1:215–226

Thurlbeck WM, Henderson JA, Fraser RG, Bates DV (1970b) Chronic obstructive lung disease. A comparison between clinical, roentgenologic, functional and morphologic criteria in chronic bronchitis, emphysema, asthma and bronchiectasis. Medicine (Baltimore) 49:81–145

Thurlbeck WM, Pun, R, Toth J, Frazer RG (1974) Bronchial cartilage in chronic ob-structive lung disease. Am Rev Respir Dis 109:73–80

Ulmer WT, Reichel G (1970) Zur Epidemiologie der chronischen Bronchitis und deren Zusammenhang mit der Luftverschmutzung. Dtsch Med Wochenschr 95:2549–2554

Watanabe S, Mitchell M, Renzetti AD Jr (1965) Correlation of structure and function in chronic pulmonary emphysema. Am Rev Respir Dis 92:221–227

Weibel ER (1963) Morphometry of the lung. Springer, Berlin Göttingen Heidelberg

Weibel ER (1973) Stereological techniques of electron microscopic morphometry. In: Hayat MA (ed) Principles and technics of electron microscopy. van Nostrand Reinhold, New York (Biological applications, vol 3, p 237)

Weibel ER, Vidone RA (1961) Fixation of the lung by formalin steam in a controlled state of air inflation. Am Rev Respir Dis 84:856–861

Wheeldon EB, Pirie HM (1974) Measurement of bronchial wall component in young dogs, adult normal dogs and adult dogs with chronic bronchitis. Am Rev Respir Dis 110:609–615

Wierich W (1976) Die Ventilationsleistung isolierter Lungen in verschiedenen Lebens-altern unter Berücksichtigung verschiedener Auswertungsmethoden, speziell unter Anwendung der Methode nach Heusingen. Pneumologie (Suppl) 183–191

Wierich W, Hartung W (1978) The resistances within the bronchial pathway during forced expiration in isolated lungs. XXVIIe Congrès de l'Association Internationale de Bronchopneumologie, Toulouse, 4–6 mai 1978

Williams MH Jr, Cane C (1965) Expriatory and inspiratory flow rates in chronic obstructive pulmonary disease. Dis Chest 48:262–264

Wilson AG, Massarella GR, Pride NB (1974) Elastic properties of airways in human lungs post mortem. Am Rev Respir Dis 110:716–729

Wright BM, Slavin G, Kreel L, Callan K, Sandin B (1974) Postmortem inflation and fixation of human lungs. A technique for pathological and radiological correlations. Thorax 29:189–194

Wright RR (1960) Bronchial atrophy and collapse in chronic obstructive pulmonary emphysema. Am J Pathol 37:63–77

Wright RR, Stuart CM (1965) Chronic bronchitis with emphysema: A pathological study of the bronchi. Med Thorac 22:210–218

Wyatt JP, Fischer VW, Sweet HC (1964) The pathomorphology of the emphysema complex. Am Rev Respir Dis 89:533–560

Primary and Secondary Pulmonary Hypertension in Childhood: A Clinicopathological Reappraisal

S.G. HAWORTH

I. Introduction

In adults and older children with pulmonary hypertension the sequence of structural changes occurring in the pulmonary circulation and the relation between structural and haemodynamic change is well recognised, following the classical studies of *Heath* and *Edwards* (1958). However, in infants and young children this is not so, and the relation between structural and functional change in the immature lung is different from that seen in adult life. Recently, improved understanding of pulmonary hypertension in childhood has resulted from (a) studies on the normal development of the pulmonary circulation; (b) the application of quantitative morphometric techniques to the study of pulmonary vascular structure, an approach which is essential in a growing organ in health or disease; (c) improved clinical care in the perinatal period, bringing to light the problem of failure of the pulmonary circulation to adapt normally to extra-uterine life when the heart is normal; and (d) improved techniques of angiographic and haemo-dynamic evaluation, which permit a more accurate correlation between pulmonary vascular structural and haemodynamic change in children with congenital heart disease.

We have not solved the two main problems: assessing the reversibility of pulmonary vascular disease and treating the disease medically. It is not always possible to predict with certainty the reversibility of pulmonary vascular change, either from the lung biopsy or from the haemodynamic findings alone, even assuming one can infer the structural change from the functional change, which is frequently a bold step. Also, when pulmonary vascular change either causes pulmonary hypertension or is so excessive that it no longer has a beneficial effect, medical treatment is difficult because there is no safe and selective pulmonary vasodilator drug available, except possibly oxygen.

To progress further it will be necessary to (a) clarify the normal development of the pulmonary circulation, particularly during the critical phase of adaptation to extra-uterine life; (b) understand the precise sequence of structural change occurring in the hypertensive immature lung; and (c) learn more about the cellular response to pulmonary hypertension in the immature lung and about the molecular pharmacology of pulmonary vascular smooth muscle.

In pulmonary hypertension, attention is generally focussed on the muscular peripheral pulmonary arteries, but this is not the only segment of the pulmonary circulation to be affected. The structure of the main pulmonary artery, the large elastic pulmonary arteries and the pulmonary veins changes when arterial pressure is increased. Structural change alters the mechanical properties of vessel walls, and because the entire pulmonary vascular bed and the heart function as a unit, changes in the mechanical properties of each part of the pulmonary circulation will alter the physical characteristics of the system. The relation between structural change and vascular impedance, resistance, capacitance and pulse-wave velocity has been explored more thoroughly in the systemic than in the pulmonary circulation, but the matching of the mechanical and physical characteristics of the pulmonary circulation with those of the heart is even more critical in the pulmonary than in the systemic circulation. This approach of viewing the heart and pulmonary circulation as a structural and functional unit has practical implications: when children with congenital heart disease undergo surgery the haemodynamic conditions change, and we should be able to predict the effect of such a change on the heart and damaged pulmonary vascular bed in the postoperative period and in later life.

II. Methods of Preparation and Quantitative Analysis Used in Studying Pulmonary Vascular Morphology

1. Preparation of Lung Tissue

In studying a *postmortem lung specimen,* the technique used to prepare the lung depends on the questions to be answered. In the study of pulmonary hypertension, points of interest include the arterial and venous branching patterns from the hilus to the alveolar wall, the volume proportion of total lung tissue occupied by the arterial or venous systems, the presence of arterial tortuosity, narrowing or occlusion of the vessel lumen, arterial size, arterial wall structure, the number of intra-acinar arteries and veins and the size and wall structure of the pulmonary veins. The best results are often achieved by using a combination of techniques. These include injection of the pulmonary arterial or venous circulation with a radio-opaque contrast medium, radiographic examination, dissection of the fixed specimen and histological examination including serial reconstruction of the arterial pathways.

For precise measurement of vessel size, wall thickness and vessel number, the system must be distended before fixation. Injection of one system ensures easy identification of both arteries and veins.

Injection of the pulmonary arterial (or venous) system with a warm radio-opaque barium sulphate—gelatin mixture permits both arteriographic study and histological examination, as the injection mixture solidifies at room temperature, allowing the material to be cut for histological preparation (*Elliott* and *Reid* 1965; *Davies* and *Reid* 1970). The pressure at which the mixture should be injected is controversial. All the specimens in one laboratory should be prepared in the same manner for purposes of comparison, but they can be injected either at the same arbitrary pressure, or at the pressure believed to be present in the pulmonary circulation during life. Because the pulmonary arterial pressure may not be known, or may only have been measured some time before death, it is perhaps preferable to inject all lungs, normal and abnormal, at the same pressure. Similarly, all lungs are best fixed by injection through the airways at the same pressure, using buffered formalin. By injecting at a pressure of 100 cm H_2O, all arteries with an internal diameter greater than $10-15$ μm are filled but not ruptured. The medium fills the arteries of the alveolar wall but does not pass through the capillary bed. A less viscous medium containing a smaller quantity of gelatin than is recommended does pass through the capillary bed, and interpretation of pulmonary vascular structure is then more difficult. Because the vessels are distended, the elastic laminae are flattened, and the external diameter and medial thickness can be measured accurately. This injection technique has many advantages, but unfortunately the cells are damaged by heating the specimen, and it is advisable to take some tissue for routine preparation before injecting the lung.

Alternatively, the pulmonary arteries and the airways can be injected with a fixative such as glutaraldehyde in cacodylate or phosphate buffer which gives better preservation of cellular detail but less satisfactory vascular distension for accurate quantitative morphometry (*Gil* and *Weibel* 1969; *Meyrick* and *Reid* 1979). This injection technique is suitable for experimental studies when electron-microscopic examination is the most important objective. For most purposes, paraffin-embedded sections are adequate, but for study of cellular detail and for analysis of the wall structure of elastic arteries, 1-μm-thick Araldite-embedded sections stained with toluidine blue are preferred.

Corrosion casts are not usually helpful in studying the hypertensive lung. This technique can be used to examine the relation between two or more vascular systems, and anastomoses between pulmonary and bronchial arterial circulation may be demonstrated (*Liebow* et al. 1947, 1950), but in pulmonary hypertension it is the changes in the wall structure which are of particular interest, and with this technique the evidence is dissolved during the preparation of the cast. Also, if connections between the pulmonary and bronchial arterial circulations are to be sought, then the combination of arteriography and serial reconstruction is generally the most satisfactory approach.

2. Lung Biopsy Technique and Fixation

In order to identify the structures microscopically, the alveoli must not be collapsed. The biopsy is therefore taken with the lung inflated and fixed in the inflated state. Two clamps are placed across the lung, an incision is made between them, and one clamp remains attached to the biopsy until it has been immersed in fixative. For light-microscopic examination, buffered formalin is a satisfactory fixative.

For electron-microscopic examination, the biopsy is immersed in 2.5% glutaraldehyde in cacodylate buffer (pH 7.2) for 10 min. The clamp is then released and the tissue allowed to fix for another 2 h; 2-mm-square blocks of tissue are then cut and processed in the usual way for electron-microscopic study.

3. Radiological Techniques

A radiograph of the whole injected lung and of 0.5-cm-thick lung slices, taken under standardised conditions, is generally sufficient to demonstrate the arterial or venous branching pattern, the density of the background haze, stenoses and obstruction of the vessel lumen, and anastomoses between pulmonary arteries and between pulmonary and bronchial arteries when the connections are enlarged. Stereoscopic techniques can avoid confusing overlapping phenomena and can "separate" vessels from one another (*Ljungquist* 1963; *Robertson* 1968). If measurements are to be taken, conditions must be standardised with respect to the focus-to-object and object-to-film distances, and for stereoscopic examination the distance between the corresponding points in the specimen at the two exposures must be known.

4. Lung Weight and Volume

The weight of the unfixed fresh specimen and the volume of the fixed lung should be compared with age and size-matched controls.

5. Selection of Blocks of Tissue for Microscopic Study

The source of every block of tissue taken from the lung should be carefully documented. Particularly in congenital heart disease, there may be regional differences in pulmonary perfusion, in venous drainage or in both, and the structural changes demonstrated in the lung will be meaningless unless the source of the tissue is known. When pulmonary vascular change is secondary to chronic lung disease, as in cystic fibrosis, there are regional differences in parenchymal lung damage. When there are no regional abnormalities in either perfusion or lung damage, the lungs are cut into 0.5-cm-thick slices and blocks are selected by a stratified random sampling technique using a transparent numbered grid (*Dunnill* 1962). Ten blocks are taken from large lungs, and as many as possible from the smaller specimens.

6. Volume Proportions of Different Tissues or Structures Whithin the Lung

Point-counting techniques are used to demonstrate the volumes of normal and abnormal tissue in an organ, or to detect an alteration in volume of a tissue which is normally present (*Dunnill* 1962). The technique depends on the principle proposed by the geologist *Delesse* (1847), which states that in a complex mineral the areal proportions of a section of the mineral are equivalent to the volume proportions. In vascular studies, macroscopic and microscopic point-counting is generally used to determine the volume proportion of arteries and to assess growth by calculating the number of alveoli in the lung (*Dunnill* 1962; *Reid* 1975).

7. Techniques of Quantitative Morphometric Analysis of Pulmonary Vascular Structure by Light Microscopy

In the normal child the lung is remodelled with growth, and the size, number and composition of different structures in the lung changes with age (*Hislop* and *Reid* 1972, 1973). In the abnormal lung, therefore, each structural feature must be compared with that of age-matched controls from tissue prepared and analysed in the same manner. There are two problems to overcome in any structural analysis of the pulmonary circulation: identification of arteries and veins, and the quantitative analysis, rather than subjective impression, of structural change in disease.

a) Identification of Pulmonary Arteries

The intrapulmonary arteries cannot be identified according to size, because size changes in the normal lung with growth and may also change in disease. The large elastic arteries are identified by counting the number of generations which separate them from the hilus, counting the segmental artery as the first generation, and their wall structure is determined by their position in the lung (*Hayward* and *Reid* 1952; *Elliott* and *Reid* 1965; *Hislop* and *Reid* 1973). An elastic artery is defined as a pulmonary artery with seven or more concentric elastic laminae between internal and external laminae, and elastic arteries extend from the hilus to the seventh arterial generation. The structure of a transitional artery is intermediate between that of an elastic artery and that of a muscular artery and consists of four to seven elastic laminae within the media. Such arteries extend over two or three arterial generations. Beyond this point the arteries contain four elastic lamellae or less and are muscular; this type extends into the acinus. Arteries accompany airways, and within the acinus the arteries continue to branch with the airways and therefore can be identified on microscopic examination according to the type of airway they accompany — either terminal or respiratory bronchioli, alveolar ducts or alveolar walls. The wall structure of the intra-acinar arteries may be muscular, partially muscular or non-muscular, and the proportion of each structural type changes with growth and varies in disease.

The term "arteriole" is best avoided, as it is open to different interpretations based on size, structure and function or a combination of attributes.

b) Assessment of Arterial Size

On the postmortem arteriogram the length of the axial pathway is determined and the lumen diameter of the vessel is measured at the hilus and at 25% intervals along the axial pathway to the periphery of the lung. Microscopic measurement of the external diameter of arteries accompanying the peripheral airways gives a complete assessment of arterial size in the lung.

c) Microscopic Examination of Elastic Wall Structure

The thickness of the media is measured using a calibrated eyepiece graticule, the number of elastic fibres intersecting the graticule is counted and from these measurements interlamellar distance is calculated. The thickness, regularity, length and orientation of the elastic fibres is noted and abnormal fragmentation is sought.

d) Assessment of Pulmonary Arterial Muscularity

Arterial muscularity can be determined by a variety of techniques.

α) Medial Thickness Related to External Diameter of an Artery

In a large and unselected population of vessels, the medial thickness and external diameter of all arteries are measured, and the percentage arterial medial thickness is calculated:

$$\frac{2 \times \text{medial wall thickness}}{\text{external diameter}} \times 100.$$

The arteries are grouped according to external diameter, and the mean percentage medial thickness is calculated for each size range (*Davies* and *Reid* 1970). Mean percentage arterial medial thickness can be determined easily and accurately, particularly in injected material, and can be related to haemodynamic measurements of pulmonary arterial pressure and vascular resistance. Expressing medial thickness differently, the mean arterial lumen to wall ratio has been used by many workers (*Dammann* and *Ferencz* 1956; *Könn* and *Storb* 1960). In the normal lung, the relation between percentage arterial medial thickness and size is constant, but in disease it may be affected not only by increase in muscle, but by abnormalities in arterial size. The measurements of the size of arteries accompanying peripheral airways will ensure correct interpretation of arterial medial thickness relative to size.

To overcome the problems of arterial dilatation and of contraction in the undistended lung, the area of muscle present can be determined either by using a planimetric technique to study individual arteries (*Naeye* 1961a) or by establishing the cross-sectional area of the media from measurements of medial width and external diameter (*Wagenvoort* 1960). The second approach has the advantage that the total muscle mass per unit area of lung is estimated for a large population of vessels. Other analytical techniques include the linear intercept method for determining an index of medial muscle tissue in the lung (*Weibel* 1962).

β) Population Counts

In pulmonary hypertension the relation between wall structure and size is altered and muscle is present in smaller arteries than those in which it is normally seen. This effect of pulmonary hypertension is ascertained by assessment of the structural type (muscular, partially muscular or non-muscular) and the external diameter of *all* arteries within a given area of lung tissue (*Reid* 1967).

γ) Structure of Arteries Accompanying Peripheral Airways

In pulmonary hypertension, muscle cells differentiate in more peripheral intra-acinar arteries than is normal. This can be detected by determining the proportion of arteries which have a muscular, partially muscular or non-muscular structure at terminal bronchiolar, respiratory bronchiolar, alveolar duct and alveolar wall level.

Thus arterial muscularity is usually assessed by determining percentage arterial medial thickness and the extent to which muscle has differentiated along the arterial pathway, as judged by both size and position of the artery in the lung field.

e) Assessment of Number of Intra-acinar Arteries

The number of intra-acinar arteries can be reduced in pulmonary hypertension. The number of alveoli and of arteries less than 200 μm in diameter are counted in 25 microscopic fields chosen at random from all the sections cut from the lung. The number of arteries per unit area or unit volume of the lung can be determined; the ratio of alveoli to arteries is calculated to overcome any difference in the degree of inflation in different lungs.

In the assessment of arterial muscularity and intra-acinar arterial size and number the results in different parts of the lung should be compared, since only if there are no significant regional differences can all the results be pooled and assumed to represent the whole lung.

f) Assessment of Pulmonary Veins

In the normal lung, the veins are unlike arteries because the outer limit of the media is not delineated by an external elastic lamina, but when the muscle hypertrophies, the vein comes to resemble an artery and is said to be "arterialised" (*Wagenvoort* 1970). Wall thickness is measured from the internal elastic lamina to the outer edge of the most peripheral muscle cell or elastic lamina, and percentage vein wall thickness is calculated as for the arteries. As for the arteries, the number of veins per unit area of lung and the ratio of alveoli to veins can be determined.

g) Assessment of Right Ventricular Hypertrophy

In pulmonary hypertension the amount of muscle increases in the pulmonary vascular bed and also in the systemic venous ventricle, normally the right ventricle. In the normal heart the septum is considered as a part of the left ventricle, and therefore hypertrophy of the right ventricle is indicated by a decrease in the ratio:

$$\frac{\text{weight of the left ventricle} + \text{septum}}{\text{weight of the right ventricle}}$$

(*Fulton* et al. 1952). During fetal life the left ventricle and septum together are heavier than the right ventricle, but the right ventricle forms a greater proportion of the total ventricular weight than it does in the child or adult. The "adult" heart weight ratio of 2.3:1 to 3.3:1 is normally reached by 4 months of age (*Recavarren* and *Arias-Stella* 1964).

8. Techniques of Preparation of Lung Tissue for Electron Microscopy

In addition to preparing small pieces of "living" lung tissue for electron-microscopic study, in experimental animals the lungs can be fixed in the distended state (*Gil* and *Weibel* 1969; *Meyrick* and *Reid* 1979). Glutaraldehyde (2.5% in cacodylate buffer, pH 7.2) is injected simultaneously into the pulmonary trunk and trachea after tying off the pulmonary veins.

9. Techniques of Quantitative Morphometric Analysis by Electron Microscopy

In addition to a descriptive assessment of the electron micrograph, point-counting and other stereological methods can be applied to determine the areal and volume proportions of organelles within the cytoplasm, the different types of extracellular ground substance and other features (*Weibel* 1970; *Meyrick* and *Reid* 1980a). Such techniques are also used to study alveolar surface area, the pulmonary and membrane diffusion capacities and the problem of "folding" of the capillary network in the lung.

Sophisticated electron-micrographic analysis is always combined with light-microscopic studies on larger amounts of tissue.

III. Normal Development of the Pulmonary Circulation

Pulmonary hypertension can have a more devasting and permanent structural effect on the pulmonary circulation in childhood than in adult life because the lung is immature. The normal lung continues to develop after birth, and pulmonary hypertension not only changes wall structure but is associated with a reduction in the size and number of intra-acinar arteries. As the child continues to grow, cardiac output increases, and failure to increase the capacity of the peripheral pulmonary circulation to accommodate even a normal increase in flow further compromises the pulmonary circulation, emphasizing the vulnerability of children with congenital heart disease, pulmonary hypertension and an abnormal increase in pulmonary blood flow.

Thus we need to understand how the pulmonary circulation grows and develops in the normal child.

1. Development of the Arterial System

a) Branching Pattern

The arteries and airways develop together. The pre-acinar arterial and airway branching pattern is complete by the 16th week of gestation, whereas the intra-acinar arteries develop relatively late in fetal life and after birth, together with the alveolar ducts and alveoli (Fig. 1) (*Hislop* and *Reid* 1972, 1973). Some arteries run alongside the airways and branch with them, others arise from the main pathway and pursue a more direct course to the respiratory epithelium (Fig. 2). With little respect for semantics, arteries branching with the airways have been called conventional arteries, and those that do not, supernumerary arteries. The adult ratio of supernumerary to conventional arteries, approximately 3:1, is achieved by the 12th week of gestation, before airway branching is complete, and by 19 weeks the pre-acinar arteries are as numerous as in the adult, with approximately 21 conventional and 58 supernumerary vessels. Although the supernumerary arteries are always smaller than adjacent conventional arteries, they account for 40% of the cross-sectional area of arterial side branches in the adult.

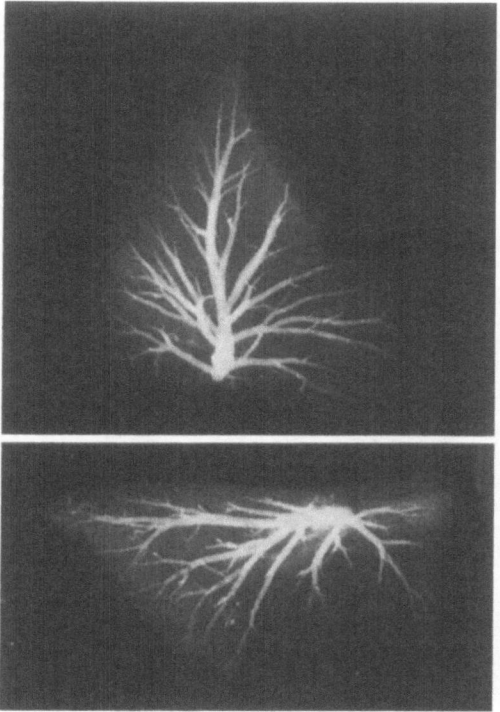

Fig. 1a. Postmortem arteriogram of a normal fetus of 19 weeks gestation. The pre-acinar arteries are all present. By permission of Dr. *A. Hislop.* × 0.95

After birth, multiplication of intra-acinar arteries keeps pace with alveolar multiplication, occurring most rapidly during the first 3 years. Conventional arteries develop as more alveolar ducts appear, up to about 18 months of age, whereas supernumerary arteries increase in number up to 8 years as new alveoli form. More supernumerary arteries develop within the acinus than along the pre-acinar pathway. Arteries multiply as the alveoli develop and the ratio of alveoli to arteries is similar throughout childhood, but the number of arteries per unit area decreases as the alveoli increase in size.

b) Arterial Wall Structure

In the adult, arterial wall structure is determined both by external diameter and by position in the lung (*Brenner* 1935; *Elliott* and *Reid* 1965). In the fetus, the distribution of elastic tissue is determined by position. It extends gradually along the arterial pathway to reach the adult level, the seventh generation, by the 19th week of gestation (*Hislop* and *Reid* 1972). In the small arteries structure depends on diameter, the muscle giving way to a partially muscular structure which in turn gives way to a non-muscular structure at the same diameter as in the adult lung, but at a more proximal part of the arterial pathway. Even at birth, relatively few intra-acinar arteries contain muscle cells. Muscle extends gradually along the arterial pathway to reach the alveolar wall vessels in late adolescence (*Hislop* and *Reid* 1973). During childhood, development of

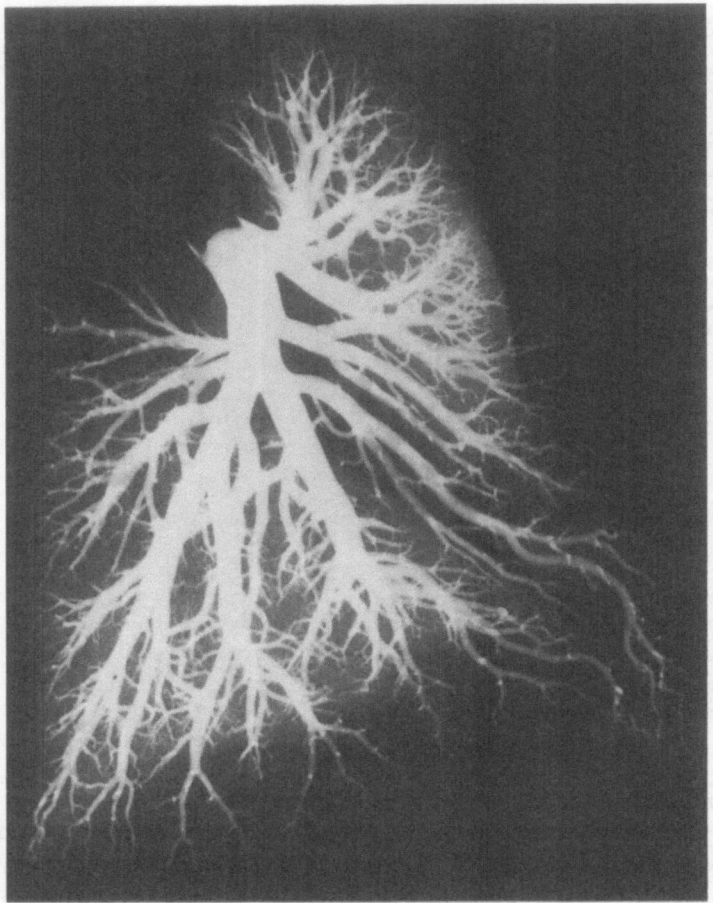

Fig. 1b. Postmortem arteriogram of a normal fetus of 40 weeks gestation. By permission of Heinemann Medical Books Ltd. × 0.95

smooth muscle cells lags behind the increase in arterial diameter, so that the intra-acinar arterial bed remains less muscular in childhood than in adult life. To the cardiologist, this structural difference between the child and adult lung has important practical implications. In lung biopsy, the presence of muscle in arteries more peripheral than those in which it is normally seen, with respect to age, is an important early indication of the structural response of the pulmonary circulation to pulmonary hypertension.

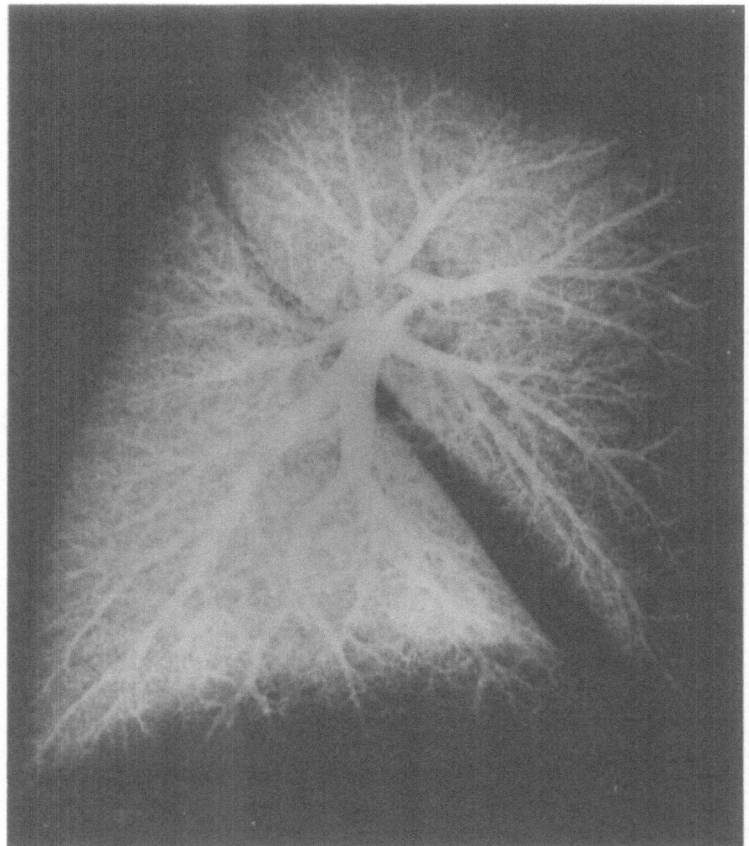

Fig. 1c. Postmortem arteriogram of a normal 18-month-old child. A dense background haze has appeared since birth, due to filling of newly formed intra-acinar arteries. × 0.95

c) Development of the Intrapulmonary Venous System

The pre-acinar drainage pattern of the fetus is similar to that of the adult and is complete halfway through gestation, development of the pulmonary veins corresponding to that of the pulmonary arteries. After birth, new veins develop in the intra-acinar region. Medial thickness when related to external diameter is the same in the newborn infant as in the adult (*Hislop* and *Reid* 1973).

d) Blood-Gas Barrier

In the human fetus, from 28 weeks gestation onwards the thickness of the potential blood-gas barrier is the same as in the adult (*Lauweryns* and *Rosan* 1970) and from this age at the latest it can support respiration. The blood-gas barrier may be only

104

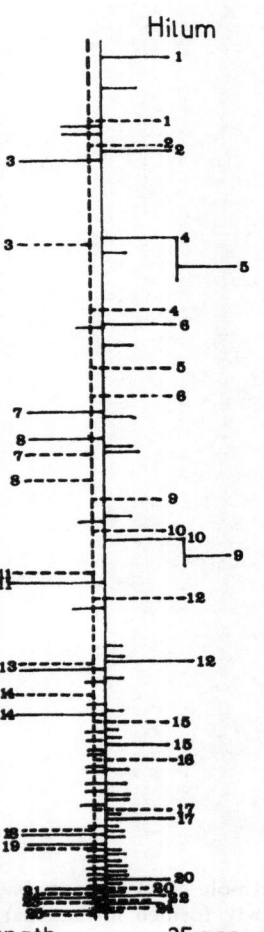

Hilum

Fig. 2. Reconstruction of the posterior basal artery and airway of the left lower lobe in a 19-week fetus. The airway branches and their accompanying conventional arteries are numbered. Also shown are 58 supernumerary arteries. ——, artery; - - - - -, airway. By permission of *Thorax*

Actual length
16 mm

25 generations
58 supernumeraries

0.001 mm thick. Recent studies on basement membrane development in fetal rat lungs show that the epithelial and endothelial basement membranes of the alveolar-capillary wall are synthesized independently and appear at different times during fetal lung development (*Grant* et al. 1981). As the alveolar-capillary wall matures and becomes thicker, the two basement membranes come into opposition and fuse focally. The epithelium makes the principal contribution to the basement membrane of the alveolar capillary wall at birth.

e) Development of Bronchial Arteries

It used to be thought that bronchial arteries developed early in fetal life, either from the peribronchial plexus surrounding the primitive lung buds (*Weibel* 1959) or from early segmental arteries arising from the aorta, of which only the lower vessels persisted as bronchial arteries (*O'Rahilly* et al. 1950). More recently, *Boyden* studied a 41-mm embryo (1970a) and a 12-week fetus of 85 mm (1970b) and found bronchial arteries growing from the aorta itself or from the right or left posterior intercostal rami of the aorta. It was concluded that these arteries arise de novo between the 9th and 12th weeks of intra-uterine life. They form a secondary arterial system, implanted relatively late upon the peripheral coats of the bronchial tree and large pulmonary vessels, which is not completed much before term (*Boyden* 1970b). As bronchial arteries grow down the bronchial tree, they keep pace with the development of cartilage.

2. Adaptation to Extra-uterine Life

At birth, the lung suddenly becomes responsible for the oxygenation of the newborn baby. The pulmonary arterial pressure has been measured in neonates of many species, including man (*Dawes* 1968), but there is relatively little information on the normal structural changes occurring in the pulmonary circulation during this time. We know only that the reduction in pulmonary arterial pressure is associated with a reduction in pulmonary arterial smooth-muscle mass (*Naeye* 1961a). Quantitative studies on the lungs of two children showed that the muscularity of the small pulmonary arteries had fallen to the low adult level by 3 days of age, whereas the reduction in muscularity in the larger arteries occurred more slowly, reaching the adult level by 4 months of age (Fig. 3). By this time the weight of the right ventricle relative to that of the left had also fallen to that seen in adult life (*Hislop* and *Reid* 1973). Studying normal adaptation to extra-uterine life in the human is difficult, because haemodynamic measurements are not made on healthy babies. Also, many malformations associated with early postnatal death, such as anencephaly (*Naeye* et al. 1971), renal abnormalities (*Hislop* et al. 1979) and rhesus incompatibility (*Chamberlain* et al. 1977) are associated with abnormal lung development.

Studies on the pig lung suggest that the functional changes occurring in the pulmonary circulation during the first 2 weeks of life follow a similar time course to those in the human infant (*Haworth* and *Hislop* 1981).

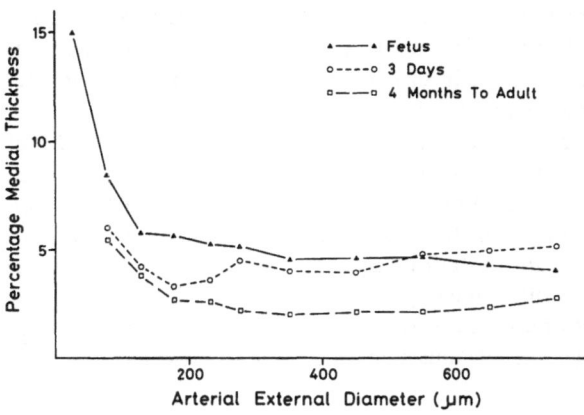

Fig. 3. Mean percentage arterial medial thickness in man related to external diameter (μm) in the normal fetus, at 3 days, and at 4 months to adulthood

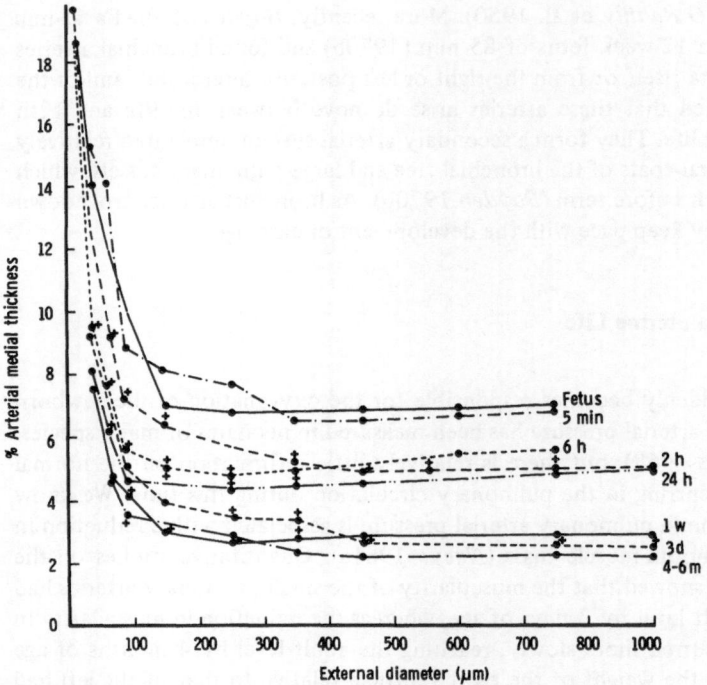

Fig. 4. Mean percentage arterial medial thickness in the pig related to external diameter (μm), in groups of animals, from fetal life to 6 months. +, values which are significantly less than those of the preceding younger age group. By permission of *Cardiovascular Research*

The first structural change seen in the pig lung after birth appears in the nonmuscular and partially muscular arteries of the precapillary bed and consists of dilatation and recruitment. During fetal life the number of arteries per unit area of lung counted microscopically is low, but it increases immediately after birth, presumably due to the dilatation of arteries previously too small to discern by light-microscopic examination and too small to fill with the injection mixture. The intra-acinar arteries increase rapidly in size, being larger than in fetal life by 5 min after birth and becoming significantly larger at terminal bronchiolar level by 12–24 h. This early change is probably due to dilatation, further increase in size being growth. Alveolar duct arteries are significantly larger than in fetal life at 1 week of age.

The percentage arterial medial thickness falls gradually after birth, and by 2 h of age has become significantly different from that found at birth, in arteries of nearly all size ranges (Fig. 4). Arteries less than 250 μm in diameter have almost reached a normal mature adult level by 24 h of age. In the larger vessels, medial thickness shows a significant reduction between 24 h and 3 days of age, after which it does not change significantly. The early reduction in percentage medial thickness is probably due largely to dilatation of arteries, but particularly after 24 h, arteries which are identified by their accompanying airway become less muscular during the first week of life, indi-

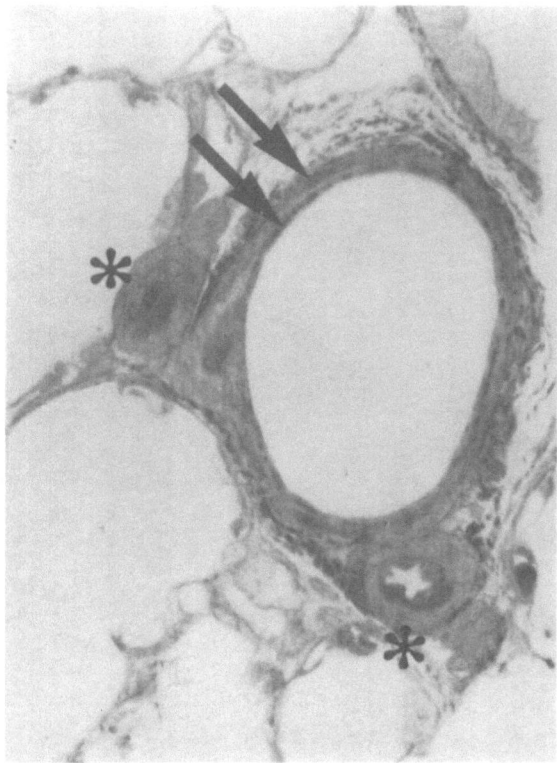

Fig. 5. Muscle cells lie between *arrows* indicating internal and external elastic laminae. In the two smaller non-muscular arteries (∗), endothelial cells almost or totally occlude the lumen. By permission of *Cardiovascular Research.* Toluidine blue, × 600

cating a loss of differentiated smooth muscle cells. For example, at alveolar duct level the proportion of partially muscular arteries decreases as that of non-muscular arteries increases during the first 4 days of life.

In fetal life, it is not only the muscular arteries which are thick-walled. The non-muscular and partially muscular arteries also have thick walls, since between the endothelial cells and the single elastic lamina is a layer of cells which probably includes pericytes or intermediate cells (Fig. 5). In adult animals of other species, these cells are known to differentiate into smooth muscle cells in the presence of hypoxic pulmonary hypertension. In the newborn pig, during the first week of life small thick-walled arteries become less conspicuous and the proportion of arteries having a mature, thin-walled, non-muscular or partially muscular structure increases.

In the pig, as in the human, the blood-gas barrier is extremely thin at birth (Fig. 6). The alveolar walls are slender, consisting of single capillary sheets with a minimum of connective tissue.

In summary, in the pig the changes in the pulmonary arterial circulation after birth consist of three overlapping phases:

1. Dilatation and recruitment of small arteries within the acinar region begins during the first 5 min and is associated with a reduction in pulmonary arterial pressure. These changes, associated with a loss of arterial muscle, continue during the first 24 h.

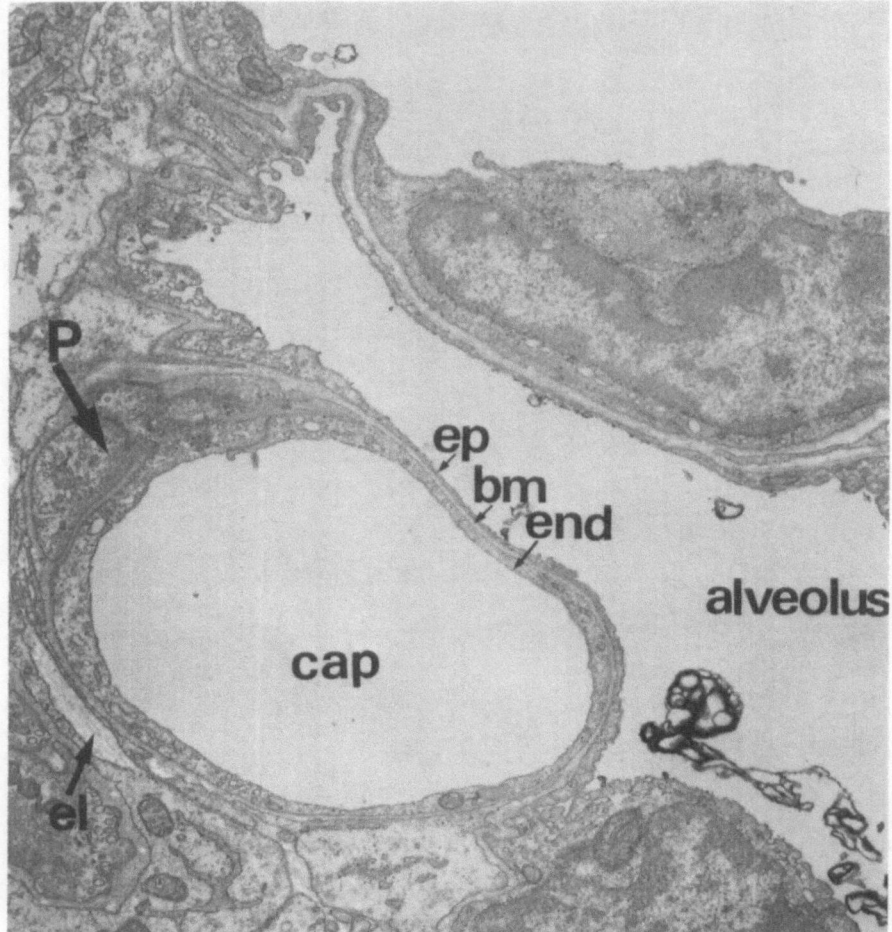

Fig. 6. Electron micrograph of the alveolar region of a newborn pig aged 4 h. *cap*, capillary; *ep*, epithelial cell, cell process of type 1 pneumonocyte; *bm*, basement membrane; *end*, endothelial cell; *el*, elastin; *P*, pericyte

2. Between 24 h and 2 weeks, a significant reduction in the amount of arterial muscle is associated with a reduction in pulmonary systemic vascular resistance ratio from 0.58 to 0.18.

3. Functionally, the pulmonary circulation appears mature at rest by 2 weeks, but growth and remodelling of the pulmonary arteries continues until an adult pattern is reached by 6 months of age.

3. Remodelling of the Pulmonary Circulation with Growth

In the fetus, the pulmonary trunk resembles the aorta (*Heath* et al. 1959). The media is similar to that of the aorta and consists of a regular pattern of alternating smooth muscle fibres and elastic laminae. After birth, the thickness of the pulmonary trunk media decreases gradually until at about 8 months of age the pulmonary trunk to aorta ratio is about 0.6:1; this level is maintained throughout life. By 4 months of age the elastic fibres are fragmented and swollen and consist of short thick rods, sometimes with clubbed ends. An adult appearance is established by the end of the 2nd year of life. Slender and thick rod-like elastic fibres are widely separated by muscle bundles. The smallest branches of the vasa vasorum can penetrate to the centre of the media.

In the human infant, the length and diameter of the pre-acinar arteries increases in a curvilinear fashion with age and with lung volume (*Hislop* and *Reid* 1977a). The diameter of the intra-acinar arteries shows a similar curvilinear increase with age. The rate of increase in length and diameter slows down after 18 months of age, probably because the rapid phase of intra-acinar arterial multiplication is over by then.

Libi-Sylora et al. (1968) divided the lung into two structural and functional components: the proximal elastic arteries, serving as a reservoir, and the distal muscular arteries, comprising a muscular segment. They suggested that with growth an increase in capacity of the pulmonary circulation is achieved mainly by an increase in size of the elastic reservoir, and that a predominantly vasomotor structure is transformed into one in the form of an elastic reservoir.

Multiplication of intra-acinar arteries keeps pace with alveolar multiplication, occurring most rapidly during the first 3 years of life.

4. Functional Implications of Structural Change in Pulmonary Circulation During Growth

In adapting to extra-uterine life, the pulmonary circulation changes in two ways, because the dimensions of the system and the composition of the vessel walls change simultaneously. As the lumen diameter and the number of arteries being perfused increases, the capacity of the system rises. As the composition of the arterial walls from the pulmonary valve to the respiratory epithelium alters, so the mechanical properties of the arterial walls change. The functional effect of these structural changes is to increase pulmonary blood flow, to alter the pattern of flow at birth and to lower pulmonary vascular resistance and characteristic impedance during the first 2 weeks of life.

Studies on the fetal lamb have shown that blood flows forwards in the pulmonary arteries only during early systole, when velocity is high, because of the high resistance maintained by thick-walled peripheral pulmonary arteries (*Rudolph* et al. 1977). In late systole, flow velocity decreases. Administration of acetylcholine to the fetal lamb lowers resistance and extends forward flow throughout systole, as occurs in the normal lamb after birth.

110

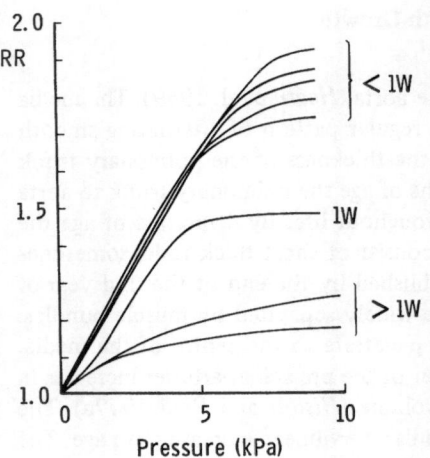

Fig. 7. Change in relative radius *(RR)* in animals of different ages related to pressure. By permission of Churchill Livingstone

Thus far, attention has been focussed on the structural changes in the peripheral pulmonary arteries. Studies on the systemic arterial circulation, however, show that it is simplistic to regard large elastic arteries as passive conduits. In the lung, the proximal elastic arteries account for around 30% of the total impedance of the circulation, as compared with 5%–10% for the large elastic arteries of the systemic circulation *(Berry* et al. 1981). Recent studies on the static elastic properties of the intrapulmonary arteries of the immature pig have shown that after birth the pulmonary arteries along the proximal two-thirds of the arterial pathway become less distensible as the pulmonary arterial pressure falls *(Berry* et al. 1981). The relationship between the change in radius and distending pressure is described as *functional* stiffness of a vessel. In Fig. 7 the relationship between change in relative radius in groups of animals of different ages relative to pressure changes with age. The curves fall into two main families: those from animals aged 2 days or less, in which the vessel remains relatively distensible up to a pressure of 6.7 kPa; and those from animals aged 2 weeks to 4 months, in which the gradient has attained its final value above 2.7 kPa. Data from the 1-week group falls between the two extremes. Thus structural and functional changes in the large elastic arteries and the peripheral intra-acinar pulmonary arteries appear to follow a similar time course, both segments of the pulmonary arterial pathway having largely completed the process of adaptation to extra-uterine life by 2 weeks of age.

At birth, the pulmonary arterial pressure is about 6.0 kPa. The comparatively high distensibility of the pulmonary arteries at this pressure will minimise the pulsatile component of cardiac work. By 2 weeks of age the pressure decreases to 1.3 kPa and the greater distensibility at high pressures is no longer necessary.

The form of the pressure-radius curve in the pulmonary circulation is similar to that seen in the systemic arterial circulation. With increase in pressure, the increase in radius becomes progressively less, and at least in the systemic circulation this is thought to represent progressive recruitment of collagen fibres *(Berry* and *Greenwald* 1976). The elastic properties of the material composing the vessel walls are measured as the *structural* stiffness of the wall, the circumferential elastic modulus. Values for the structural stiffness of the elastic pulmonary arteries of the newborn pig are similar to those of the aorta in adult animals, suggesting similarities in mechanical behaviour (*S.G. Haworth,* personal observations). Structural similarities between the pulmonary trunk and the aorta during fetal life, when both vessels are exposed to the same pressure, are well recognised (*Heath* et al. 1959). In newborn pigs, structural stiffness increases significantly between 4 h and 2 weeks of age.

As the child grows, so the cardiac output increases, but the progressive growth and remodelling of the pulmonary vascular bed ensures that pulmonary vascular resistance does not rise. Proximal to the arterial pathways of the microcirculation, resistance is mainly determined by lumen diameter, and total pulmonary vascular resistance is determined by the number of resistance pathways arranged in parallel. With growth, not only does arterial size increase, but the number of peripheral arterial pathways also increases, thus ensuring a progressive rise in capacity of the peripheral pulmonary vascular bed during childhood.

IV. Persistent Pulmonary Hypertension

Persistence of the fetal circulation implies failure of the pulmonary circulation to adapt normally to extra-uterine life. Pulmonary vascular resistance remains elevated and right-to-left shunting persists across the ductus arteriosus and/or the foramen ovale. The heart is anatomically normal. Since it was first described in 1969, persistent fetal circulation has been recognised with increasing frequency as a cause of neonatal cyanosis (*Gersony* et al. 1969; *Siassi* et al. 1971; *Brown* and *Pickering* 1974).

Persistent fetal circulation is associated with perinatal hypoxia in 80% of cases. It is seen less frequently in term babies following a normal delivery and is called idiopathic persistence of the fetal circulation, because no "trigger" factor has been identified (*Gersony* 1973). The clinical course is variable. Most infants improve gradually during the first week of life, but there may be little or no response to pulmonary vasodilator drugs such as tolazoline, and the mortality is high, 25%–30% (*Gersony* et al. 1969; *Brown* and *Pickering* 1974; *Levin* et al. 1976). Less commonly, persistent pulmonary hypertension occurs in babies born to mothers taking prostaglandin synthetase inhibitors (*Manchester* et al. 1975). It is postulated that prostaglandin synthetase inhibitors such as aspirin and indomethacin can cause constriction or premature closure of the ductus arteriosus and thus produce severe prenatal pulmonary hypertension. In two studies of babies born to mothers taking indomethacin, ten of a total of 39 babies had persistence of the fetal circulation, and two died (*Csaba* et al. 1978; *Rubatelli* et al. 1979). The offspring of sheep and rats given indomethacin show constriction of the ductus arteriosus and structural changes in the lungs similar to those in babies with persistent fetal circulation (*Levin* et al. 1979; *Harker* et al. 1981).

Persistent fetal circulation is also a feature of the respiratory distress syndrome, pulmonary hypoplasia, the aspiration syndromes, severe parenchymal lung disease and congenital diaphragmatic hernia, probably as a result of impaired oxygenation. It is also associated with polycythaemia.

1. Idiopathic Persistent Pulmonary Hypertension

The application of quantitative morphometric techniques to the injected and uninjected pulmonary arterial circulation of postmortem lung specimens shows an increase in peripheral arterial muscularity (Fig. 8a,b) (*Wagenvoort* and *Wagenvoort* 1970; *Haworth* and *Reid* 1976). Measurement of percentage arterial medial thickness, population counts relating structure of the vessel wall to external diameter, and examination of

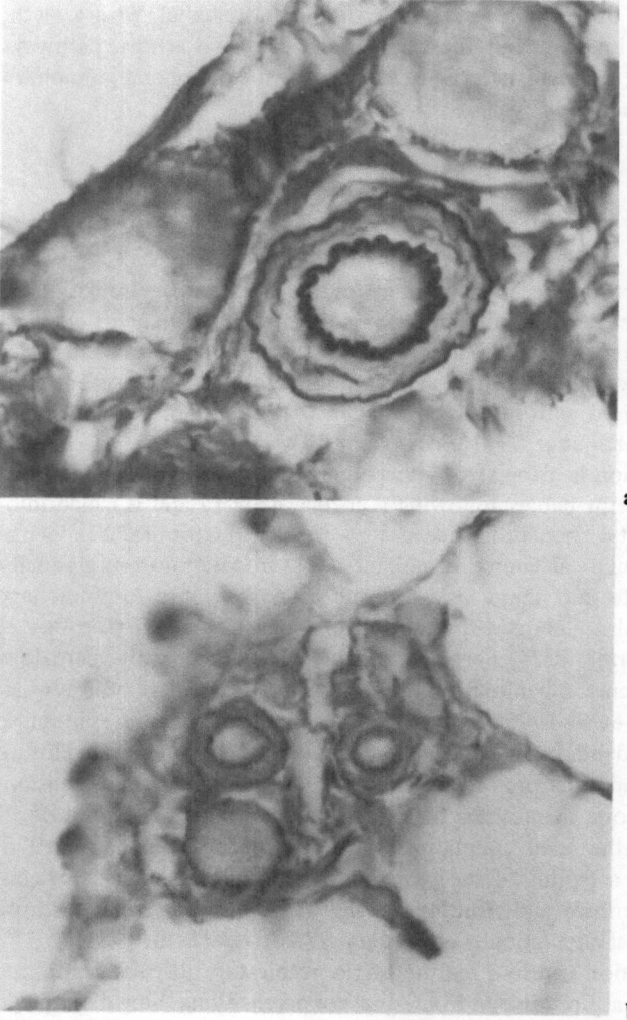

Fig. 8. Photomicrographs of the lung of a child with persistent pulmonary hypertension and an anatomically normal heart dying at 5 months of age, showing thick-walled muscular arteries **a** accompanying an alveolar duct, **b** within the alveolar walls and **c** non-muscular arteries with little or no lumen. × 500

the structure of arteries identified by the type of airway they accompany show the presence of mature smooth muscle cells in smaller and more peripheral intra-acinar arteries than normal (*Haworth* and *Reid* 1976). Arteries which in the normal lung are non-muscular or only partially muscularised are surrounded by a thick coat of muscle cells. The larger arteries with an external diameter greater than 150 μm generally show an increase in the amount of muscle present, but the response is more variable, probably due to differences in the duration of pulmonary hypertension. Serial sections of the arterial pathway show progressive encroachment on the lumen by smooth muscle cells and enlarged swollen endothelial cells until in the small precapillary arteries, the lumen is occluded (Fig. 8c). Whether or not some of these vessels are occluded from birth, or indeed are never recruited into the pulmonary circulation, is not clear, but if this does happen, then it probably induces a secondary increase in intra-acinar arterial muscle. No intrinsic abnormality of lung growth has been demonstrated. Airway and alveolar development are normal, as is the pre-acinar arterial branching pattern, and a full complement of intra-acinar arteries is present in babies dying soon after birth.

The increase in muscularity is probably due initially to failure of the vessels to adapt normally to extra-uterine life and subsequently to postnatal development of muscle in response to the presence of pulmonary hypertension. An excessive amount of muscle might develop in the intra-acinar arteries before birth, but there is no apparent reason for this to happen. There is no clinical evidence of intra-uterine hypoxia in such cases. The pulmonary circulation might, however, develop abnormally before birth in the presence of a normal intra-uterine environment. This could happen if the pulmonary circulation is abnormally sensitive to the hypoxic environment of fetal life, responding by excessive vasoconstriction and then by hypertrophy of muscle. After birth, sensitivity to hypoxia is known to vary considerably in different individuals (*Naeye* 1965). Alternatively, increased muscularity in these cases may represent a chance excessive growth of muscle which, after birth, initiates the vicious circle of maintained pulmonary arterial pressure, leading to further hypertrophy of arterial muscle.

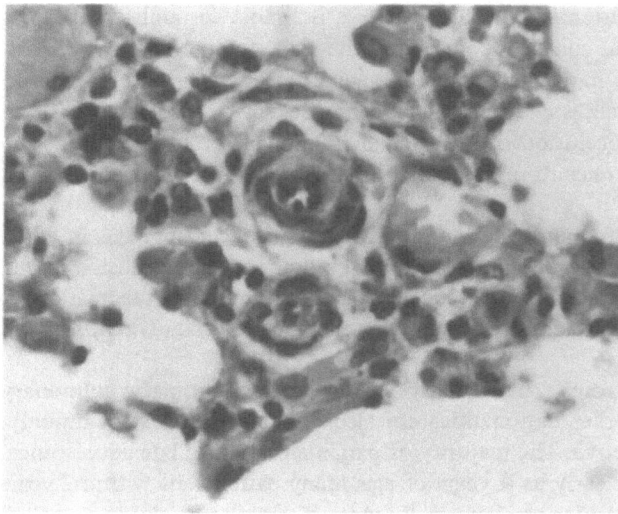

Fig. 8c

2. Relation Between Persistent Pulmonary Hypertension and "Primary" Pulmonary Hypertension in Children and Adults

In 1970, *Wagenvoort* and *Wagenvoort* described 110 cases of pulmonary hypertension of unknown aetiology which they called "vasocontrictive" because of the type of morphological change in the lungs. Thirty-nine of the patients were less than 15 years old, the youngest being 4 days old. The structural changes were age-related. In infants and young children, the small pulmonary arteries showed only medial hypertrophy, but with increase in age, percentage arterial medial thickness decreased and percentage intimal thickness increased. Intimal proliferation and lamellar concentric fibrosis, dilatation lesions and plexiform lesions appeared in older patients. Because medial hypertrophy was the only early lesion found, a vasoconstrictive mechanism was proposed, the pulmonary circulation being affected at or soon after birth. More recent studies on normal adaptation of the pulmonary arterial circulation to extra-uterine life and on the lungs of babies dying in the first months of life with persistent pulmonary hypertension support this hypothesis. We do not know, however, whether vasoconstriction is indeed the first abnormality or is a response to an elevated pulmonary arterial pressure, perhaps caused by failure of dilatation or recruitment of intra-acinar arteries at birth.

If pulmonary hypertension is present from birth, the media of the pulmonary trunk retains the aortic configuration of elastic fibres normally present at birth (*Heath* et al. 1959). In some adult patients with primary pulmonary hypertension, the pulmonary trunk has an aortic configuration, but in most it does not, suggesting that pulmonary hypertension is not usually present from birth (*Wagenvoort* and *Wagenvoort* 1977). This does not, however, imply that the pulmonary arterial circulation has adapted to extra-uterine life and grown normally in all patinets. The pulmonary vascular reserve is large and the pulmonary arterial pressure may have fallen initially, despite a persistent reduction in capacity of the intra-acinar pulmonary arterial circulation.

Primary pulmonary hypertension in older patients is almost certainly multifactorial, the clinical and structural changes representing the final common pathway. Postmortem arteriography shows narrowing of the pre-acinar arteries and a loss of background haze. In adults as well as children this appearance can be associated with an increase in muscularity and occlusion of intra-acinar pulmonary arteries, without the more advanced changes of concentric lamellar intimal fibrosis and plexiform lesions (*Anderson* et al. 1973).

In children, primary pulmonary hypertension affects males and females in equal numbers, but in adults, females predominate. Familial pulmonary hypertension is well described, is generally a spontaneous occurrence, but is sometimes an autosomal dominant inheritance of a single genetic trait and may present in childhood (*Thompson* and *McRae* 1970).

Indian children suffer from a particularly vicious form of primary pulmonary hypertension. Children of other nationalities are also affected, but less commonly. The clinical picture is distinctive. The majority of patients present in late adolescence, although they can present as early as 4 years of age. Many patients die within 2 years of diagnosis, a few surviving as long as 10 years. Pulmonary vascular change is described as grade IV–VI, using the Heath and Edwards classification (*Subramanian* et al. 1974). In patients from Sri Lanka, Wallooppillai and Wagenvoort found the picture of plexigenic pulmonary arteriopathy (*Wagenvoort* and *Wagenvoort* 1977). There is generally no familial incidence or evidence of collagen disorder, coagulation defect, eosinophilia or thrombo-embolism.

3. Drug-Associated Persistent Pulmonary Hypertension

The injected pulmonary arteries in the lungs of two term infants whose mothers had taken either salicylates or indomethacin during pregnancy showed an increase in pulmonary arterial medial width/external diameter ratio (*Levin* et al. 1978). The infant with long-term exposure to salicylates had a constricted ductus arteriosus, and in this case the number of peripheral pulmonary arteries per unit area of lung tissue was reduced. Administration of indomethacin to pregnant sheep and rats is associated in the offspring with ductal constriction or closure, pulmonary arterial medial hypertrophy, and in the rat, "newly muscularised arterioles" (*Levin* et al. 1979; *Harker* et al. 1981). Also in the rat, the ratio of capillary mass to saccular wall mass is decreased, suggesting a decreased surface for gas exchange and an increase in pulmonary vascular resistance.

4. Perinatal Hypoxia in Babies Born at Sea Level

In the majority of babies dying with perinatal hypoxia, interpretation of the structural changes in the pulmonary circulation is complicated by the immaturity of the lung and the effects of alveolar collapse and disease. However, in a group of babies born at term in whom the lungs were well expanded, hypoxia was associated with failure of the intra-acinar arteries to adapt normally to extra-uterine life (*Haworth* 1979). In the normal lung at birth, the intra-acinar arteries dilate, and there is a rapid reduction in both smooth muscle mass and in the thickness of the subendothelial layer of non-muscular arteries. These changes are always readily apparent by 24 h of age. In the hypoxic babies dying during the first 32 h of life, the appearance of the intra-acinar arteries, percentage arterial medial thickness and mean arterial external diameter were similar to that in the fetus at term.

5. Effect of Altitude on Adaptation to Extra-uterine Life

The weight of the right ventricle and the muscularity of the pulmonary arterial circulation are similar in babies born at altitude and in those born at sea level (*Arias-Stella* and *Recavarren* 1962). After birth, however, pulmonary arterial muscularity in babies born at altitude does not decrease at the same rate or reach the same low level as in those born at sea level (*Arias-Stella* and *Saldana* 1962; *Naeye* 1961b). From the age of 1 month, the peripheral pulmonary arteries show medial hypertrophy as compared with the normal at sea level. This difference represents an adaptive phenomenon, not disease, but there is evidence to suggest that the incidence of primary pulmonary hypertension in childhood is greater at altitude than at sea level (*Koury* and *Hawes* 1963; *Berthrong* and *Cochran* 1955). Recently the problems associated with adaptation to extra-uterine life have been studied by exposing newborn pigs to an hypoxic environment at a low barometric pressure of 380 torr (*S.G. Haworth*, personal observations). Animals were exposed to the hypoxic environment for 2—5 days at various ages, from birth to 14 days. The younger the animal, the more severe were the abnormalities produced. Animals exposed to hypoxia from birth showed an elevated percentage arterial medial thickness, although it was generally less than is seen in fetal life. Also the proportion of non-muscular and partially muscularised arteries with a thick sub-endothelial layer remained high, as in fetal life. By 3 days of age, "new" muscle cells developed in normally non- or partially muscularised arteries. Older animals showed a less marked increase in muscularity, even those exposed to hypoxia at 2 days of age, emphasizing the extreme vulnerability of the intra-acinar pulmonary arterial circulation at birth.

V. Thrombo-embolic Pulmonary Hypertension

In children thrombo-embolic pulmonary hypertension is usually iatrogenic or due to schistosomiasis. It is a complication of intravenous hyperalimentation, catheterisation of the umbilical vein in the newborn and ventriculovenous shunts for hydrocephalus (*Emery* and *Hilton* 1961; *Emery* 1962; *Noonan* and *Ehmke* 1963; *Firor* 1972). Showers of emboli are discharged from the tip of the catheter, become lodged in elastic or muscular pulmonary arteries and gradually occlude a large proportion of the pulmonary vascular bed.

Schistosomiasis is a parasitic infection of tropical areas produced by schistosomes, or blood flukes, which are parasitic in man. The ova of *Schistosoma haematobium* are more often found in the lungs, but pulmonary vascular lesions are more frequently caused by *Schistosoma mansoni* (*Shaw* and *Ghareeb* 1938). Pulmonary hypertension is probably caused by embolic obstruction by ova, an allergic response to the ova and vasoconstriction, followed by plexigenic pulmonary arteriopathy (*Wagenvoort* and *Wagenvoort* 1977). The pulmonary vascular morphology is well reviewed by *Wagenvoort* and *Wagenvoort* (1977). Impacted *Schistosoma* ova may remain in the arterial lumen, causing a granulomatous reaction within the vessel. More often, they penetrate the arterial wall, a granuloma is found outside the lumen, and focal interstitial fibrosis occurs. The granulomata contain foreign body giant cells, mononuclear cells, eosinophils and calcified remnants of the ova, and possibly result from an immunologic reaction of the delayed hypersensitivity type. Hyalin or fibrin thrombi are present in the peripheral pulmonary arteries. Necrotising arteritis may occur near impacted ova and is thought to be an allergic response to the ovum. The morphological features of plexigenic pulmonary arteriopathy, medial hypertrophy, concentric-lamina intimal fibrosis and plexiform lesions may develop in areas of lung tissue not apparently infested by ova. A vasoconstrictor agent has been invoked to explain plexigenic pulmonary arteriopathy in schistosomiasis, because vasoconstrictive lesions often appear also in the liver. Many patients with *Schistosoma* pulmonary hypertension and cardiac failure have hepatic cirrhosis, portal hypertension and portal-systemic anastomoses.

VI. Pulmonary Hypertension in Lung Disease

Chronic lung disease can lead to sustained pulmonary hypertension, particularly when associated with hypoxia. Structural changes develop in the intrapulmonary arteries, and the right ventricle hypertrophies. "Hypertrophy of the right ventricle resulting from diseases affecting the function and/or structure of the lung, except when these pulmonary alterations are the result of diseases that primarily affect the left side of the heart or of congenital heart disease" is how a WHO committee (1961) defined cor pulmonale. This definition is unsatisfactory for the purist. Only the pathologist can diagnose right-ventricular hypertrophy, but a clinical assessment of right-ventricular hypertrophy may be at least as accurate as a pathological assessment. Moreover, to the clinician "cor pulmonale" describes a clinical entity. The term is best avoided.

In children who develop pulmonary hypertension secondary to lung disease, the lung is generally normal at birth. When pulmonary hypertension develops, the structure of the developing pulmonary circulation is altered, and although an increase in pulmonary arterial muscularity is generally reversible, other changes, such as a reduction in the number of arteries, may not be. Also, chronic lung diesease in childhood damages the airways and alveoli while they are still developing. Permanent alterations in airway structure probably alter the structure of the arteries accompanying the affected airways. Thus lung diesease in childhood may have a long-term effect on the pulmonary circulation.

Pulmonary hypertension can result from a variety of lung disorders. The commonest causative disease in adults is chronic bronchitis, and in children in Europe and the United States it is probably cystic fibrosis. Heart failure may also complicate scoliosis in childhood. As in adults, extensive small-airway and alveolar disease occurring in bronchiolitis, fibrosing alveolitis and the collagen disorders can lead to pulmonary vascular change and hypertension, but this is not common in childhood. Chronic upper airways obstruction due to large tonsils and adenoids is a well-recognised cause of pulmonary hypertension and right heart failure in children, but there is a rapid improvement following surgery and no evidence of permanent pulmonary vascular damage.

The pulmonary arterial circulation is frequently involved in hypoplastic lung disorders, but the respiratory signs dominate the clinical picture. In the lungs of babies dying with congenital diaphragmatic hernia, rhesus isoimmunisation, renal dysplasia or agenesis or a single lung, the airway and arterial branching pattern is incomplete, and hence the number of alveoli and intra-acinar arteries is reduced (*Ryland* and *Reid* 1975; *Hislop* and *Reid* 1976a; *Chamberlain* et al. 1977; *Hislop* et al. 1979). Pulmonary arterial muscularity is generally greater than normal in these children, most of whom die in early infancy. Children who survive with a hypoplastic lung are probably more vulnerable to respiratory tract infections and hypoxic vasoconstriction than normal children.

1. Cystic Fibrosis

In the majority of patients with cystic fibrosis the respiratory signs overshadow the cardiac, and many die with extensive lung disease without developing right ventricular hypertrophy. In some patients, however, pulmonary hypertension and right heart failure are an important feature of the disease. On the electrocardiogram right axis deviation usually indicates an abnormally heavy right ventricle at autopsy, but the absence of electrocardiographic changes does not preclude the presence of right ventricular hypertrophy (*Ryland* and *Reid* 1975). In the lung, quantitative morphometric analysis of injected postmortem specimens shows a reduction in size of the pre-acinar arterial lumen diameter, an increase in pulmonary arterial muscularity and a reduction in number of intra-acinar arteries; the changes are more severe when the right ventricle is hypertrophied. *Ryland* and *Reid* (1975) studied the hearts and lungs of 36 children aged between 5 and 12 years who died with cystic fibrosis. They found that in arteries smaller than 1000 μm in diameter, percentage arterial medial thickness was increased in proportion to the degree of right-ventricular hypertrophy, significantly so in arteries 25–75 μm in diameter. Population counts showed the presence of muscle in smaller arteries than normal. Intimal change was patchy, developed in the most severely diseased parts of the lung, and was most common in patients with right ventricular hypertrophy, as was thickening of the walls of small pulmonary veins.

The pulmonary arterial changes were most severe in the most diseased parts of the lungs, which were presumably the most hypoxic. All cases showed extension of muscle into smaller arteries than normal and an increase in wall thickness of normally muscularised arteries, features common to almost all types of pulmonary hypertension irrespective of aetiology. The differentiation of smooth muscle cells in the non-muscular arteries of the precapillary bed is, however, one of the earliest structural changes seen in experimental hypoxia. The first change to occur in experimental animals exposed to hypoxia is swelling of the endothelial cells, which occlude the lumen. In children with cystic fibrosis the reduction in number of intra-acinar arteries is probably due to loss of arteries during acute infective hypoxic episodes, which cause further damage to parts of the lung which are already diseased. Also, the intra-acinar arteries might fail to multiply normally, although this is unlikely since the majority of children with cystic fibrosis develop severe respiratory disease after the first 3 years of life, after the period of most rapid arterial development.

2. Scoliosis

As in cystic fibrosis, in the majority of children with scoliosis the lung is probably normal at birth, but with progressive spinal deformity the space available for lung growth diminishes. In addition, repeated respiratory-tract infections may further compromise lung growth. When scoliosis is severe, signs of pulmonary hypertension and right ventricular hypertrophy frequently develop, and cardiac failure may supervene. Morphological studies on the lungs of patients dying with scoliosis show a reduction in the number of alveoli, some of which are emphysematous and others atrophied, the changes being distributed irregularly throughout the lung according to the distortion of the thoracic cage (*Davies* and *Reid* 1971). In the pulmonary circulation, the size of the pre-acinar arteries is appropriate to the volume of the lung and hence these vessels are small for age. There are many reports of an increase in peripheral arterial muscularity in scoliosis (*Bergofsky* et al. 1959; *Naeye* 1961c; *Davies* and *Reid* 1971). *Naeye* (1961c) used a planimetric technique to demonstrate an increase in medial muscle area in the lungs of nine patients who had had signs of pulmonary hypertension. *Davies* and *Reid* (1971) using an injection technique, found an increase in percentage arterial medial thickness and extension of muscle into smaller and more peripheral arteries than normal in two cases with right ventricular hypertrophy, but not in two cases without right ventricular hypertrophy.

It seems that scoliosis prevents normal multiplication and growth of the alveoli and may cause atrophy of the alveoli, thereby decreasing the surface area available for gas exchange and causing extensive areas of lung to be poorly ventilated and hypoxic. Hypoxia probably explains the increased pulmonary arterial muscularity in patients with scoliosis.

VII. Pulmonary Hypertension in Acquired Heart Disease

In developing countries, rheumatic heart disease is a common cause of severe pulmonary hypertension in childhood. In a study of 100 Indian patients with mitral stenosis, 42 patients were less than 20 years of age (*Tandon* and *Kasturi* 1975). The more severe structural changes in the lungs were seen in the younger patients (Fig. 9). As in adult patients with mitral stenosis, the structural changes consist chiefly of medial hypertrophy of the pulmonary arteries, development of muscle in smaller arteries than normal, intimal thickening of peripheral pulmonary arteries and capillarities, thickening of the walls of lymphatics, hypertrophy of the pulmonary veins and "arterialisation" of the small veins (*Wagenvoort* 1970). Generalised thickening and fibrosis of the alveolar walls is often particularly severe in children with mitral stenosis. The more advanced changes of obliterative pulmonary vascular disease are less common.

Following mitral valvotomy, clinically the pulmonary arterial pressure appears to fall. Many children, however, suffer repeated attacks of carditis and can develop severe pulmonary vascular disease (Fig. 9).

VIII. Pulmonary Hypertension in Congenital Heart Disease

Clinical practice has change in paediatric cardiology during the past 10 years. With improvements in surgical technique and in the management of cardiopulmonary bypass and cardioplegia, many children now undergo surgery during the first month of life. Not surprisingly, the structural changes in the lungs of very young infants with pulmonary hypertension are not like those seen in older patients. The pulmonary

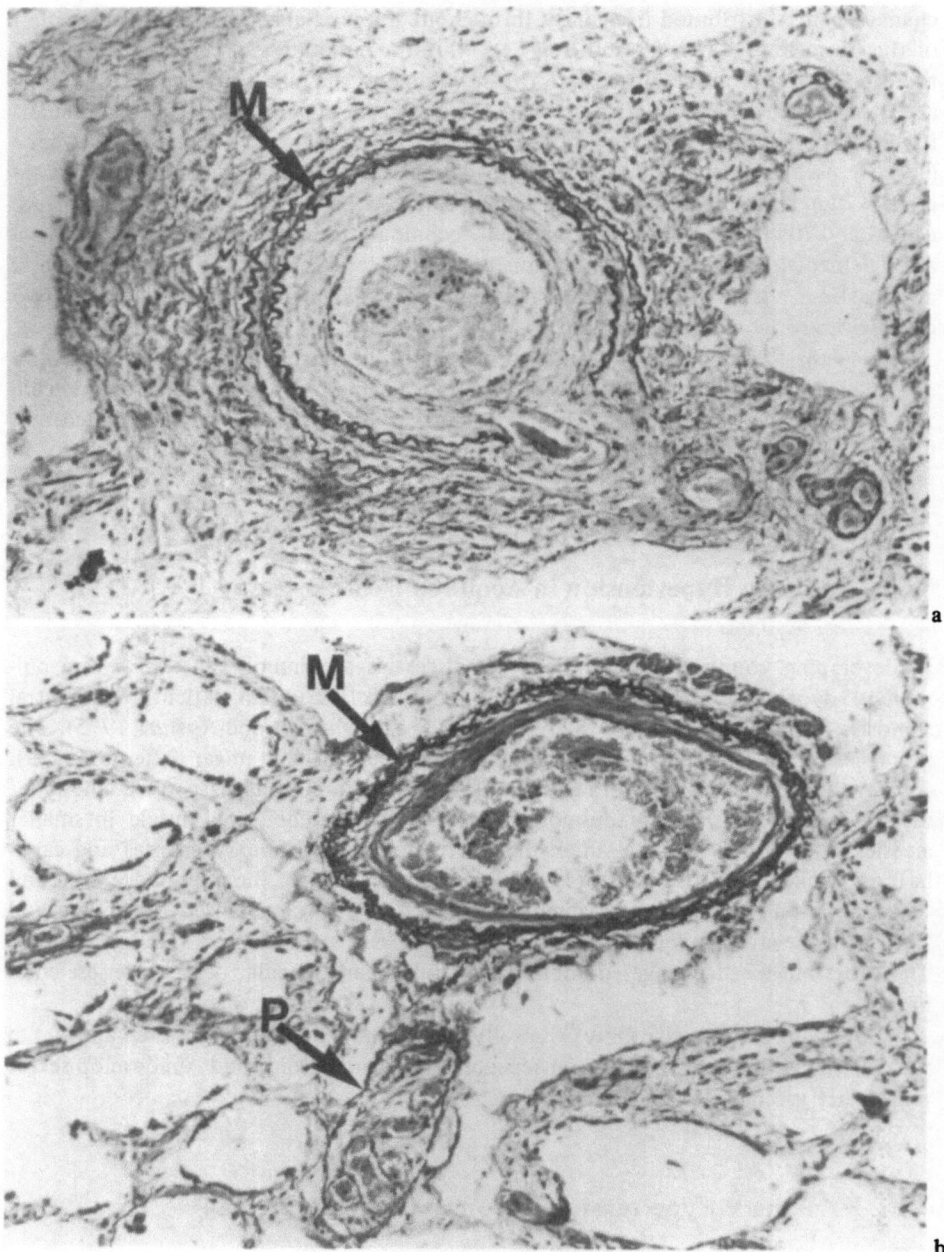

Fig. 9a—c. Photomicrographs of the lung of an Indian child with severe mitral stenosis who died at 9 years of age. **a** Small pre-acinar artery, showing atrophy of the media *(M)*, and circumferential intimal proliferation. × 125. **b** Respiratory bronchiolar artery showing medial atrophy and intimal fibrosis, with a branch containing a plexiform lesion *(P)*. × 300. **c** Alveolar duct artery showing severe medial atrophy. × 500. The alveolar septa are abnormally thick

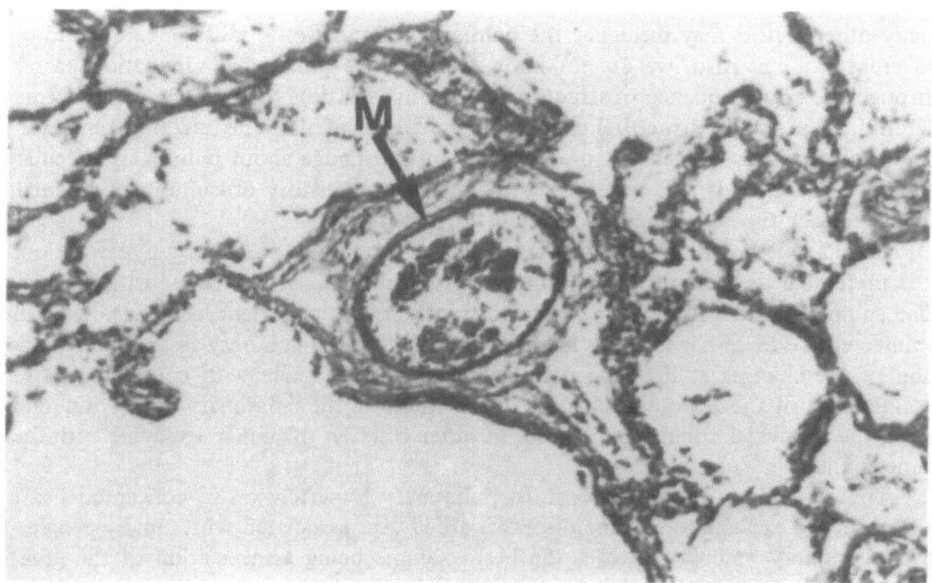

Fig. 9c

circulation is normally remodelled after birth, and thus the emphasis has shifted from descriptive pathology of established disease to study of the effect of pulmonary hypertension on the growth and development of the pulmonary circulation.

Increasingly, the optimal time for surgical intervention is a compromise between the surgical problems encountered in operating on a young infant with a small heart but little pulmonary vascular change and the risks involved in operating on an older, larger patient with more advanced pulmonary vascular change. We are now more concerned with the prevention of pulmonary vascular obliterative disease than previously, because it has become feasible to act on information obtained. We ought to be able to predict not only the immediate outcome of an operation, but also the reversibility of the pulmonary vascular changes present at the time of surgery. Unfortunately, however, the natural history of pulmonary vascular change in the different types of congenital heart disease is still not completely understood.

In most studies on the pulmonary vasculature in which structural change is related to measurements of the pulmonary arterial pressure and resistance, patients of different ages with different types of cardiac abnormalitiy are grouped together. The same values of pulmonary arterial pressure and resistance may, however, result from different intracardiac abnormalities and be associated with a different structural response within the lung. For example, a child with an atrioventricular canal may have pulmonary arterial pressure and resistance similar to that in one with total anomalous pulmonary venous return with obstruction to venous return, but the structural changes in the lung are unlikely to be the same. In different anomalies, pulmonary blood flow and pressure, the magnitude of the bronchial arterial supply, haematocrit, possible obstruction to pulmonary venous return, a stenotic or incompetent mitral valve and many other factors may influence the pulmonary circulation in different ways and to different extents. Also, we do not know whether the pulmonary circulation passes through the same sequence of structural change in each type of anomaly, what factors determine the rate of structural change, or the length of time the lung may remain in one stage of disease. Given our present state of knowledge about pulmonary vascular disease in childhood, it is wiser to study the natural history of pulmonary vascular change in each type of anomaly separately.

Because of the complexity of the structural response to pulmonary hypertension, it is preferable to base studies on pulmonary vascular change associated with any car-diac anomaly on the findings in whole postmortem lung specimens, using injected and uninjected tissue, rather than relying solely on the findings in biopsy tissue. Interpreta-tion of the changes at the lung periphery can only be made with confidence after examination of the structural changes in the whole of the pulmonary circulation, and often the bronchial circulation as well, in other children of similar age dying with the same anomaly.

The variability of the response to pulmonary hypertension in congenital heart disease defies explanation. Some disorders are always associated with rapidly progres-sive pulmonary vascular disease, the best example being transposition of the great arteries with ventricular septal defect. Other abnormalities are sometimes associated with pulmonary vascular disease, such as a large ventricular septal defect. In other abnormalities, pulmonary vascular disease develops later in adult life or not at all. "Individual susceptibility" is said to explain the variable response seen in many types of congenital heart disease. This term includes a variety of functional and structural differences in susceptible individuals. The list of possibilities is long, including an excessive amount of pulmonary vascular smooth muscle present from birth, an exces-sive tendency to vasoconstrict, and a reduction in size and number of intra-acinar arteries. In animals, variation in the propensity to vasoconstrict has been related to genetically determined differences in the medial thickness of the muscular pulmonary arteries (*Grover* et al. 1963).

In general, patients with post-tricuspid shunts — such as ventricular septal defect, large patent ductus arteriosus, atrioventricular canal, aortopulmonary window or truncus arteriosus — are more likely to develop pulmonary hypertension and severe pulmonary vascular disease than those with a pretricuspid shunt, such as an atrial septal defect. Only a minority of patients with a secundum atrial septal defect develop severe pulmonary hypertension, and those not usually before the 3rd decade of life.

1. Structure of the Main Pulmonary Artery and Elastic Pulmonary Arteries

In the presence of severe pulmonary hypertension, the lumen diameter of the main pulmonary artery is frequently larger than that of the aorta. When pulmonary hyper-tension is present from birth, the relative wall thickness of the main pulmonary artery remains similar to that of the aorta, and the elastic laminae tend to remain long and continuous, as in fetal life. The main pulmonary artery retains its "aortic configuration" in most but not all patients (*Wagenvoort* and *Wagenvoort* 1977). Aneurysmal dilation of the main pulmonary artery is not uncommon in children with severe pulmonary hypertension and is sometimes associated with bacterial endocarditis. Yellow streaks or patches of atheroma may be found in the extrapulmonary and elastic intrapulmonary arteries and are more common in some malformations than in others. Atheromatous change is particularly common in the presence of a large ductus arteriosus.

2. Compression of the Airways

Large, dilated pulmonary arteries frequently compress the main and lobar bronchi in children with high pulmonary blood flow, with and without pulmonary hypertension. In infants with severe pulmonary hypertension, this leads to the familiar clinical problem of recurrent collapse of different lobes or segments of lung. Not infrequently, the respiratory complications of congenital heart disease constitute an indication for corrective surgery in infancy. After operation, the deformity of the bronchi may persist for some time, and in some patients prolonged compression appears to be associated with bronchomalacia.

3. Classification of Pulmonary Vascular Change in Congenital Heart Disease

In their classic paper on pulmonary vascular disease published in 1958, *Heath* and *Edwards* classified pulmonary vascular change into six grades, arranged in order of increasing vascular damage. The structural features of each grade were related to measurements of pulmonary arterial pressure, resistance and flow and to the outcome of surgery. The structural changes associated with each grade were:

Grade I   Medial hypertrophy
Grade II   Medial hypertrophy with cellular intimal proliferation
Grade III   Progressive fibrous occlusion
Grade IV   Progressive generalised arterial dilatation with the formation of complex dilatation lesions
Grade V   Chronic dilatation with numerous dilatation vessels throughout the lung and pulmonary haemosiderosis
Grade VI   Fibrinoid necrosis of the media

Grades I–III indicate a "high-resistance, high-reserve", pulmonary vascular bed which is still labile (*Edwards* 1957). The pulmonary arterial pressure and pulmonary blood flow are high and the direction of the shunt is left to right. Grades V–VI indicate a "high-resistance, low-reserve" pulmonary vascular bed which is no longer labile, because the lumen of many of the arteries is occluded. Pulmonary arterial pressure is higher than in patients with Grades I–III pulmonary vascular disease, flow is low and the direction of the shunt is predominantly right to left. Grade IV represents a transitional stage. However, although Grades I–III reflect a succession of structural changes, Grades IV–VI probably do not. *Wagenvoort* and *Wagenvoort* (1977) believe that necrotising arteritis can precede the development of plexiform lesions. Certainly many changes such as necrotising arteritis, plexiform lesions or dilatation lesions may be seen alone or in combination with other changes. *Wagenvoort* and *Wagenvoort* (1977) found that none of these lesions carried a more severe prognosis than the others. Therefore in the individual patient, this classification cannot replace a careful description of all the structural changes seen.

The majority of patients studied by *Heath* and *Edwards* were older children with an atrial or ventricular septal defect or a patent ductus arteriosus. Excluded from consideration were three infants in whom the pulmonary arterial pressure was higher than expected for the severity of structural change, only medial hypertrophy being noted.

Recent studies have shown that in young children with pulmonary hypertension, the pulmonary arterial circulation fails to grow and develop normally (*Haworth* et al. 1977). Therefore not only pulmonary arterial muscularity but also arterial size and intra-acinar arterial number are measured and compared with values obtained from normal age-matched controls. Abnormalities in arterial wall thickness, size and number are associated with changes in the appearance of the arterial wall. Unfortunately, however, the Heath and Edwards classification of structural change cannot be applied without modification in young children, and it is preferable to avoid all attempts at classification and simply to describe what is seen. Other workers have subdivided the Grade I pulmonary vascular disease described by *Heath* and *Edwards* into Ia, Ib and Ic, representing respectively differentiation of muscle in smaller and more peripheral arteries than is normal, an increase in medial thickness of normally muscularised arteries and a reduction in number of intra-acinar arteries (*Rabinovitch* et al. 1978). However, to be workable this classification presupposes that these are the only changes present in the specimen and that we understand how and why arterial number is reduced — which we do not. Again, it is better to record the findings precisely, knowing that eventually a more accurate and comprehensible picture of the response of the pulmonary circulation will emerge, both in the individual patient and in other patients with similar clinical and haemodynamic findings.

A classification system is often useful in describing the principal structural abnormalities in tissue, particularly when relating structural to functional change. It is, however, important when examining tissue to keep one's mind open to all possibilities, rather than to seek features which will fulfill certain criteria.

In postmortem tissue, the structure of the entire pulmonary arterial and venous systems can be studied, from the pulmonary valve and left atrium to the respiratory epithelium. In a biopsy, only the end of the pre-acinar pathway and the intra-acinar vessels are examined, but the same techniques of quantitative morphometric analysis and description of wall structure are used to study both tissue procured at autopsy and that obtained by biopsy. These techniques may be summarised as follows:

Quantitation
Percentage arterial medial thickness
External diameter of intra-acinar arteries
Alveolar/arterial ratio
Qualitative studies
Description of structural changes in:
    Pre-acinar arteries
    Terminal bronchiolar arteries

Respiratory bronchiolar arteries
Alveolar duct arteries
Alveolar wall arteries
Veins

The use of quantitative morphometric techniques to analyse pulmonary vascular structure facilitates the early detection of pulmonary vascular change. The descriptive, qualitative assessment is required to explain the quantitative changes in both early and advanced disease, in addition to observing the effect of pulmonary hypertension on the composition of the vessel wall.

4. Appearance of Structural Changes in the Muscular Pulmonary Arteries in Pulmonary Hypertension

a) Medial Hypertrophy

The media is composed of a dense layer of circumferentially arranged smooth muscle cells interspersed with thin elastic fibres (Fig. 10a). Longitudinal muscle bundles may develop in contact with the external elastic lamina and, less commonly, internal to the internal elastic lamina. The internal elastic lamina is thickened, and in uninjected tissue is often crenellated. The adventitial coat appears more dense than normal and is composed largely of thick collagen fibres. Because these vessels are often tortuous, multiple cross-sections of the same vessel may be seen on microscopic examination.

b) Cellular Intimal Proliferation

In pulmonary hypertensive congenital heart disease cellular intimal proliferation is usually concentric. Initially the cells are arranged loosely perpendicular to the intima, but gradually the cell layer becomes more compact. Occasionally cells are seen penetrating the internal elastic lamina, suggesting that they originated in the media. Electron microscopy showed that the proliferating cells in the intima have the characteristics of smooth muscle cells (*Wagenvoort* and *Wagenvoort* 1977). Occasionally, mucopolysaccharides are deposited in this layer.

c) Intimal Fibrosis

Gradually, collagen fibres and then elastic fibres are deposited in the cellular intimal layer. The extent to which elastin is deposited varies (compare Figs. 9b and 10b). Intimal fibrosis has a compact, lamellar appearance and may completely occlude the arterial lumen.

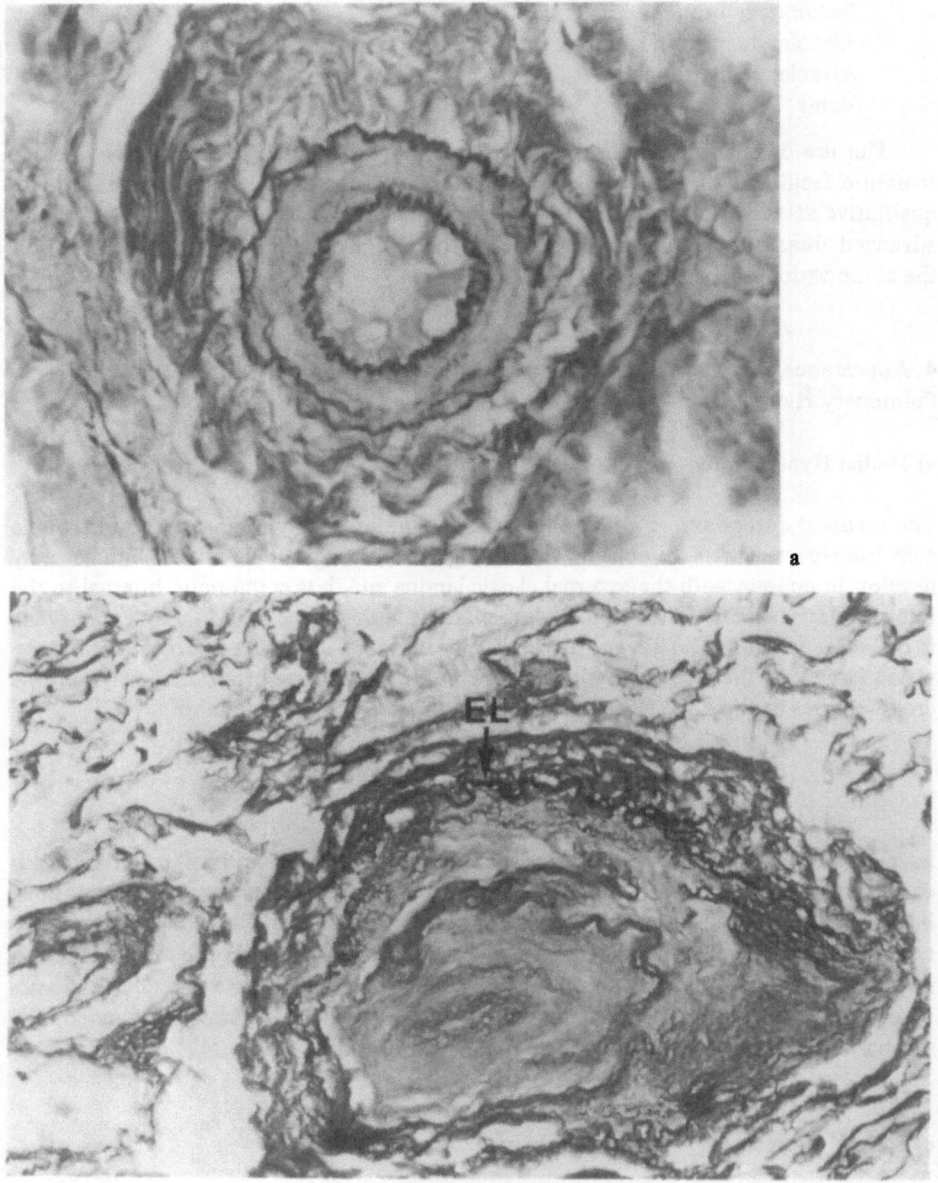

Fig. 10a—c. Photomicrographs from three patients dying with transposition of the great arteries. **a** Severe medial hypertrophy in a respiratory bronchiolar artery in a child aged 3 months. × 500. **b** Occlusive circumferential intimal fibrosis lying within a disrupted external elastic lamina *(EL)*, in a 31-year-old patient. × 120. **c** Thin media *(M)*, intimal fibrosis *(IF)*, and long thin-walled vein-like branches in a child aged 11 months

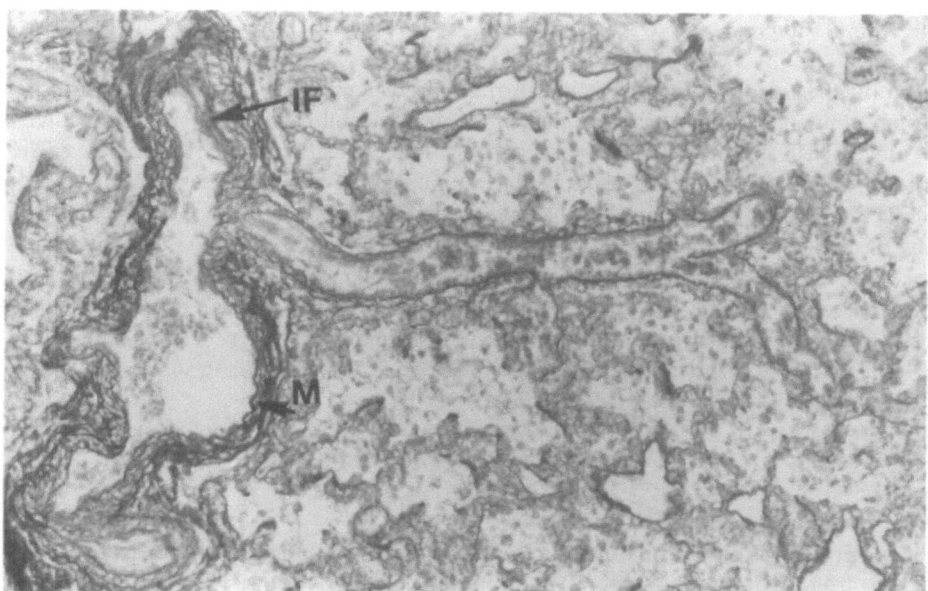

Fig. 10c

d) Generalised Arterial Dilatation and Formation of Dilatation Lesions

Chronic pulmonary hypertension leads to thinning and to atrophy of the media. Medial atrophy and dilatation is associated with, and is probably the result of narrowing or obliteration of the parent artery by intimal fibrosis. Also, the lumen of such thin-walled branches is frequently severely narrowed at the origin from a still patent parent vessel. In this situation, thinning of the media may represent "disuse atrophy" distal to an obstructive lesion. By contrast, in larger thick-walled arteries with a thin media and intimal proliferation, ultrastructural examination reveals necrotic smooth muscle cells embedded in an increased amount of collagen and elastin. Care is sometimes needed to distinguish between the atrophied media of the hypertensive artery and a normal vessel (Fig. 9c). Finally, the media may disappear, leaving a thin-walled vein-like dilated artery. Thin-walled arteries branching within the alveolar walls are frequently seen in children with severe pulmonary hypertension, but the angioma-like mass, the "angiomatoid" lesion, is rare (Fig. 10c).

e) Haemosiderosis

Haemosiderin is produced by disintegrated erythrocytes after rupture of small blood vessels or diapedesis. It accumulates in macrophages, then called siderophages, and is deposited in the vessel wall and connective tissue of the lung. It is generally most severe in cases of long-standing pulmonary hypertension.

f) Fibrinoid Necrosis of the Media

Fibronid necrosis is generally found in the muscular pre- and intra-acinar arteries. In severe pulmonary hypertension, a part of the arterial wall becomes necrotic, the nuclei of the smooth muscle cells disappear and fibrin is deposited in the necrotic area. The affected part of the wall has an acellular, homogenous, opaque appearance, is eosino-philic and stains bright pink with haematoxylin. The media is swollen and the internal and external elastic laminae tend to bulge. Fibrinoid necrosis may excite an inflamma-tory response with infiltration by polymorphonuclear leucocytes. The inflammatory response often extends into the adventitia and surrounding alveolar tissue. The entire circumference of the vessel may be affected, generally over a short segment of the arterial pathway. When the entire circumference is involved, a fibrin clot is usually present.

g) Plexiform Lesion

Plexiform lesions are complex lesions found only in the lung, and occur in the intra-acinar arteries of patients with severe pulmonary hypertension. The incidence of the lesion varies considerably in different cases. *Wagenvoort* (1973) has made detailed studies of this type of pulmonary vascular change. The lesion arises from an artery showing medial hypertrophy, often with concentric lamellar fibrosis. The branch is dilated, parts of its wall are necrotic and the lumen is large and filled with strands of proliferating intimal cells separated by a plexus of narrow channels (Fig. 9b). Distally, arteries arising from a plexiform lesion are thin-walled. The plexiform lesion is thought to be located between a high-pressure vessel and the alveolar wall arteries in which the pressure is not elevated. Plexiform lesions are not anastomotic channels, multiple angiomas or congenital malformations of the pulmonary arteries.

Mature plexiform lesions are rare in infancy, but arteries showing the early features of the lesion have been reported in children between 3 weeks and 4 months of age.

5. Lung Biopsies in Children with Congenital Heart Disease

a) Assessment of Lung Biopsies by Light Microscopy

For many years, the assessment of pulmonary vascular disease using lung biopsy in young children with congenital heart disease proved to be a disappointing exercise. Biopsies were generally taken only from the most severely ill children in whom the structural changes of severe obstructive pulmonary vascular disease tended to confirm the clinical impression of inoperability. Once it became apparent, however, that the influence of pulmonary hypertension on the growth and development of the pul-monary circulation could be assessed in terms of arterial size, number and muscularity, interest was renewed. The problems associated with biopsying the lung include:

1. The state of preservation of the biopsy tissue.
2. The distribution of structural change in the lung. Are those changes present in the biopsy representative of those in the entire pulmonay circulation?

3. Assessment of the different types of pulmonary vascular change (for example, intimal proliferation in some and fibrosis in other vessels).

When the biopsy is taken from the inflated lung and fixed with the airways distended, alveolar collapse does not occur and structures can be identified easily. In adults, the distribution of pulmonary vascular change can vary throughout the lung, the lower lobes generally being more severely affected than the upper lobes (*Harrison* 1958). In young children, however, extensive postmortem studies have not demonstrated regional differences in structural change when there are no regional differences in pulmonary perfusion. In one study designed specifically to detect regional differences in structure, none were found (*Haworth* and *Reid* 1978). In a group of children with ventricular septal defect and pulmonary hypertension, there were no significant differences in percentage arterial medial thickness, intra-acinar arterial size and number, appearance of the vessels in the subpleural, central, anterior and posterior regions of

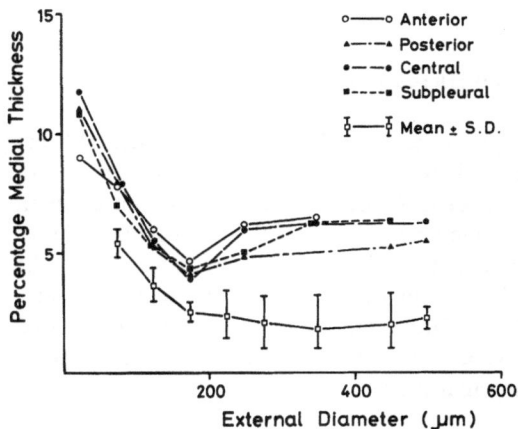

Fig. 11. Mean percentage arterial medial thickness (mean ± SD) related to external diameter (μm) in four sections from the lower left lobe of an infant with a ventricular septal defect, showing in all sections a similar increase in medial thickness above normal (□——□) and extension of muscle into smaller arteries above normal. By permission of the *British Heart Journal*

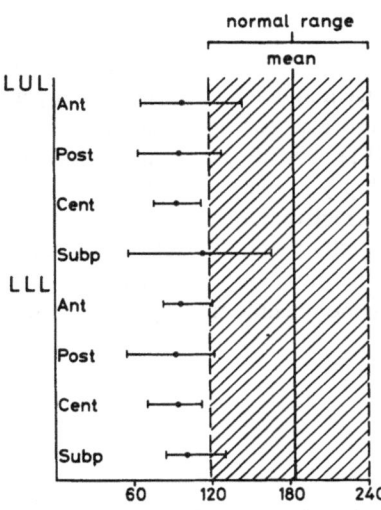

Fig. 12. External diameter (μm) of arteries accompanying respiratory bronchioli in each section of tissue from the left upper lobe *(LUL)* and left lower lobe *(LLL)*, showing in all sections a similar reduction in size in comparison with the normal of the same age.—●—, mean and range in each section of tissue. By permission of the *British Heart Journal*

the same lobe, or between contralateral lobes or lungs of the same patient (Figs. 11 and 12. Also, 1 cm² of lung tissue was sufficient for a satisfactory assessment of pulmonary vascular structure. When taking a lung biopsy, the lingula is best avoided. Even in the normal lung, the intra-acinar pulmonary arteries tend to have a thicker muscle coat than those in other parts of the lung (*Heath* and *Best* 1958). In both adults and children with pulmonary hypertension, muscularity may be greater in the lingula than elsewhere in the lung.

In giving opinion on an individual biopsy, the combination of measurement and description of structural change provides a system of internal control. To take an obvious example, if the percentage of arterial medial thickness is normal, does this mean that the arterial wall is in fact normal, or is the muscle coat atrophied? If the alveolar/arterial ratio indicates a reduction in arterial numbers, can one see occluded vessels? This system ensures more thoughtful analysis, demanding as it does a structural explanation for the measured changes in each biopsy.

b) Examination of Lung Biopsy by Electron Microscopy

Electron-microscopic examination of lung biopsies from children with congenital heart disease is not a routine procedure, and is unlikely to become one unless electron microscopy of lung biopsy proves to be useful for diagnostic management purposes, as in renal biopsies. A recent electron-microscopic examination of the intra-acinar arteries of eight children with pulmonary hypertension clarified the characteristics of the cells seen by light microscopy, forming a thick layer beneath the endothelium of non-muscular arteries (*Meyrick* and *Reid* 1980c). These cells are relatively undifferentiated smooth muscle cells, called pericytes when found in non-muscular arteries, intermediate cells when present in the non-muscular regions of a partially muscular artery.

c) Examination of Lung Biopsies Using Frozen Material

Analyses of pulmonary vascular change using frozen lung biopsy material has been advocated in children in whom there are clinical and haemodynamic doubts about operability and in whom the pulmonary arterial pressure was not measured during the cardiac catheterisation study (*Rabinovitch* et al. 1981). The surgeon takes the biopsy and then waits in the operating theatre until the biopsy is analysed and the decision taken whether or not the patient can undergo corrective surgery. In deciding the feasability of doing a corrective procedure, it is generally preferable not to use frozen material to make a rapid decision, but to take an open lung biopsy, stain it appropriately and then discuss the structural, clinical and haemodynamic findings again before making a final decision.

6. Effect of Pulmonary Hypertension in Different Types of Congenital Heart Disease

In studying the effects of pulmonary hypertension on the structural development of the pulmonary circulation, it is convenient to consider how pulmonary hypertension affects a lung at various stages of its development during (a) fetal life, (b) adaptation to postnatal life and (c) the childhood years. Such a division is obviously artificial, since problems arising at one time will have repercussions in later life, but it is a helpful approach.

a) Fetal Life

Children with atresia or critical stenosis of the aortic valve and an intact ventricular septum are born with abnormal intra-acinar arteries (*Naeye* 1962; *Haworth* and *Reid* 1977a). In this condition, the entire cardiac output is ejected into the pulmonary artery, and the body is perfused by the ductus arteriosus. Probably to ensure normal systemic perfusion in the developing fetus, pulmonary vascular smooth muscle hypertrophies. The medial coat of arteries becomes extremely thick and abnormally muscularised, and muscle develops in smaller and more peripheral arteries than is normal. Also, in some patients the number of intra-acinar arteries per unit area of lung is increased, and these vessels are also heavily muscularised. Vein wall thickness is also increased. The majority of patients with aortic atresia or critical stenosis die soon after birth, but a minority in whom the aortic valve is stenosed and the left ventricle relatively well developed undergo aortic valvotomy as an emergency procedure. In such children, a greater proportion of the arterial pathway is muscularised than normal and the muscle coat is extremely thick, suggesting an increased tendency to react to vasoconstricting factors such as acidosis and hypoxia. The reactivity of the pulmonary vascular bed makes the management of perioperative period at least as critical as the operation itself.

In the presence of excess muscularity of the intra-acinar arteries, adaptation to extra-uterine life probably occurs more slowly than is normal.

b) Adaptation to Extra-uterine Life

Even when the pulmonary circulation is probably structurally normal at birth, adaptation to extra-uterine life may fail to occur normally in the presence of congenital heart disease associated with pulmonary hypertension. In children with transposition of the great arteries, pulmonary vascular structure in those with an intact septum and a normal pulmonary arterial pressure soon differs from that seen in those with a ventricular septal defect and pulmonary hypertension.

In children with transposition and intact ventricular septum, the intra-acinar arteries have a thick coat of relatively undifferentiated cells and of muscle at birth, as normal, but then the pulmonary arterial pressure falls and pulmonary arterial wall thickness is reduced. Figure 13 shows the percentage arterial medial thickness related to external diameter in the injected postmortem lung specimens of five children, compared with normal. Muscularity was high in the child dying during the 1st day of

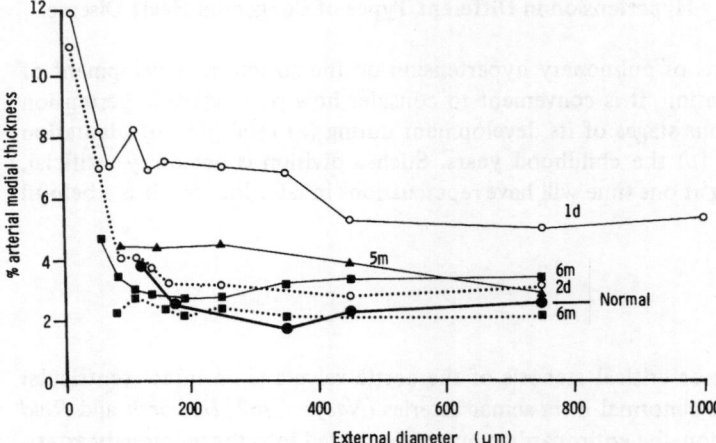

Fig. 13. Transposition of the great arteries with intact ventricular septum: mean percentage arterial medial thickness related to external diameter (μm) in injected postmortem material

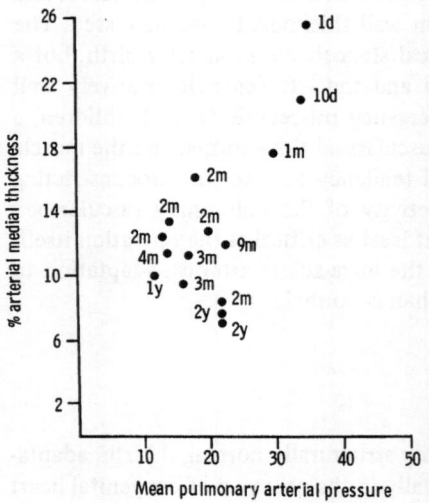

Fig. 14. Transposition of the great arteries with intact ventricular septum: mean percentage arterial medial thickness in arteries 50–100 μm in diameter related to mean pulmonary arterial pressure in lung biopsy material

life, but normal in the child dying during the 2nd day. In a series of lung biopsies, muscularity was high on the first day, but by 2 months of age the mean pulmonary arterial pressure was generally less than 22 mmHg and the percentage arterial medial thickness was less than 14%, and was normal with respect to age in each child (Fig. 14). Intimal proliferation was uncommon, occurring in only two of 20 patients, the younger of these two being 17 months of age.

Children with transposition of the great arteries and an intact ventricular septum who have a large patent ducuts arteriosus fare badly if the ductus is not closed: they

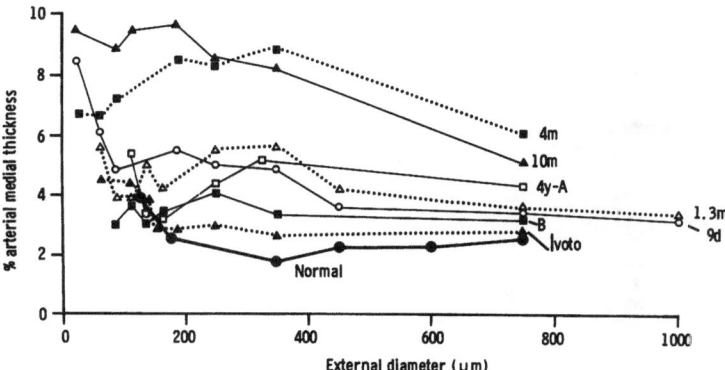

Fig. 15. Transposition of the great arteries with ventricular septal defect *(TGA VSD):* mean percentage arterial medial thickness related to external diameter (μm) in injected post-mortem material. *A,* medial atrophy, *B,* pulmonary arterial band; *lvoto,* left ventricular outflow tract obstruction

frequently develop severe obliterative pulmonary vascular disease during the first year of life.

Unlike children with transposition and an intact ventricular septum, in those with a ventricular septal defect, pulmonary arterial pressure and muscularity increase with age. By 2 months, the intra-acinar arteries, including the majority of alveolar wall arteries, are entirely surrounded by a thick medial layer. It is tempting to suppose that these muscle cells differentiate from the thick subendothelial cell layer present at birth, but we do not know that this is so. The adventitia appears thicker and more compact than normal, and the collagen stains as a thick dense layer surrounding the media. Post-mortem injection studies showed an increase in percentage arterial medial thickness, except in 2 patients who had obstruction to pulmonary outflow (Fig. 15). Muscle was also present in smaller arteries than normal in the children aged 9 days to 10 months. In one child aged 4 years, the percentage arterial medial thickness was significantly increased in arteries larger than 300 μm in diameter but was normal in the smaller vessels where the medial coat was atrophied.

In series of lung biopsies taken from children with transposition of the great arteries and ventricular septal defect, the mean pulmonary pressure increased with age (Fig. 16). Percentage arterial medial thickness was high in all children less than 7 months of age. By 1 year, however, the percentage arterial medial thickness decreased. In none of the biopsies did arterial wall structure appear normal, even in the youngest child, aged 2 months. The structural changes were more advanced in the peripheral than the proximal arteries. In respiratory bronchiolar arteries, from the 2nd month a layer of muscle cells with a complete internal elastic lamina surrounded the lumen of these normally thin-walled, partially muscular vessels (Fig. 10a). In children aged 9 months or more, the media of these arteries appeared thin and intimal fibrosis was present, sometimes occluding the lumen (Fig. 10c). In the alveolar duct and alveolar wall arteries, the first change seen at 2 months of age was thickening of the subendothelial layer, and many arteries were thick-walled and entirely muscularised. By

134

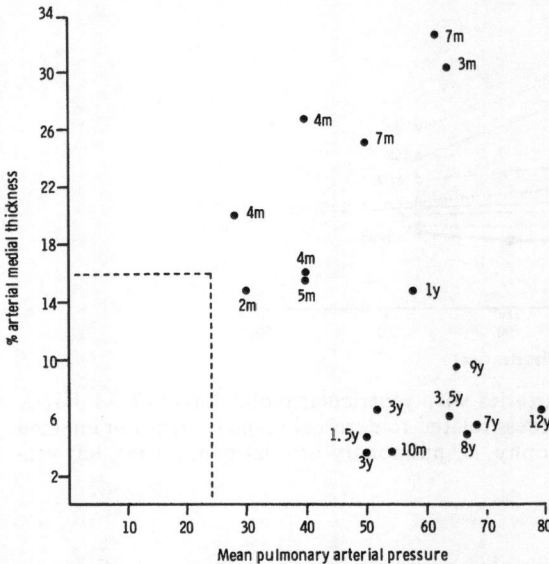

Fig. 16. Transposition of the great arteries with ventricular septal defect *(TGA VSD):* mean percentage arterial medial thickness in arteries 50−100 μm in diameter related to mean pulmonary arterial pressure in lung biopsy material. Note that the scale of the vertical axis is different from that in Fig. 14, and that the results in patients older than 10 days of age in Fig. 14 fit into the area indicated by the interrupted lines in this figure

9 months of age, however, many of the alveolar duct and alveolar wall arteries had a thin media, intimal fibrosis sometimes occluded the lumen, and dilated thin-walled vein-like arteries branched within the alveolar walls (Fig. 10c).

In a series of 200 lung biopsies from children with transposition of the great arteries, *Newfeld* et al. (1974) showed that of those with an intact ventricular septum only 8.4% had more than Grade II pulmonary vascular disease, using the *Heath* and *Edwards* classification (1958). By contrast, in the presence of a ventricular septal defect, 40% had more than Grade II pulmonary vascular disease and of those aged 1 year or older, 75% had Grade IV disease. In this study, the individual arteries in the biopsy were not identified and all were described by one grade of pulmonary vascular disease. However, the structural changes in children with transposition and a ventricular septal defect at 1 year of age are more severe than those described in the preceding paragraph, where generalised vascular dilatation, particularly plexiform lesions, was uncommon at this age.

Less commonly, severe pulmonary vascular disease develops in children with transposition of the great arteries and an intact ventricular septum who do not have a patent ductus arteriosus. A higher haematocrit causing multiple small pulmonary thromboses is a possible initiating factor, but more recently, the bronchial arterial circulation has been incriminated. Angiographic studies indicate that the bronchial circulation is enlarged in children with transposition as compared with the normal child, particularly in patients with an intact septum. Using micro-angiopathic and histological techniques,

Robertson (1968) demonstrated a considerably increase in size of the bronchial arteries and of the bronchopulmonary arteries in 10 children of less than 2 months of age with transposition of the great arteries and an intact ventricular septum. In the normal lung, bronchopulmonary arteries become narrowed and obliterated in early infancy and can rarely be detected either histologically or by micro-angiography after the immediate neonatal period (*Wagenvoort* and *Wagenvoort* 1967; *Robertson* 1968). *Aziz* et al. (1977) suggested that the low arterial oxygen tension of the systemic arterial blood flowing into the pulmonary vascular bed and also into the vasa vasorum encouraged vasoconstriction and thus medial hypertrophy. Equally, the bronchial arterial circulation may cause harm by increasing the pressure and flow of blood entering the intra-acinar arteries.

Patients with transposition of the great arteries with severe pulmonary vascular disease and a high resistance can be helped by a palliative Mustard operation, with creation of a ventricular septel defect if the ventricular septum is intact. The systemic arterial oxygen saturation increases and physical activity improves.

Obstruction to pulmonary venous return can produce severe pulmonary hypertension in the newborn and young infants with total anaomalous pulmonary venous return. Children with an infradiaphragmatic type of pulmonary venous return usually develop obstruction soon after birth, but when the connection is to a supradiaphragmatic site, obstruction can also develop at this time. The clinical and pathological findings suggest that children with a supradiaphragmatic type of connection have a large left-to-right shunt before obstruction develops (*Haworth* and *Reid* 1977b). In a group of children aged 21 days to 3 months, postmortem arteriography showed arterial dilatation and the right ventricle was dilated and hypertrophied. The septum was markedly hypertrophied and bowed into a left ventricle of normal size. In contrast, in pulmonary venous return to an infradiaphragmatic site, obstruction probably developed soon after birth and prevented an abnormal increase in pulmonary blood flow. In a group of children aged 8 days to 1 month, neither the pulmonary arteries nor the right ventricle were dilated.

The lungs of children with either type of connection showed an increase in medial thickness and extension of muscle into smaller and more peripheral intra-acinar arteries than normal. In patients with a supradiaphragmatic type of connection, the severity of arterial medial hypertrophy correlated inversely with the magnitude of the pulmonary to systemic flow ratio, increasing as pulmonary blood flow fell. None of these cases showed intimal proliferation. The intra-acinar arteries appeared to have multiplied normally. Only in one child aged 2 months was the number of arteries reduced, suggesting a secondary reduction in arterial number resulting from severe pulmonary hypertension. In all cases, the vein wall thickness was increased and the small veins were "arterialised." Microscopic examination also showed enlarged capillaries, perivascular oedema and dilated lymphatic channels, and eosinophilic material within the alveoli suggested pulmonary oedema. These changes were more severe in children with total anomalous pulmonary venous return of the infradiaphragmatic type than in those with the supradiaphragmatic type. In all cases, the alveolar walls appeared thickened.

c) The Childhood Years

Many cardiac malformations do not cause concern immediately after birth, although it is probable that the structural abnormalities in the lungs of older children originate at birth. This is particularly true of children with a large isolated ventricular septal defect. It used to be thought that a high level of resistance was caused by pulmonary vascular disease in which obliterative changes in small pulmonary arteries gradually reduced the cross-sectional area of the pulmonary vascular bed. However, during the first few years of life obliterative changes of the kind seen in older patients rarely occur, suggesting that at this young age a different mechanism is associated with a high pulmonary arterial pressure, and in some cases with an elevated resistance.

The application of quantitative morphometric techniques to the analysis of structural changes in the lungs of nine children dying between 3 months and 4 years of age with a large ventricular septal defect showed that the presence of pulmonary hypertension interferes with the growth and development of the pulmonary circulation (*Haworth* et al. 1977). The pre-acinar arteries were not dilated and showed an increase in medial thickness. Within the acinus arterial muscularity was increased, as judged by an increase in percentage medial thickness of normally muscularised arteries and by the presence of muscle in smaller and more peripheral arteries than normal (Fig. 17). The vein wall muscularity was also increased and the small veins were arterialised (*Wagenvoort* 1970). The intra-acinar arteries were abnormally small, generally being similar to the normal at birth (Fig. 18). Postmortem arteriography showed a reduction in the density of the background haze, suggesting a reduction in the number of intra-acinar arteries (Fig. 19). This was confirmed by counting microscopically the number of arteries per unit area of lung tissue.

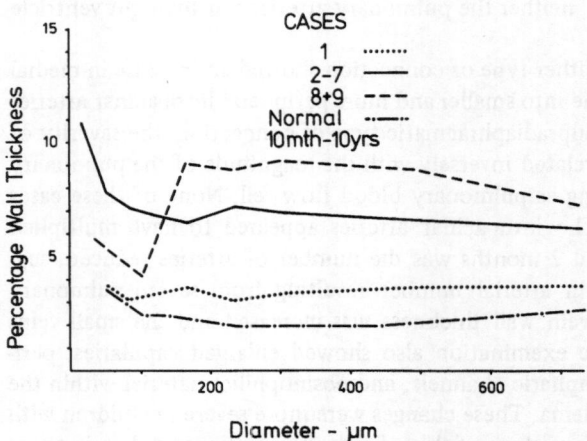

Fig. 17. Mean percentage arterial medial thickness related to external diameter (μm), showing in all cases medial hypertrophy, and in infancy the presence of muscle in smaller arteries than is normal. ———, infants less than one year; – – –, children aged 3 and 4 years; ······, child aged 3 months; –·–··–, normal. By permission of the *American Journal of Cardiology*

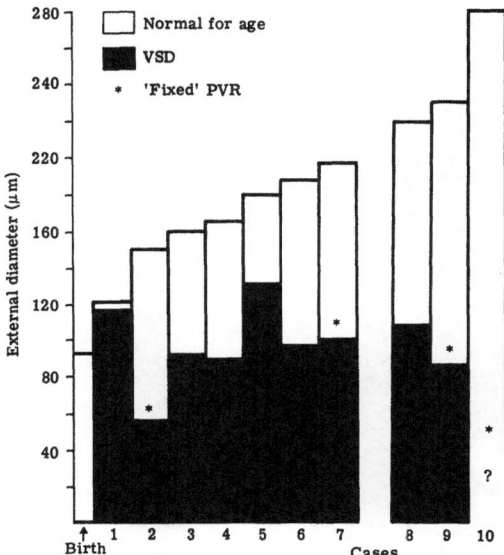

Fig. 18. Mean external diameter (μm) of arteries accompanying respiratory bronchioli in the normal infant at birth and in nine children with a ventricular septal defect *(VSD)*, showing growth failure of the intra-acinar arteries. Arteries in patients with a "fixed" pulmonary vascular resistance *(PVR)* did not differ structurally from those of the other patients. Case 10 died aged 10 years with obliterative pulmonary vascular disease, and destruction of the intra-acinar vessels made accurate quantitation impossible. By permission of the *American Journal of Cardiology*

The sequence of change in the arterial wall has been studied more closely in a series of lung biopsies taken from 38 children with a ventricular septal defect. The earliest structural change seen was thickening of the subendothelial layer of the alveolar duct and alveolar wall arteries during the first 3 months of life, and in slightly older children, the presence of differentiated smooth muscle in these vessels. In children of more than 3 months of age, the alveolar arteries were partially or entirely surrounded by a thick media. During the first 9 months of life, normally muscularised arteries at the end of the pre-acinar pathway and within the acinus showed an increase in percentage arterial medial thickness. Intimal proliferation appeared in the pre-acinar and intra-acinar arteries of several children aged 9 months or more. Medial atrophy with intimal fibrosis was present in the alveolar duct and alveolar wall arteries of two children less than 1 year of age, but such changes were uncommon before the age of 4 years.

Measurements of increased muscularity and of decreased arterial number, and also the type of structural change in the arterial wall at each airway level, can be related to measurements of pulmonary arterial pressure and resistance (Fig. 20). These findings help explain several surgical reports that following correction of a large ventricular septal defect, resistance falls to normal more frequently in patients operated upon before the age of 2 years (*Dushane* et al. 1972; *Friedli* et al. 1974). There is then still sufficient time for the pulmonary circulation to grow and develop, at least to an extent to allow it to function normally. In older patients, an equally high resistance may fall, but not to a normal level. In addition, patients with a normal resting pressure frequently have an inappropriate increase in pressure on exercise (*Hallidie-Smith* 1968). This suggests a permanent reduction in the capacity of the pulmonary circulation, and although this is usually attributed to obliterative pulmonary vascular disease, it is more probably related to a permanent failure of the intra-acinar arteries to multiply and grow normally. At least in childhood, obliterative changes are probably superimposed

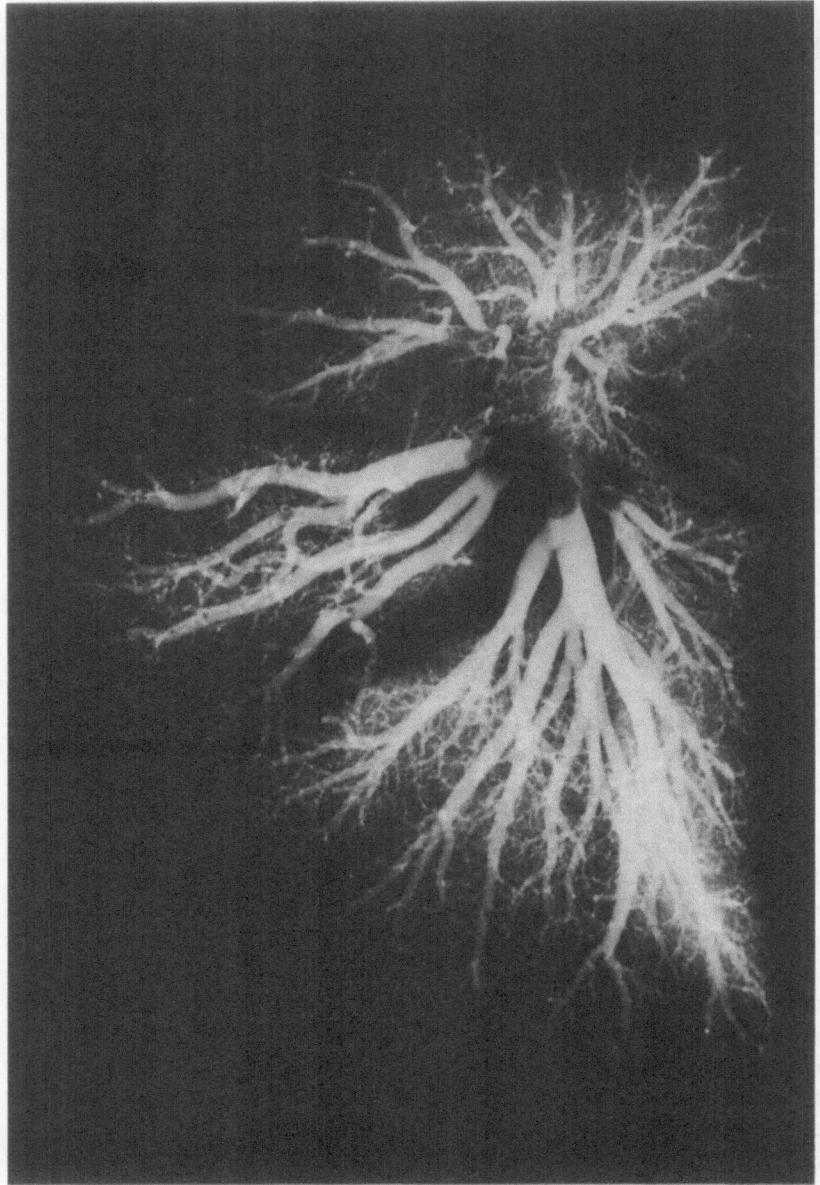

Fig. 19. Postmortem arteriograms **a** from a 9-month-old child with a ventricular septal defect and **b** from a normal child of the same age. × 1. By permission of the *American Journal of Cardiology*

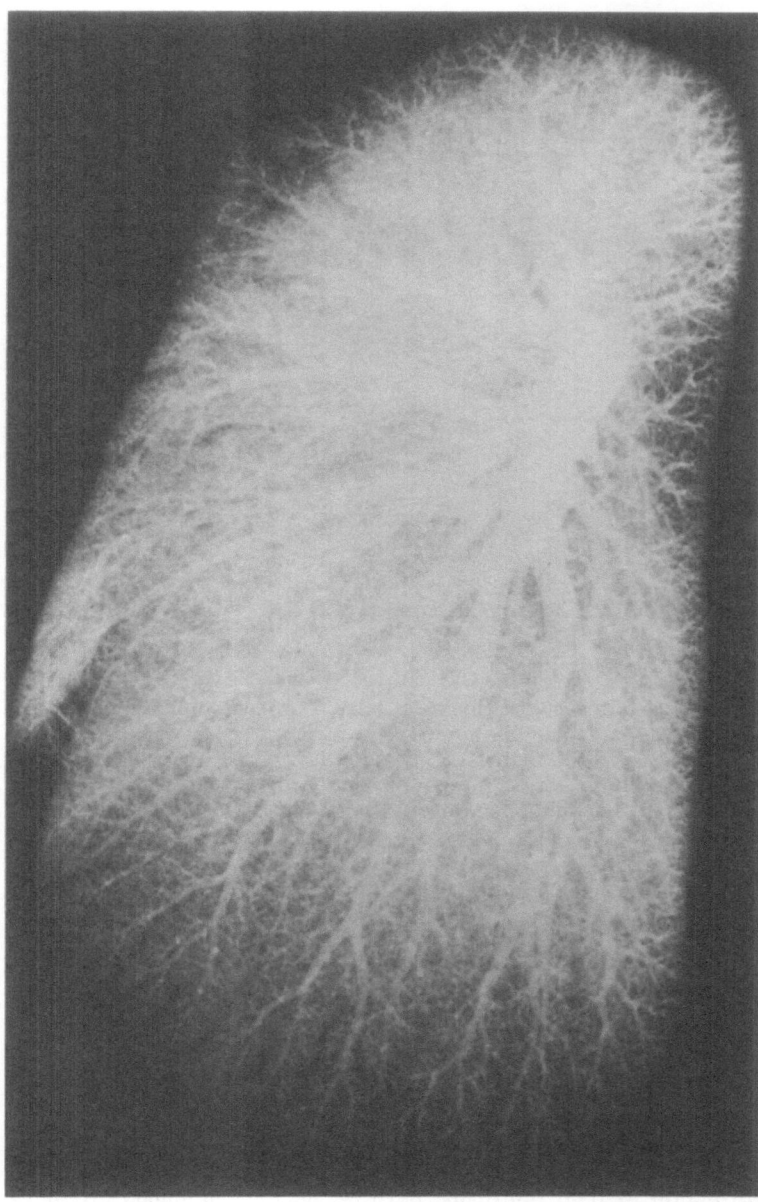

Fig. 19b

on an incompletely developed circulation. The reduction in intra-acinar arterial development helps explain why young infants have a higher resistance than one might expect from the degree of structural change assessed qualitatively, since the vessel walls shows only medial hypertrophy; however, medial hypertrophy is not the only abnormality and it is necessary to quantify pulmonary vascular structure in order to obtain a complete picture.

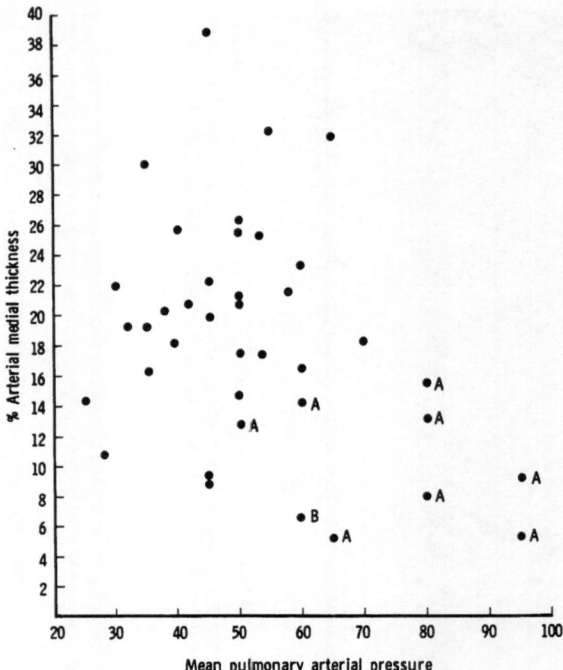

Fig. 20. Mean percentage arterial medial thickness related to mean pulmonary arterial pressure in lung biopsy material from children with a ventricular septal defect, showing an increased wall thickness greater than 10% in most cases and a low wall thickness due to medial atrophy in those whose mean pulmonary arterial pressure exceeded 60 mmHg. *A*, medial atrophy; *B*, pulmonary arterial band

When a ventricular septal defect is not closed and the pulmonary arterial pressure remains high, then obliterative pulmonary vascular disease develops, with intimal proliferation and fibrosis, followed by atrophy of the media which leads to dilatation. Fibrinoid necrosis, arteritis and the formation of plexiform lesions develop to a variable extent.

7. Pulmonary Hypertension as a Result of Aortopulmonary Anastomosis

Children with obstruction to right ventricular outflow, such as pulmonary atresia or tetralogy of Fallot, may need a palliative operation to increase the flow of blood to the lung before undergoing corrective surgery. An anastomosis is created between a pulmonary artery and either a systemic artery or the aorta itself. In a minority of patients the pulmonary blood flow is excessive, and occasionally patients die in severe cardiac failure during the first week after operation. In such children the lungs are congested, the vessels and capillaries are distended, the alveolar walls appear thickened and there is evidence of pulmonary oedema (*Ferencz* 1960). Children with a low pulmonary blood flow are particularly vulnerable to a sudden increase in flow, because many are born with abnormally thin-walled intra-acinar arteries (*Naeye* 1961d; *Haworth and Reid* 1977c). In pulmonary atresia, these arteries are also smaller and fewer in number than normal (*Haworth and Reid* 1977c). Thus the capacity of the pulmonary vascular bed is below normal and the arteries are probably unusually fragile when suddenly exposed to an increase in flow (and if the shunt is large, to an increase in pressure). Despite reduction in medial thickness at birth, however, if the child dies 2 or 3 weeks after the operation, then medial hypertrophy of the muscular pulmonary arteries with extension of muscle into smaller arteries than normal can be demonstrated. The lungs of patients surviving longer with pulmonary hypertension due to an aortopulmonary anastomosis show the structural changes associated with cardiac defects and pulmonary hypertension.

The type of aortopulmonary anastomosis influences the development of pulmonary hypertension. A Waterston anastomosis between the right pulmonary artery and ascending aorta is associated with a relatively high incidence of pulmonary hypertension. A shunt may become kinked, and severe pulmonary vascular disease develops in the lung with an excessive blood flow. In a Blalock-Taussig shunt, an anastomosis between the subclavian artery and the ipsilateral pulmonary artery is associated with a lower incidence of pulmonary hypertension, but the percentage arterial medial thickness of the pulmonary arteries on the same side as the shunt is frequently greater than in the other lung, and greater than normal even when the pressure is not elevated.

8. Pulmonary Hypertension with Uneven Distribution of Pulmonary Blood Flow

The pathologist must obtain all the available clinical, haemodynamic and angiographic information before examining a postmortem specimen or analysing a lung biopsy on a patient in whom the pulmonary blood supply does not come entirely and exclusively from the right ventricle. In pulmonary atresia with a ventricular septal defect and major aortopulmonary collateral arteries arising from the aorta, each lobe or even bronchopulmonary segment may be connected to a different collateral artery or to a central pulmonary artery connected to other collateral vessels (*Haworth and Macartney* 1980). The structure of the intra-acinar arteries depends on the flow and pressure of blood at which they are perfused, and therefore the arteries in some bronchopulmonary segments may show pulmonary vascular obstructive disease whereas in others the structure suggests a reduction of flow. Particularly when analysing a lung biopsy from such a patient, it is important to know the proportion of lung which is connected to the same source of blood supply as the biopsy, in order to know the proportion of the pulmonary vascular bed which the biopsy represents.

IX. Experimental Pulmonary Hypertension

Animal models are used to study the sequence of structural changes which develop in the lung in the presence of pulmonary hypertension and to study the pathogenesis of pulmonary hypertension. In the majority of children with congenital heart disease and a markedly increased pulmonary blood flow, the pulmonary arterial pressure is elevated from birth. Unfortunately, it is difficult to produce severe pulmonary hypertension in experimental animals by increasing pulmonary blood flow, even in newborn animals. The reserve capacity of the pulmonary vascular bed is enormous.

In adult animals, anastomosing a systemic to an extrapulmonary artery met with little success, but anastomosing a systemic to a lobar or more distal intrapulmonary artery produced a greater increase in pressure (*Ferguson* and *Varco* 1955; *Dammann* et al. 1959; *Hawe* et al. 1972). Despite the pulmonary vascular resistance being higher in the newborn than in the mature lung, a systemic-pulmonary anastomosis in puppies and in 1-month-old pigs produced little increase in pressure (*Richardson* et al. 1961; *Rendas* et al. 1979). A pneumonectomy in puppies produced an increase in pressure in some studies, but not in others (*Rudolph* et al. 1961; *Massion* and *Schilling* 1964). In newborn calves, ligation of the right pulmonary artery caused an increase in pressure in some animals, but ligation of the left pulmonary artery did not (*Vogel* et al. 1967). In all these experimental studies only the early structural response to pulmonary hypertension, an increase in pulmonary arterial medial thickness, developed, but the more advanced obliterative lesions seen in sustained pulmonary hypertension did not occur. Following an aortopulmonary anastomosis in the pig lung, the application of quantitative morphometric techniques showed that a moderate increase in pulmonary arterial blood flow and pressure was associated with an increase in medial thickness and extension of muscle into smaller and more peripheral arteries than normal, as occurs in children with similar haemodynamic findings (*Rendas* et al. 1979).

Recently, ligation of a pulmonary artery in the pig at birth was associated with failure of the intra-acinar arteries in the contralateral lung to adapt normally to extra-uterine life, despite a normal postnatal reduction in pulmonary arterial pressure (*Haworth* et al. 1981). The relative wall thickness of intra-acinar arteries less than 250 μm in diameter remained elevated after birth, and the medial thickness in the larger muscular arteries increased with time, pulmonary hypertension developing at 5–6 months of age. Thus, doubling the pulmonary blood flow at birth prevented normal adaptation in the smallest and most peripheral pulmonary arteries, followed by a secondary increase in muscularity in more proximal vessels and a gradual increase in pulmonary arterial pressure.

The nature of the cellular changes occurring in pulmonary hypertension has been studied more closely in mature rats exposed to hypoxia. Right-ventricular hypertrophy, an increase in medial thickness and the presence of muscle in smaller arteries than normally is generally reported. In addition, *Hislop* and *Reid* (1976a) reported a reduction in pre-acinar arterial size and in the number of intra-acinar arteries. Ultrastructural studies show that the earliest changes occur in the non-muscular arteries of the precapillary bed and in the capillaries of the alveolar wall (*Meyrick* and *Reid* 1978). In the normal rat lung, the non-muscular section of the partially muscular arteries

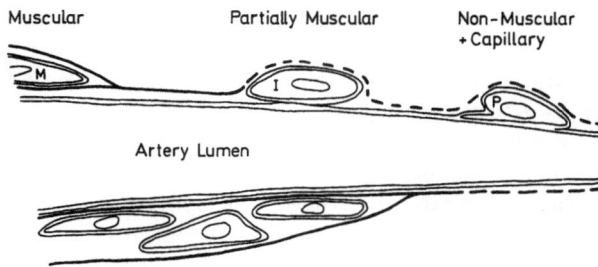

Fig. 21. The precapillary region of the rat pulmonary artery. *M*, smooth muscle cell; *I*, intermediate cell; *P*, pericyte. By permission of Dr. *B. Meyrick*

contains a cell which lies internal to a single elastic lamina, has its own basement membrane and contains myofilaments, but unlike a mature muscle cell has no dense bodies and its basement membrane is adjacent to and often fused with the basement membrane of the overlying endothelial cell (Fig. 21) (*Meyrick* and *Reid* 1979). This cell is termed "intermediate" because it is intermediate in structure and in terms of its position along the arterial pathway, between the mature smooth muscle cell of muscular arteries and the pericyte of non-muscular arteries. The pericyte lies internal to the basement membrane of the endothelial cell.

Both cell types contain smooth muscle myosin. On exposure to an hypoxic environment, from the 2nd day of exposure the volume of the intermediate cells and pericytes is increased and they differentiate, the pericyte into an intermediate cell and the intermediate cell into a mature smooth muscle cell (*Meyrick* and *Reid* 1980a). Mitoses occur in the differentiating cells after about 5 days exposure to hypoxia. After about 10 days in a hypoxic environment an internal elastic lamina is deposited and the vessel is either partially or entirely surrounded by a muscle coat.

Within the newly muscularised arteries, the endothelial cells increase in size and number, so that the endothelial layer doubles in thickness (*Meyrick* and *Reid* 1980a). The ribosomes, rough endoplasmic reticulum and Golgi apparatus hypertrophy. The subendothelial layer becomes thickened with oedema, and microfibrillar basement-membrane-like material is found focally within the subendothelial layer. The enlarged endothelial cells, subendothelial layer and new muscle cells encroach on the lumen of the small precapillary vessels and may even occlude the lumen. These ultrastructural findings help explain the reduction in number of intra-acinar arteries first noted on the light-microscopic studies.

Within the more proximal muscular arteries, medial thickness increases rapidly on exposure to hypoxia, chiefly due to hypertrophy of the smooth muscle cells with an increase in extracellular collagen (*Meyrick* and *Reid* 1980b). Muscle cell mitoses are not prominent; the labelling index is doubled after 14 days exposure to hypoxia. There is an increase in the amount of ground substance, and the extracellular connective tissue, collagen fibres, elastin and microfibrils increases. The internal elastic lamina doubles in thickness and oedema-like fluid appears. The adventitia is also doubled in thickness. The fibroblasts show an early burst of mitotic activity, the cells hypertrophy and extracellular connective tissue increases, particularly collagen.

Increase in activity of muscle fibres produces hypertrophy of the muscle cell. Hypoxia is a potent vasoconstrictor agent and in the experimental animal has been useful in clarifying the early structural response to prolonged vasoconstriction. More severe pulmonary vascular damage is effected by ingestion of the seed of *Crotalaria spectabilis*, a monocrotaline derivative (*Heath* and *Smith* 1978). In rats, ingestion of *Crotalaria spectabilis* causes evaginations of smooth muscle cells in both small muscular pulmonary arteries and in veins. These evaginations are devoid of myofilaments and organelles, suggesting sustained vasoconstriction. In the arteries, however, necrosis of medial cells occurs, probably due to intense vascular spasm. Such necrosis stimulates infiltration of the tissues with neutrophil polymorphs. From the thrombus occluding the arterial lumen in many vessels, fibrin appears to be forced into the intima and is deposited beneath the endothelium. Further penetration into the arterial wall is largely prevented by the internal elastic lamina. An increased amount of ground substance separates the medial cells. Within the media, myofibroblasts and vasoformative reserve cells are present. Vasoformative reserve cells are thought to represent a differentiated smooth muscle cell identical or similar to the myointimal cell, which migrates from the media into the intima and dedifferentiates into a cell which shares the structural characteristics of a fibroblast and a muscle cell (*Buck* 1961; *Stein* et al. 1969; *Heath* and *Smith* 1978).

Thus pulmonary hypertension induced by various means – increasing pulmonary blood flow, exposure to hypoxia or ingestion of *Crotalaria spectabilis* seeds – produces a uniform response of differentiation of precursor smooth muscle cells into a muscle cell and an increase in thickness of the media. More detailed ultrastructural studies on hypoxic animals show that increased medial thickness is due to an increase in cell size, rather than number, that the endothelial cells show a significant increase in both size and number and that there is much deposition of connective tissues in the subendothelial layer and within the media and adventitia. Prolonged vasoconstriction appears to cause fibrinoid necrosis of the arterial wall subsequent to ingestion of *Crotalaria spectabilis*.

In the rat, hypoxia of 14 days duration permanently alters the structure of the pulmonary arterial circulation (*Meyrick* and *Reid* 1980a, b; *Hislop* and *Reid* 1977b). On recovery from hypoxia, medial thickness decreases considerably but does not usually return to a normal level, many newly muscularised arteries persist, the number of intra-acinar arteries remains below the normal level and the amount of scleroprotein, particularly collagen, remains greater than normal.

X. Reversibility of Pulmonary Vascular Disease

The structural effects of lowering the pulmonary arterial pressure in children with congenital heart disease is rarely seen, because although the lung is frequently biopsied before or during the operation, it is rarely biopsied afterwards. However, after banding the pulmonary artery to reduce the pulmonary arterial pressure and flow, medial hypertrophy regressed and cellular intimal proliferation generally showed deposition of collagen-rich fibrous tissue which retracted towards the media, increasing lumen diameter (*Dammann* et al. 1961; *Wagenvoort* and *Wagenvoort* 1977). Cases showing obstruction of the arterial lumen in the first biopsy showed similar changes in the second. In the presence of more advanced lesions, such as necrotising arteritis and plexiform lesions, the clinical prognosis is less optimistic, but the fate of these lesions is unknown (*Wagenvoort* and *Wagenvoort* 1974). Medial atrophy and dilatation is associated with, and probably the result of, narrowing or obliteration of the lumen of the parent artery by intimal fibrosis and is therefore associated with fixed organic obstruction of the pulmonary vascular bed. Such changes are probably not reversible.

The early structural response to pulmonary hypertension in children with congenital heart disease is similar to that seen in the hypoxic experimental rat. In the rat, on recovery from hypoxia a reduction in pulmonary arterial pressure is associated with a permanent increase in the amount of connective tissue in the subendothelial layer, media and adventitia of the arteries and a permanent reduction in intra-acinar arterial number. Thus although children whose lungs show only medial hypertrophy largely comprise the group of patients thought to have a "labile, high-reserve, pulmonary bascular bed", they probably have an abnormal pulmonary vascular bed after corrective surgery. Doubtless, the older the patient, the greater the degree of residual permanent change.

In young infants, the perioperative period may be particularly hazardous. In many children, excessively thick-walled muscular arteries and large endothelial cells narrow the lumen considerably, making the baby vulnerable to hypoxia and acidosis, which encourage vasoconstriction. Also, cardiopulmonary bypass damages the capillary endothelium, causing occlusion of the lumen (*Parker* et al. 1972; *Utsonomiya* et al. 1977). Remembering that similar changes can cause the death of some babies with persistent pulmonary hypertension and a normal heart, the risk of operating on such children can be significant, although the long-term outlook is good.

In the presence of advanced obliterative change, the pulmonary arterial pressure and resistance tend to remain elevated after surgery, and the prognosis is less satisfactory (*Heath* et al. 1958). Such patients comprise the group said to have a "fixed, high-resistance, low-reserve pulmonary vascular bed." Generally, such children are older, more than 4 years of age in the original series described by *Heath* et al. (1958). However, infants with a similar degree of structural change also have a poor prognosis, as occurs in transposition of the great arteries with ventricular septal defect.

Clinically and pathologically, the majority of patients fall between the two extremes. The prognosis must depend on a combination of factors, which include the lumen diameter of pre- and intra-acinar arteries, the number of patent intra-acinar arteries and the wall thickness and composition of the arterial walls from the pulmonary trunk to the capillary bed. The relationship between these factors is not understood. We do not know, for example, to what extent a reduction in arterial size and number can lead to further structural damage to the arterial wall. The fate of the pulmonary circulation depends on the extent to which the cross-sectional area of the pulmonary vascular bed is diminished. Equally important is the mechanical behaviour of the structurally altered system. If the pulmonary circulation cannot function normally, then after corrective surgery the process of pulmonary vascular destruction can be self-perpetuating.

Attempts to assess the potential reversibility of pulmonary vascular disease clinically during the cardiac catheterisation study are based on the premise that if the only structural change in the pulmonary vascular bed is an increase in muscularity, then the circulation will respond to vasodilator substances such as oxygen and tolazoline. The relief of vasoconstrictor tone will lower pulmonary vascular resistance, increase the magnitude of the left-to-right shunt and frequently lower the pulmonary arterial pressue. Failure to achieve this response implies fixed, organic obstruction of the pulmonary circulation. In practice, however, it is often difficult to predict pulmonary vascular structure in this manner, particularly after the first year of life. Children with Down's syndrome are particularly difficult to assess. They suffer from upper airways obstruction, which may contribute to the increased pulmonary vascular resistance determined at cardiac catheterisation. The pathologist will then find less pulmonary vascular damage on the lung biopsies than expected for the increase in pulmonary arterial pressure and resistance.

One of the major differences between the lungs of the infant and the adult is the speed with which muscle hypertrophies. In clinical management, emphasis must be on the prevention of pulmonary vascular disease. When the natural history of the cardiac abnormality is that of rapidly progressive pulmonary vascular disease, as in transposition of the great arteries with ventricular septal defect, or univentricular heart without pulmonary outflow tract obstruction, then the child should undergo either corrective surgery or banding of the pulmonary artery by 4 months of age. Where the natural history of pulmonary vascular disease is less aggressive, as in a ventricular septal defect, the abnormality should be corrected before 1 year of age if the pulmonary arterial pressure remains high.

This discussion has been restricted to the problem of preventing pulmonary vascular disease in patients with congenital heart disease, because in other children with pulmonary hypertension, the only possible treatment is medical and this is unsatisfactory. Long-term administration of oxygen to patients with pulmonary hypertension, aimed at relieving vasoconstrictor tone, is employed with increasing frequency. The results in adult patients with hypoxic lung disease due to chronic bronchitis are encouraging. Long-term administration of pulmonary vasodilator drugs has been disappointing.

XI. Future Studies

The aims of future studies will include a greater understanding of (a) the natural history of pulmonary vascular disease in children with congenital heart disease, (b) the mechanical behaviour of the pulmonary circulation in relation to structural change and (c) the functional relationship between different types of cells present in the vessel wall.

In children with congenital heart disease and pulmonary hypertension, only the results of long-term follow-up studies on children who have had a lung biopsy will help, eventually, to predict the clinical course in other children. In order to study the relation between structure and function, the clinical, haemodynamic and lung biopsy data are now correlated using computer-assisted analysis. An experimental model of pulmonary hypertension from birth is needed to help understand the evolution of the different types of structural change seen in pulmonary hypertension and their effect on the mechanical behaviour of the system, and to study the fate of the structural lesions and the mechanical properties of the vessels after reducing the pulmonary arterial pressure.

In this chapter the pulmonary veins have received only cursory attention. In pulmonary hypertension, vein wall muscularity frequently increases in the presence of a normal left atrial and left ventricular diastolic pressure. The pathogenesis and functional significance of these changes deserves further study. In pulmonary hypertension, arterial medial thickness increases. In the systemic arterial circulation, medial hypertrophy is associated with an increase in resting tone, and spontaneous contractions of myogenic origin develop which do not occur in the normotensive state (*Brann* et al. 1981). The amount of connective tissue also increases when pulmonary arterial pressure rises, as also occurs in systemic arteries in systemic hypertension. In the growing rat with systemic hypertension, the systemic arteries show a reduction in stiffness as the scleroprotein content increases (*Berry* and *Greenwald* 1976). This response is thought to be adaptive, to maintain the difference between the high-impedence peripheral vascular bed and the low-impedance origin of the aorta in order to minimise cardiac work. Preliminary studies on the static mechanical properties of the lungs in hypertensive children suggests that a similar adaptation occurs during the first 6 months of life.

Recent studies have emphasized the close functional relationship between the media and endothelium. In the systemic circulation, the contractile activity of the media is partly dependent on the overlying endothelial cells (*Furchgott* and *Zawadzki* 1980). Also, the endothelium of systemic arteries contains a heparin-like substance which inhibits proliferation of smooth muscle cells, and damage to the endothelium can lead to medial hypertrophy, both at and at some distance from the site of injury (*Guyton* et al. 1980). Such a mechanism may be important in the pathogenesis of pulmonary vascular disease.

The developing pulmonary circulation in health and disease should be studied in its own right, rather than its behaviour being inferred from studies on either the adult pulmonary circulation or the systemic circulation.

Acknowledgement. I am grateful to Dr. Luis Becu for his expert assistance in the preparation of this chapter.

References

Anderson EG, Simon G, Reid L (1973) Primary and thrombo-embolic pulmonary hypertension. A quantitative pathological study. J Pathol 110:273–293

Arias-Stella J, Recavarren S (1962) Right ventricular hypertrophy in native children living at high altitude. Am J Pathol 41:55–64

Arias-Stella J, Saldana M (1962) The muscular pulmonary arteries in people native to high altitude. Med Thorac 19:484–493

Aziz KA, Paul MH, Rowe RD (1977) Bronchopulmonary circulation in d-transposition of the great arteries: possible role in genesis of accelerated pulmonary disease. Am J Cardiol 39:432–438

148

Bergofsky EH, Turino GM, Fishman AP (1959) Cardiorespiratory failure in kypho-scoliosis. Medicine (Baltimore) 38:263–317

Berry CL, Greenwald SE (1976) Effects of hypertension on the static mechanical properties and chemical composition of the rat aorta. Cardiovasc Res 10:437–451

Berry CL, Greenwald SE, Haworth SG (1981) Mechanical properties of the pulmonary vessels in the normal and in congenital heart disease. In: Godman MJ (ed) Paediatric cardiology 4. Churchill Livingstone, Edinburgh, pp 64–70

Berthrong M, Cochran TH (1955) Pathological findings in nine children with "primary" pulmonary hypertension. Bull Johns Hopkins Hosp 97:69–11

Boyden EA (1970a) The time lag in the development of bronchial arteries. Anat Rec 166:611–614

Boyden EA (1970b) The developing bronchial arteries in a fetus of the twelfth week. Am J Anat 129:357–368

Brann L, Halpern W, Mongeon S (1981) Spontaneous contractions and intrinsic tone in small cerebral arteries of the hypertensive rat (Abstr no 613). Fed Proc 40:340

Brenner O (1935) Pathology of the vessels of the pulmonary circulation. Part I. Arch Intern Med 56:211–237

Brown R, Pickering D (1974) Persistent transitional circulation. Arch Dis Child 49: 883–885

Buck RC (1961) Intimal thickening after ligature of arteries. Circ Res 9:418–426

Chamberlain D, Hislop A, Hey E, Reid L (1977) Pulmonary hypoplasia in babies with severe rhesus isoimmunisation: a quantitative study. J Pathol 122:43–52

Csaba IP, Sulyok E, Ertle T (1978) Relationship of maternal treatment with indo-methacin to persistent fetal circulation syndrome. J Pediatr 92:484

Dammann JF Jr, Ferencz C (1956) The significance of the pulmonary vascular bed in congenital heart disease. I. Normal lungs. II. Malformations of the heart in which there is pulmonary stenosis. Am Heart J 52:7–17

Dammann JF Jr, Baker JP, Muller WH Jr (1959) Pulmonary vascular changes induced by experimentally produced pulmonary arterial hypertension. Surg Gynecol Obstet 105:16–26

Dammann JF Jr, McEachen JA, Thompson WM Jr, Smith R, Muller WH (1961) The regression of pulmonary vascular disease after the creation of pulmonary stenosis. J Thorac Cardiovasc Surg 42:722–734

Davies G, Reid L (1970) Growth of the alveoli and pulmonary arteries in childhood. Thorax 25:669–681

Davies G, Reid L (1971) Effect of scoliosis on growth of alveoli and pulmonary arteries and on right ventricle. Arch Dis Child 46:623–632

Dawes GS (1968) Foetal and neonatal physiology. Year Book Medical Publishers, Chicago, p 167

Delesse MA (1847) Procédé mécanique pour déterminer la composition des roches. C R Acad Sci (Paris) 25:544

Dunnill MS (1962) Quantitative methods in the study of pulmonary pathology. Thorax 17:320–328

DuShane JW, Weidman WH, Ritter DG (1972) Influence of the natural history of ventricular septal defects on management of patients. Birth Defects 8:63–68

Edwards JE (1957) Functional pathology of the pulmonary vascular tree in congenital cardiac disease. Circulation 15:164–196

Elliott FM, Reid L (1965) Some new facts about the pulmonary artery and its branching pattern. Clin Radiol 16:193–198

Emery JL (1962) Pulmonary embolism in children. Arch Dis Child 37:591–595

Emery JL, Hilton HB (1961) Lung and heart complications of the treatment of hydro-cephalus by ventriculo-auriculostomy. Surgery 50:309–314

Ferencz C (1960) The pulmonary vascular bed in tetralogy of Fallot. II. Changes following a systemic-pulmonary arterial anastomosis. Bull Johns Hopkins Hosp 106: 100–118

Ferguson DJ, Varco RL (1955) The relation of blood pressure and flow to the development and regression of experimentally induced pulmonary arteriosclerosis. Circ Res 3:152–158

Firor HV (1972) Pulmonary embolization complicating total intravenous alimentation. J Pediatr Surg 7:81

Friedli B, Kidd BSL, Mustard WT, Keith JD (1974) Ventricular septal defect with increased pulmonary vascular resistance. Late results of surgical closure. Am J Cardiol 33:403–409

Fulton RM, Hutchinson EC, Jones AM (1952) Ventricular weight in cardiac hypertrophy. Br Heart J 14:413–420

Furchgott RF, Zawadzki JV (1980) The obligatory role of endothelial cells in the relaxation of arterial smooth muscle by acetylcholine. Nature 288:373–376

Gersony WM (1973) Persistence of the fetal circulation. A commentary. J Pediatr 82: 1103–1106

Gersony WM, Duc GV, Sinclair JC (1969) "PFC" syndrome (persistence of the fetal circulation) (Abstr). Circulation (Suppl III) 40:87

Gil J, Weibel ER (1969) Improvements in demonstration of lining layer of lung alveoli by electron microscopy. Respir Physiol 8:13–36

Grant MM, Roth N, Brody JS (1981) Basement membrane in fetal rat lungs (Abstr). Fed Proc 40:468

Grover RF, Vogel JHK, Averill KH, Blunt SG (1963) Pulmonary hypertension. Individual and species variation relative to vascular reactivity. Am Heart J 66:1–3

Guyton JR, Rosenberg RD, Clowes AW, Karovsky MJ (1980) Inhibition of rat arterial smooth muscle cell proliferation by heparin. In vivo studies with anticoagulant and nonanticoagulant heparin. Circ Res 46:625–634

Hallidie-Smith KA (1968) The long-term results of closure of ventricular septal defect with pulmonary vascular disease. Am Heart J 76:591–595

Harker LC, Kirkpatrick SE, Friedman WF, Bloor CM (1981) Effects of indomethacin on fetal rat lungs; a possible cause of persistent fetal circulation (PFC). Pediatr Res 15:147–151

Harrison CV (1958) The pathology of the pulmonary vessels in pulmonary hypertension. Br J Radiol 31:217–226

Hawe A, Tsakiris AG, Rastelli GC, Titus JL, McGoon DC (1972) Experimental studies on the pathogenesis of pulmonary vascular obstructive disease. J Thorac Cardiovasc Surg 63:652–669

Haworth SG (1979) Pulmonary vascular structure in persistent fetal circulation. In: Godman MJ, Marquis RM (eds) Heart disease in the newborn. Churchill Livingstone, Edinburgh (Paediatric cardiology, vol 2, pp 67–78)

Haworth SG, Hislop A (1981) Adaptation of the pulmonary circulation to extrauterine life in the pig and its relevance to the human infant. Cardiovasc Res 15: 108–119

Haworth SG, Macartney FJ (1980) Growth and development of the pulmonary circulation in pulmonary atresia with ventricular septal defect and major aorto-pulmonary collateral arteries. Br Heart J 44:14–24

Haworth SG, Reid L (1976) Persistent fetal circulation: newly recognised structural features. J Pediatr 88:614–620

Haworth SG, Reid L (1977a) A quantitative structural study of the pulmonary circulation in the newborn with aortic atresia, stenosis or coarctation. Thorax 32:121–128

Haworth SG, Reid L (1977b) Structural study of pulmonary circulation and of heart in total anomalous pulmonary venous return in early infancy. Br Heart J 39:80–92

Haworth SG, Reid L (1977c) Quantitative structural study of the pulmonary circulation in the newborn with pulmonary atresia. Thorax 32:129–133

Haworth SG, Reid L (1978) A morphometric study of regional variation in lung structure in infants with pulmonary hypertension and congenital cardiac defect: a justification of lung biopsy. Br Heart J 40:825–831

150

Haworth SG, Sauer U, Bühlmeyer K, Reid L (1977) Development of the pulmonary circulation in ventricular septal defect: a quantitative structural study. Am J Cardiol 40:781–788

Haworth SG, de Leval M, Macartney FJ (1981) Hypo- and hyperperfusion in the immature lung: pulmonary arterial development following ligation of left pulmonary artery in the newborn pig. J Thorac Cardiovasc Surg 82:281–292

Hayward J, Reid L (1952) Observations on the anatomy of the intrasegmental bronchial tree. Thorax 7:89–97

Heath D, Best PV (1958) The tunica media of the arteries in pulmonary hypertension. J Pathol Bacteriol 76:165–174

Heath D, Edwards JE (1958) The pathology of hypertensive pulmonary vascular disease. A description of six grades of structural changes in the pulmonary arteries with special reference to congenital cardiac septal defects. Circulation 18:533–547

Heath D, Smith P (1978) The electron microscopy of "fibrinoid necrosis" in pulmonary arteries. Thorax 33:579–595

Heath D, Helmholtz HF, Burchell HB, DuShane JW, Kirklin JW, Edwards JE (1958) Relation between structural changes in the small pulmonary arteries and the immediate reversibility of pulmonary hypertension following closure of ventricular and atrial septal defects. Circulation 18:1167–1174

Heath D, DuShane JW, Wood EH, Edwards JE (1959) The structure of the pulmonary trunk at different ages and in cases of pulmonary hypertension and pulmonary stenosis. J Pathol Bacteriol 77:443–456

Hislop A, Reid L (1972) Intra-pulmonary arterial development during fetal life — branching pattern and structure. J Anat 113:35–48

Hislop A, Reid L (1973) Pulmonary arterial development during childhood – branching pattern and structure. Thorax 28:129–135

Hislop A, Reid L (1976a) New findings in pulmonary arteries of rats with hypoxia-induced pulmonary hypertension. Br J Exp Pathol 57:542–554

Hislop A, Reid L (1976b) Persistent hypoplasia of the lung after repair of congenital diaphragmatic hernia. Thorax 31:450–455

Hislop A, Reid L (1977a) Formation of the pulmonary vasculature. In: Hodson WA (ed) Development of the lung. Dekker, New York, p 52

Hislop A, Reid L (1977b) Changes in the pulmonary arteries of the rat during recovery from hypoxia-induced pulmonary hypertension. Br J Exp Pathol 58:653–662

Hislop A, Hey E, Reid L (1979) The lungs in congenital bilateral renal agenesis and dysplasia. Arch Dis Child 54:32–38

Khoury GH, Hawes CR (1963) Primary pulmonary hypertension in children living at high altitude. J Pediatr 62:177–185

Könn G, Storb R (1960) Über den Formwandel der kleinen Lungenarterian des Menschen nach der Geburt. Beitr Pathol Anat 123:212

Lauweryns JM, Rosan RC (1970) The unit lobule: A revised concept of the neonatal lung. Proc 2nd European Congress on Perinatal Medicine, London. Perinatal Med 1970:259–263

Levin DL, Heymann MA, Kitterman JA, Gregory GA, Phibbs RH, Rudolph AM (1976) Persistent pulmonary hypertension. J Pediatr 89:626–630

Levin DL, Fixler DE, Morriss FC, Tyson J (1978) Morphologic analysis of the pulmonary vascular bed in infants exposed in utero to prostaglandin synthetase inhibitors. J Pediatr 92:478–483

Levin DL, Mills LJ, Weinberg AG (1979) Haemodynamic, pulmonary, vascular and myocardial abnormalities secondary to pharmacologic constriction of the fetal ductus arteriosus. Circulation 60:360–364

Libi-Sylora M, Greco J, Ferencz C (1968) Postnatal growth of the pulmonary arterial tree. Morphological characteristics. Am J Dis Child 115:191–201

Liebow AA, Hales MR, Lindskog GE, Bloomer WE (1947) Plastic demonstrations of pulmonary pathology. J Tech Methods 27:116–129

Liebow AA, Hales MR, Bloomer WE, Harrison W, Lindskog GE (1950) Studies on the lung after ligation of the pulmonary artery. II. Anatomical changes. Am J Pathol 26:177–185

Ljungquist A (1963) The intrarenal arterial pattern in the normal and diseased human kidney. Acta Med Scand (Suppl) 174:401

Manchester D, Margolis HS, Sheldon RE (1975) Possible association between maternal indomethacin therapy and primary pulmonary hypertension of the newborn. Am J Obstet Gynecol 126:467–469

Massion WH, Schilling JA (1964) Physiological effects of lung resection in adult and puppy dogs. J Thorac Cardiovasc Surg 48:239–249

Meyrick B, Reid L (1978) The effect of continued hypoxia on rat pulmonary arterial ciruclation. Lab Invest 38:188–200

Meyrick B, Reid L (1979) Ultrastructural features of the distended pulmonary arteries of the normal rat. Anat Rec 193:71–98

Meyrick B, Reid L (1980a) Endothelial and subintimal changes in rat hilar pulmonary artery during recovery from hypoxia. A quantitative structural study. Lab Invest 42:603–615

Meyrick B, Reid L (1980b) Hypoxia-induced structural changes in the media and adventitia of the rat hilar pulmonary artery and their regression. Am J Pathol 100:151–169

Meyrick B, Reid L (1980c) Ultrastructural findings in lung biopsy material from children with congenital heart defects. Am J Pathol 101:527–542

Naeye RL (1961a) Arterial changes during the perinatal period. Arch Pathol 71:121–128

Naeye RL (1961b) Hypoxemia and pulmonary hypertension. Arch Pathol 71:447–452

Naeye RL (1961c) Kyphoscoliosis and cor pulmonale: a study of the pulmonary vascular bed. Am J Pathol 38:561–574

Naeye RL (1961d) Perinatal changes in the pulmonary vascular bed with stenosis and atresia of the pulmonic valve. Am Heart J 61:586–592

Naeye RL (1962) Perinatal vascular changes associated with underdevelopment of the left heart. Am J Pathol 41:287–293

Naeye RL (1965) Children at high altitude: pulmonary and renal abnormalities. Circ Res 16:33–38

Naeye RL, Harcke HT, Blanc WA (1971) Adrenal gland structure and the development of hyaline membrane disease. Pediatrics 47:650–657

Newfeld EA, Paul MH, Muster AJ, Idriss FS (1974) Pulmonary vascular disease in complete transposition of the great arteries: a study of 200 patients. Am J Cardiol 34:75–82

Noonan JA, Ehmke DA (1963) Complications of ventriculovenous shunts for control of hydrocephalus. N Engl J Med 269:70–77

O'Rahilly R, Debson H, King TS (1950) Subclavian origin of bronchial arteries. Anat Rec 108:227–238

Parker DJ, Karp RB, Kirklin JW, Bedard P (1972) Lung water and alveolar and capillary volumes after intracardiac surgery. Circulation (Suppl I) 45:139–146

Rabinovitch M, Haworth SG, Castaneda AR, Nadas AS, Reid LM (1978) Lung biopsy in congenital heart disease: a morphometric approach to pulmonary vascular disease. Circulation 58:1107–1122

Rabinovitch M, Castaneda AR, Reid L (1981) Lung biopsy with frozen section as a diagnostic aid in patients with congenital heart defects. Am J Cardiol 47:77–84

Recavarren S, Arias-Stella J (1964) Growth and development of the ventricular myocardium from birth to adult life. Br Heart J 26:187–192

Reid L (1967) The pathology of emphysema, Appendix B. Lloyd-Luke, London

Reid L (1975) Objectivity and quantification in lung disease. Postgrad Med J 51:711–715

Rendas A, Lennox S, Reid L (1979) Aorta-pulmonary shunts in growing pigs. J Thorac Cardiovasc Surg 77:109–118

Richardson JW, Phillips CE, DeWeese JA, Manning JA, Mahoney EB (1961) Influence of pulmonary vascular maturity on response to subclavian pulmonary arterial anastomosis (Abstr). Circulation 24:1020

Robertson B (1968) The intrapulmonary arterial pattern in normal infancy and in transposition of the great arteries. Acta Pediatr Scand (Suppl) 184

Rubatelli FF, Chiazza ML, Zanardon V, Cantarott F (1979) Effect on neonate of maternal treatment with indomethacin (Letter). J Pediatr 94:161

Rudolph AM, Neuhauser EBD, Golinko RJ, Auld PAM (1961) Effects of penumonectomy on pulmonary circulation in adult and young animals. Circ Res 9:856−861

Rudolph AM, Heymann MA, Lewis AB (1977) Physiology and pharmacology of the pulmonary circulation in the fetus and newborn. In: Hodson WA (ed) Development of the lung. Dekker, New York, pp 503−505 (Lung biology in health and disease, vol 6)

Ryland D, Reid L (1975) The pulmonary circulation in cystic fibrosis. Thorax 30: 285−292

Shaw AFB, Ghareeb AA (1938) The pathogenesis of pulmonary schistosomiasis in Egypt with special reference to Ayerza's disease. J Pathol Bacteriol 46:401−424

Siassi B, Goldberg SJ, Emmanouilides GC, Higoshino SM, Lewis E (1971) Persistent pulmonary vascular obstruction in newborn infants. J Pediatr 78:610−615

Stein AA, Mauro J, Thibodeau L, Alley R (1969) The histogenesis of cardiac myxomas: relation to other proliferative diseases of subendothelial vasoformative reserve cells. In: Sommers SC (ed) Pathology annual, vol 4. Butterworths, London, p 293

Subramanian N, Bakthaviziam A, Sukamar IP, Krishnaswami S, Cherian G (1974) Primary pulmonary hypertension. A clinicopathological study of 11 cases. Indian Heart J 26:171−178

Tandon HD, Kasturi J (1975) Pulmonary vascular changes associated with isolated mitral stenosis in India. Br Heart J 37:26−36

Thompson P, McRae C (1970) Familial pulmonary hypertension. Evidence of autosomal dominant inheritance. Br Heart J 32:758−760

Utosonomiya T, Yamamoto N, Maeno M, Morioka T, Akagi M (1977) Detection of lung basement membrane degrading substance in plasma during cardiopulmonary bypass. Am J Surg 134:599−603

Vogel JHK, McNamara DG, Hallman G, Rosenberg H (1967) Effects of mild chronic hypoxia on the pulmonary circulation in calves with reactive pulmonary hypertension. Circ Res 21:661−669

Wagenvoort CA (1960) Vasoconstriction and medial hypertrophy in pulmonary hypertension. Circulation 22:535−546

Wagenvoort CA (1970) Morphologic changes in intrapulmonary veins. Hum Pathol 1: 205−213

Wagenvoort CA (1973) Hypertensive pulmonary vascular disease complicating congenital heart disease: a review. Cardiovasc Clin 5:43−60

Wagenvoort CA, Wagenvoort N (1967) Arterial anastomoses, bronchopulmonary arteries and pulmobronchial arteries in perinatal lungs. Lab Invest 16:13−24

Wagenvoort CA, Wagenvoort N (1970) Primary pulmonary hypertension: a pathologic study of the lung vessels in 156 clinically diagnosed cases. Circulation 42:1163−1184

Wagenvoort CA, Wagenvoort N (1974) Pathology of the Eisenmenger syndrome and primary pulmonary hypertension. Adv Cardiol 11:123−130

Wagenvoort CA, Wagenvoort N (1977) Pathology of pulmonary hypertension. Wiley, New York, pp 69, 87, 121−125, 166−171

Weibel ER (1959) Die Blutgefäßanastomosen in der menschlichen Lunge. Z Zellforsch 50:653−692

Weibel ER (1962) A quantitative approach to the morphologic study of the peripheral pulmonary vasculature. Med Thorac 19:208−214

Weibel ER (1970) Morphometric estimation of pulmonary diffusion capacity. Respir Physiol 11:54−75

World Health Organisation (1961) Chronic cor pulmonale. WHO Tech Rep Ser 213:6

Inflammatory Disease of the Human Lung of Definite or Presumed Viral Origin.
Cytologic and Histologic Topics

H.-E. SCHAEFER

I. Introduction

A large part, perhaps even the majority, of inflammatory diseases of the respiratory tract are caused by viral infection. The pathoanatomical changes associated with banal viral infections (common cold) of the upper respiratory tract, may be readily observed in biopsies from the nasal mucosa as documented in studies by *Hilding* (1930) and *Tyrell* and *Parsons* (1960).

Our knowledge of morphologic alterations associated with viral infections of the lung is, however, still rather limited. Biopsy of pulmonary tissue in the acute stage of uncomplicated viral infection is usually contraindicated. Information is mostly derived from experimental work, surgical specimens obtained by chance, or autopsy material from cases with fatal, that is to say, atypical outcome. The interpretation of autopsy findings is additionally hampered by the difficulties of finding postmortem virus identification. While DNA viruses may be identified correctly in post mortem material by electron microscopy or as Feulgen positive cell inclusions, infection by RNA viruses can only be diagnosed by immunohistochemical or indirect evidence from certain histologic or cytologic criteria or in a retrospective evaluation of the epidemiologic situation.

The present chapter attempts a synopsis of some observations about viral or potentially viral disease of the lung published in the literature, together with some paradigmatic findings from our own studies. These cases, with a brief comment in the legends of the illustrations, have been examined with the current methods of light and electron microscopy. A few procedures that are less common in pulmonary pathology will be explained in greater detail.

II. Special Histochemical Methods

1. Demonstration of Acid Phosphatase in Lung Tissue

Acid phosphatase (AP) is an almost ubiquitous lysosomal enzyme, whereas its tartrate-resistant form (TAP) is found only in certain definite cell types. TAP was known first as a marker enzyme of neoplastic lymphocytes in hairy cell leukemia (*Yam* et al. 1971); more recent studies have shown that TAP can also be demonstrated histochemically in macrophages (*Schaefer* et al. 1977) and in osteoclast cells (*Schaefer* 1980). TAP occurs further in the macrophages of storage disease, especially in Gaucher cells. Apparently, TAP is produced during the transformation of monocytes into macrophages in connection with the storing of ceroid or other deposits. In Gaucher's disease, even blood monocytes may contain TAP of lower activity (*Schaefer* 1981). Being largely resistant to damage by conventional paraffin embedding, TAP positive macrophages can be demonstrated even in routine paraffin sections, especially in alveolar macrophages which show particularly high TAP activity. Thus, the demonstration of TAP helps to identify beyond doubt the presence of alveolar macrophages in paraffin sections. In particular, this method will help to distinguish the alveolar macrophages found in fresh inflammatory infiltrates, from desquamated epithelia, pneumocytes, and monocytes that are just emigrating from the circulation, but not yet undergoing histiocytic transformation.

For TAP demonstration, dewaxed sections are incubated for 2.5 hrs at 37°C in a medium made as follows: 16 mg Naphthol AS-BI phosphate, dissolved in 0.5 ml dimethylsulfoxide, are mixed first with 100 ml 0.1 M acetate buffer (pH 5.6) and then with 0.8 ml hexazotized pararosaniline solution, and filtered. After incubation the sections are rinsed in tap water, counterstained with Mayer's hemalum and covered with glycerin jelly. Hexazotized pararosaniline (modified according to *Davies* and *Ornstein* 1959) is prepared as follows: 50 mg pararosaniniline hydrochloride are completely dissolved in 3 ml 1 N HCl, cooled to 0°C, and added slowly to 0.5 ml of an equally cooled 1 N NaNO$_2$ solution. This hexazotate solution is ready for use after 5 min for reaction, or may be stored frozen ($-$ 15°C) for several weeks.

Since ordinary tartrate-sensitive AP will be inactivated by prolonged fixation with formol and by embedding in paraffin, the reaction medium presented above can be used to demonstrate selectively in conventional paraffin sections, the TAP positive alveolar macrophages appearing in distinct red color within the lung tissue (Fig. 1). Tartrate-sensitive AP, however, will show a positive reaction in unfixed or lightly fixed cryostat or imprint preparations. These activities of tartrate-sensitive AP can be sup-

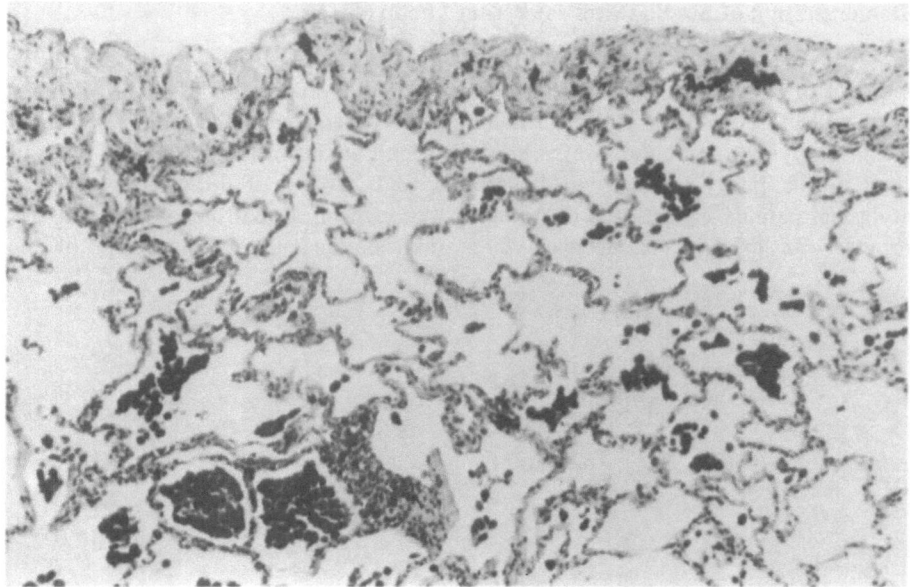

Fig. 1. Alveolar macrophages stained for TAP in a routinely formalin fixed and paraffin-embedded open lung biopsy taken from a heavy smoker. Due to their high TAP—activity the augmented macrophages appear as selectively dark stained clusters

pressed by addition of 150 mg L(+) tartaric acid plus 1.8 ml 1 N NaOH to the reaction medium.

2. Demonstration of Chloroacetate Esterase

The substrate naphthol AS-D chloroacetate can be applied to conventional paraffin sections for almost selective demonstration of neutrophilic granulocytes and tissue mast cells (*Moloney* et al. 1960). Even the cell detritus of disintegrating neutrophils show positive reactions in inflammatory infiltrates. Moreover, positive reactions are also frequently observed in pneumocystis carinii organisms. The medium we used is a modification of the method described by *Leder* (1964).

Dewaxed sections are incubated one hour at room temperature in the following medium: 3 mg naphthol AS-D chloroacetate are dissolved in 1 ml of a 9:1 mixture of dimethylsulfoxide and triton X-100, then 50 ml phosphate buffered saline (PBS) are added. Subsequently, an approximate pH of 6.5 is established by adding 0.3—0.5 ml hexazotate solution (see II.1). After a brief rinse in running water the nuclei can be counterstained with Mayer's hemalum. The stained slides are mounted and covered with glycerine jelly.

3. Demonstration of Binding Sites for Peanut Lectin (PNA)

The lectin of Arachis hypogaea (peanut antigen, PNA), possesses high binding affinity for β-D-galactose(1-3-)N-acetylgalactosamine. This sequence occupies a terminal position in glycoproteins that are specifically found at the surface of diverse types of epithelial cells, partly covered with neuraminic acids. Groups of β-D-galactose(1-3)-N-acetylgalactosamine can also be observed on the surface of endothelial cells and erythrocytes. On erythrocyte surfaces, these disaccharides are a component of the

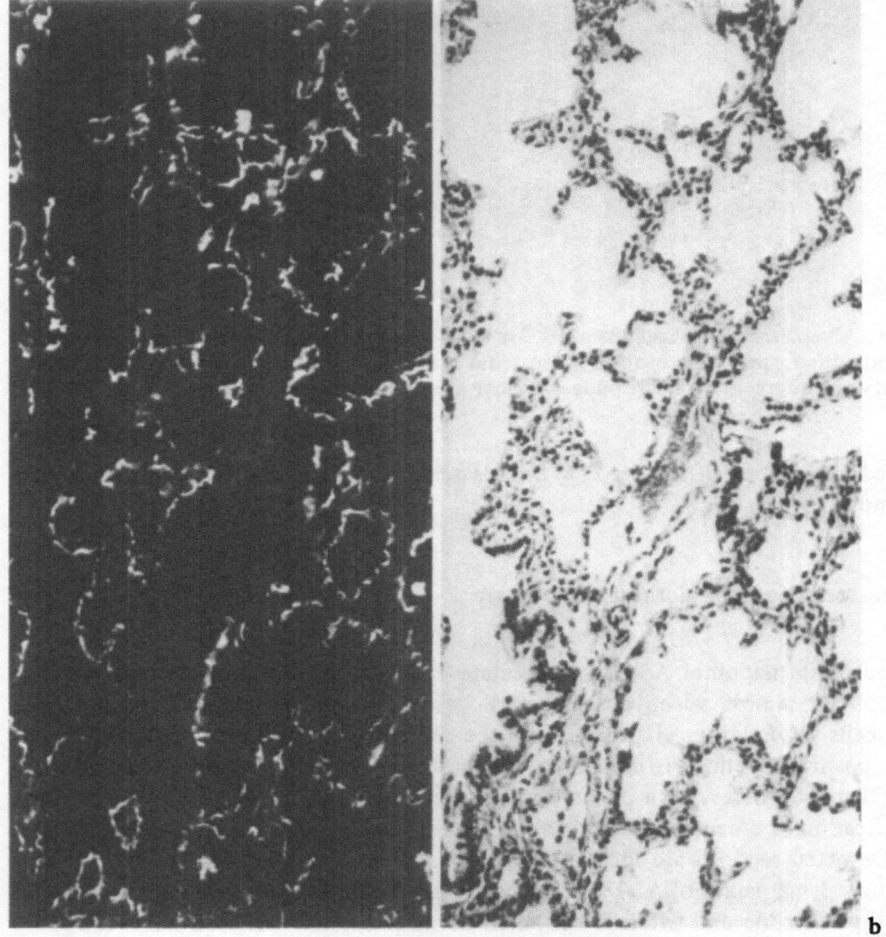

a   b

Fig. 2. a The distribution of binding sites for the peanut lectin (glycoproteins containing the terminal sequence β-D-galactose(1-3)-N-acetyl-D-galactosamine) covered by sialic acid in normal human lung tissue as visualized by fluorescence microscopy after prior neuraminidase treatment and incubation with FITC-labeled PNA (method 2.3). The non-ciliated epithelia of terminal bronchioles and type II pneumocytes exhibit the most intense fluorescence on their luminal surfaces. b Identical area as shown in a, illuminated by visible light. Nuclei are stained by Mayer's haemalum

Thomsen-Friedenreich-cryptantigen, and are normally found completely covered with neuraminic acid (*Klein* et al. 1978). Thus, these erythrocytic binding sites will react to PNA only after pretreatment with neuraminidase. On epithelial surfaces, however, free lectin receptors may be found beside other sites covered with neuraminic acid, and so these free receptors will bind PNA without previous application of neuraminidase.

Application of FITC-labeled PNA reveals positive PNA fluorescence on the surface of nonciliated lung epithelial cells, of Clara cells, and of pneumocytes; fluorescence is enhanced by pretreatment with neuraminidase. Positive reaction is also found in bronchial mucus and in mucus-producing cells. Epithelia with a microvillous surface (pneumocytes II) show stronger fluorescence than those with smooth surfaces (pneumocytes I). Ciliated epithelia always have negative reactions. The fluorescence method, demonstrating PNA receptor sites, especially after pretreatment with neuraminidase, facilitates a clear light microscopical identification of pneumocytes by means of their surface fluorescence (Fig. 2). In particular, the loss of pneumocytes with denudation of alveoli, as observed in certain viral pneumonias, can be demonstrated in a convincing fashion.

As the disaccharide structures identifiable with PNA will not be damaged by formol fixation nor by paraffin embedding, the demonstration of PNA receptors is possible in conventional paraffin as follows:

1) Dewaxed sections are briefly rinsed under running tap water, with a last rinse in aqua dest. to which a mixture of aceton and triton X-100 in equal proportions has been added (0.01 ml per 100 ml).

2) After rinsing the sections are dried, placed in a humid chamber and layered for 30 min with a solution of 0.1 I.U. neuraminidase (Vibrio cholerae) plus 5×10^{-3} M CaCl$_2$ in 0.2 M acetate buffer (pH 5.6). Subsequently the sections are again rinsed as described in 1).

3) The dried sections are again placed in a humid chamber and covered for 30 min with a solution of 0.5 mg FITC-labeled PNA in 1 ml 0.05 M sodium barbital buffer (pH 7.2).

4) Finally, the sections are again rinsed in three times renewed 0.05 M sodium barbital buffer (pH 7.2) and mounted for fluorescence microscopy with a covering of equal proportions of 85% glycerine and 0.05 M sodium barbital buffer (pH 7.2).

Free lectin receptors that are not naturally covered by neuraminic acid, are demonstrated by omitting the second step, i.e. the pretreatment with neuraminidase. Staining the nuclei with Mayer's hemalum does not impair PNA fluorescence at the cell surfaces.

III. Pulmonary Infection by DNA Viruses

Infection by DNA viruses is readily diagnosed by light and electron microscopy from morphological criteria, including the evidence of typical inclusion bodies. Their easy morphologic definition explains the historical development of modern virology from this morphologic approach. Cellular changes that were later subsumed under the term "cytomegaly" by *Goodpasture* and *Talbot* (1921), had been observed and described as "protozoal formations" as early as 1904 by *Jesionek* and *Kiolemenoglu* in the liver, lung and kidney of a child who died from syphilis at the age of 8 months. Their initial publication had stimulated a number of papers describing similar inclusions in the kidney (*Ribbert* 1904), parotid (*Löwenstein* 1907), in kidney, liver and lung (*Pisano* 1910), in bile duct epithelia (*Mouchet* 1911) and in the thyroid (*Pettavel* 1911) of newborns and infants. In 1925 *v. Glahn* and *Pappenheimer* described a case of generalized cytomegaly in a male patient of 36 yrs, postulating a viral etiology of the disease. A few years previously, *Lipschütz* (1921) had shown the agent provoking the nuclear inclusions typical of several herpes diseases to be experimentally transferable. In 1934, *Cowdry* suggested that the nuclear inclusions he would call "type A", and which were chiefly observed in herpes and varicella, could be identified as accumulated viruses. The development and perfection of electron microscopy in later years has provided an efficient tool for viral taxonomy, especially of DNA viruses, by exact morphologic criteria (review see *Almeida* 1963; *Blank* et al. 1970).

1. Pulmonary Cytomegaly

Friedman (1981) has recently emphasized the difference between subclinical infection and manifest disease. Cytomegalic cells are known to occur frequently in the salivary glands of small children (*Farber* and *Wohlbach* 1932). In certain animal species cytomegalic cells are found with great regularity in the salivary glands of obviously healthy animals: In the guinea pig, these cells were described by *Cole* and *Kuttner* (1926) at a rate of 84%, in the North American mole by *Rector* and *Rector* (1934) in 14/14 salivary glands. Cytomegaly of salivary glands is found almost regularly in apparently healthy European and Algerian hedgehogs (*Günther* and *Schaefer* 1981), and was recently observed by us also in the common shrew mouse (Crocidura russula).

The presence of cytomegalic cells in the lung is usually associated with generalized cytomegalic disease (*Seifert* and *Oehme* 1957) signalizing not only subclinical infection but genuine disease which occurs preferentially in newborns or adults with impaired immunocompetence (see review in *Dahm* 1980).

It is still uncertain whether and by what means pulmonary cytomegaly may impair pulmonary functions. Interstitial plasmacytic infiltration of the pulmonary tissue is seen, especially in those forms of cytomegalic disease that are associated with pneumocystic infection (*Hamperl* 1956; *Seifert* and *Oehme* 1957). Pulmonary cytomegaly that is not characterized by superinfections will often show inflammatory reactions of lesser intensitiy, or none at all.

Cytomegalic transformation in its early stages displays an initial proliferation of pneumocytes with increasing cellular size and the development of an intranuclear inclusion visible under the light microscope (Fig. 3), to which granular intracytoplasmic inclusions are later added (Fig. 4). Electron microscopically, the intranuclear inclusion consists of a grid-like accumulation of heterochromatin. The nucleolus is displaced from the centre by this inclusion and can be visualized in only some of the serial sections (Figs. 7–8). Within this grid of heterochromatin it is possible to identify the earliest stages of newly formed nucleocapsids which are extruded from the nucleus, and then become enveloped by a glycoprotein-rich coat within the cytoplasm (Figs.

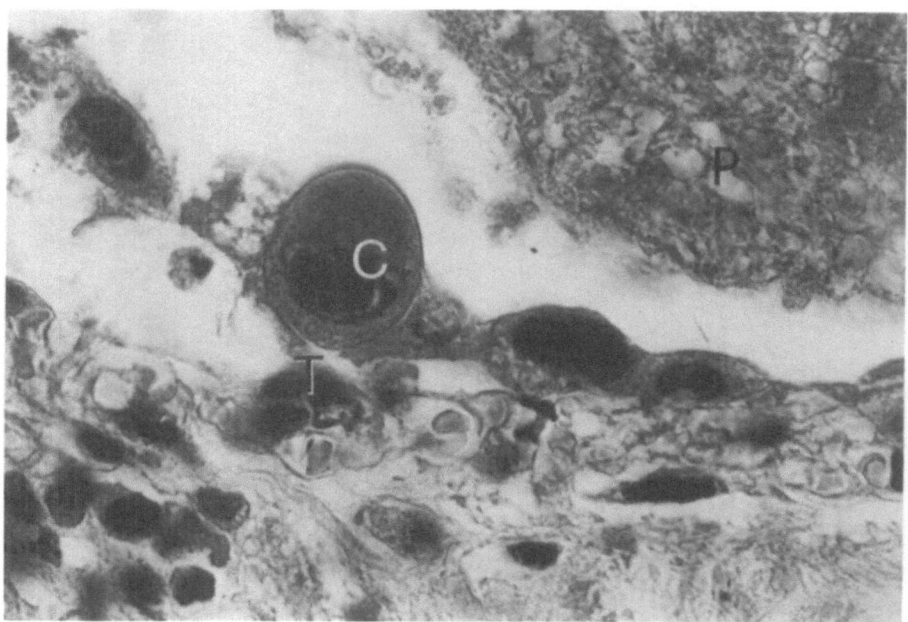

Fig. 3. Combined pneumocystis and cytomegalovirus pneumonia in a male suffering from dyskeratosis congenita Cole-Engman-Zinsser, deceased with 20 years. Beside a cluster of Pneumocystis carinii *(P)*, the development of cuboid hypertrophied pneumocytes into a cytomegalic cell *(C)* with typical nuclear and cytoplasmic inclusions can be seen. Post-mortem tissue, HE-stain

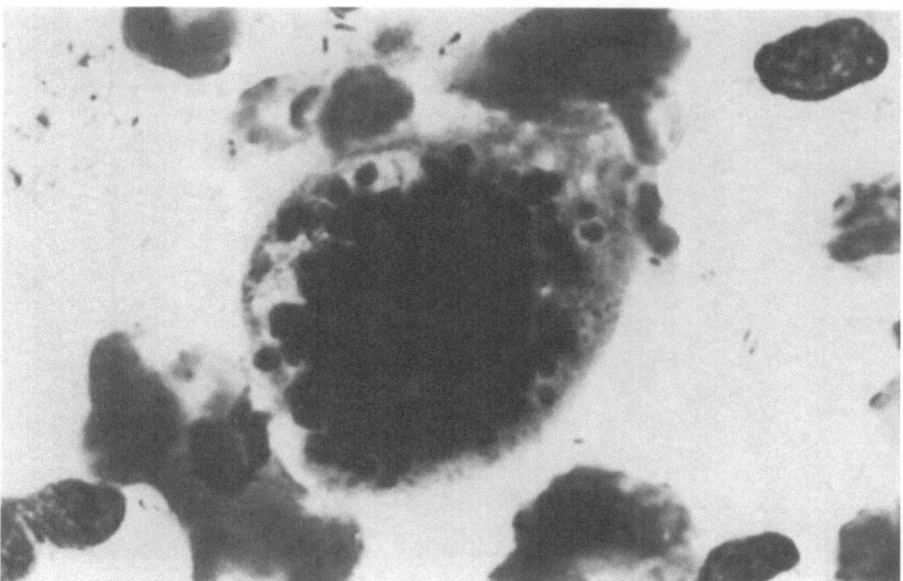

Fig. 4. Cytomegalic pneumocyte in a lung imprint. Coarse granular inclusions obscure the nucleus. Same case as in Fig. 3. May-Grünwald-Giemsa's stain

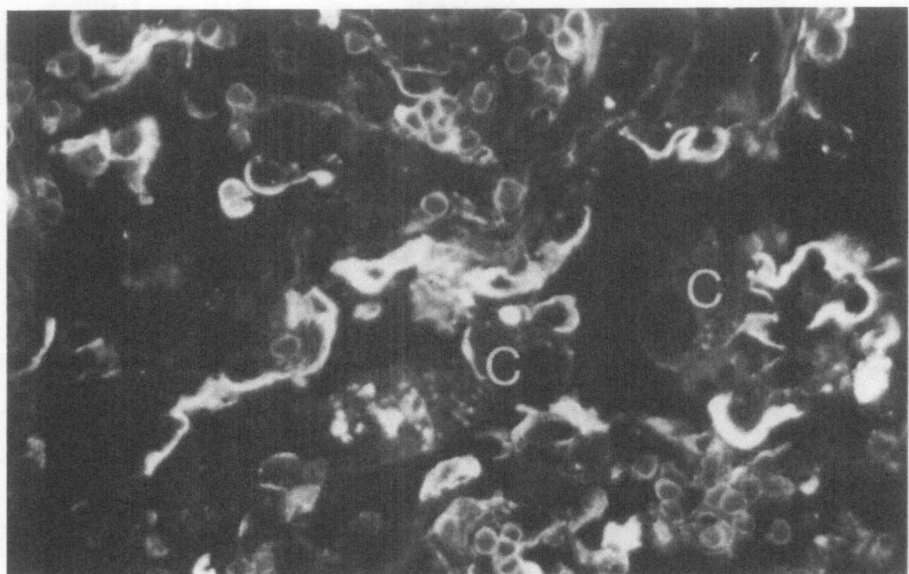

Fig. 5. PNA-binding sites (after neuraminidase treatment) in cytomegalovirus pneumonia (girl dead at the age of 14 years after rejection of a renal transplant): intense linear
fluorescence marks the surfaces of hypertrophied pneumocytes; this surface fluorescence gets lost on the way of cytomegalic transformation *(C);* early cytomegalic cells
develop a faint granular intracytoplasmic PNA-fluorescence. The circular fluorescence
corresponds to erythrocytes (PNA-binding to the Thomsen-Friedenreich-antigen)

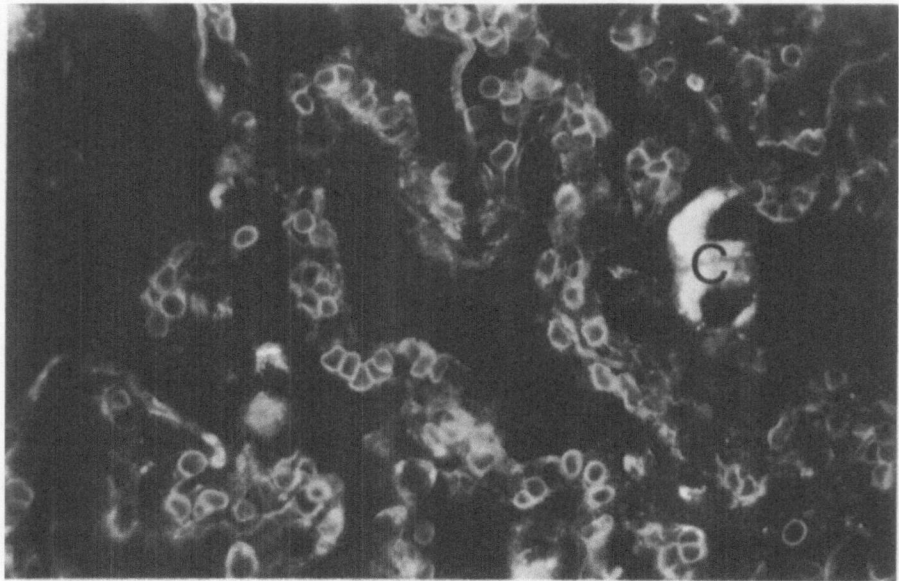

Fig. 6. The distribution of PNA-binding sites in an advanced focus of cytomegalovirus
pneumonia (same case as Fig. 5): two-full-grown cytomegalic cells *(C)* with a bright
fluorescence of intracytoplasmic granular inclusions have completely detached themselves from the alveolar wall. This process results in a complete loss of pneumocytes.
The dilated capillaries of the naked alveolar septa are engorged with erythrocytes
(circular fluorescence)

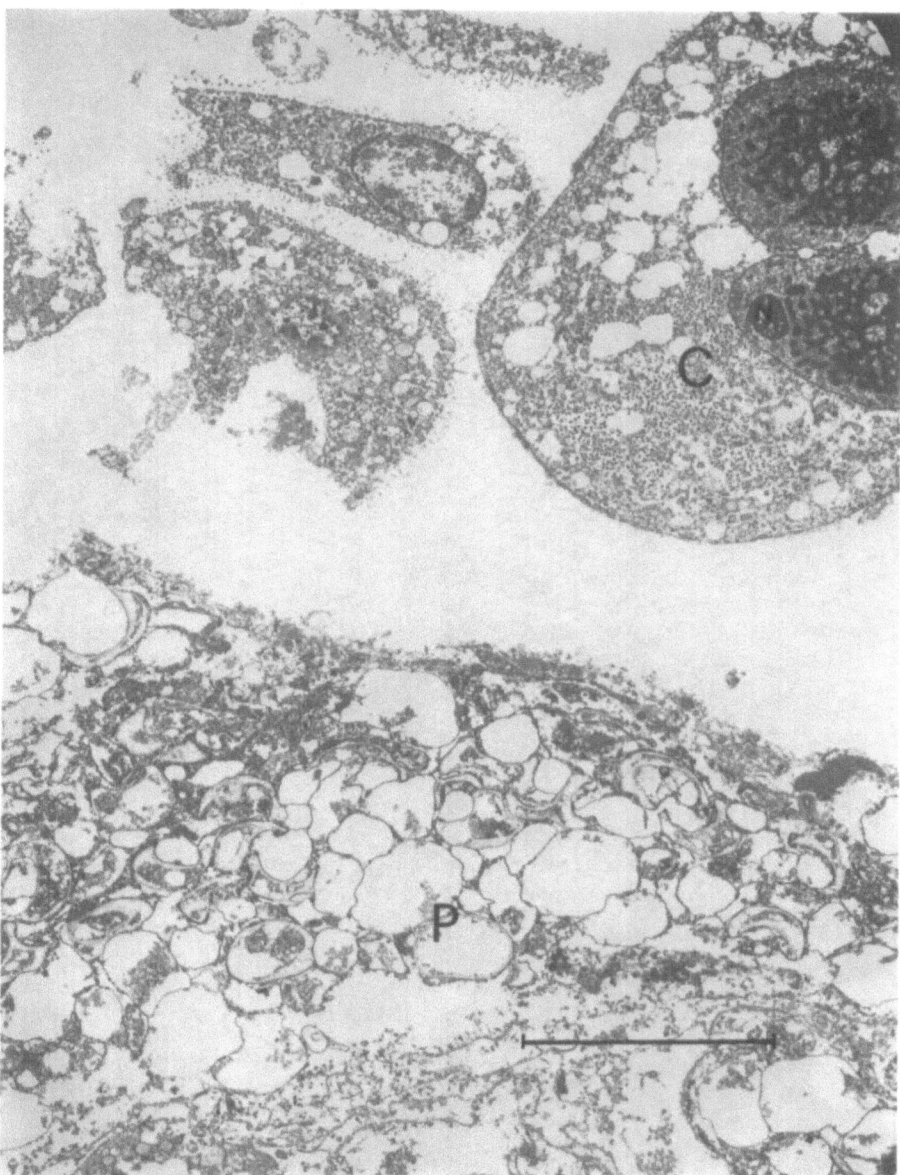

Fig. 7. Combined pneumocystis and cytomegalovirus pneumonia (same case as Fig. 3). The alveolus contains masses of Pneumocystis carinii *(P)*, detached pneumocytes and a binuclear cytoplasmic cell with mature intracytoplasmic virions *(C)*. The large grid-like intranuclear inclusion body has excentrically displaced the nucleolus *(N)*. Electron-micrograph from post-mortem tissue stained by lead citrate and uranylacetate; scale bar: 10 μm

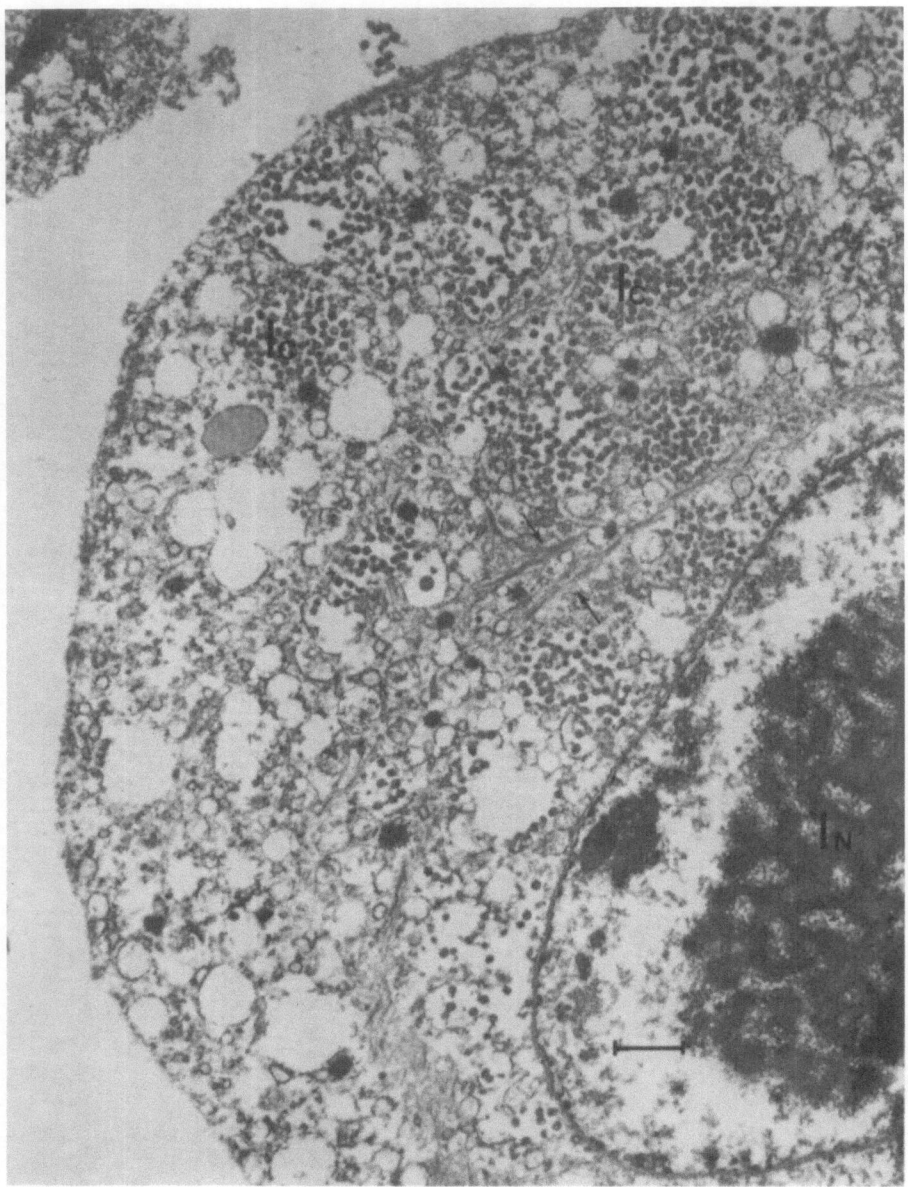

Fig. 8. Cytomegalic pneumocytes (same case as Fig. 3). The cytoplasm contains sparse tonofilaments *(arrows)* and mature virions clustering in vacuoles that correspond to the coarse granular cytoplasmic inclusions *(Ic)* as seen in the light microscope (compare Fig. 4). The nuclear inclusion body *(In)* is formed by a large grid of condensed chromatin including small circular profiles of immature nucleocapsids in its meshes. Electronmicrograph from post-mortem tissue; scale bar: 1 μm

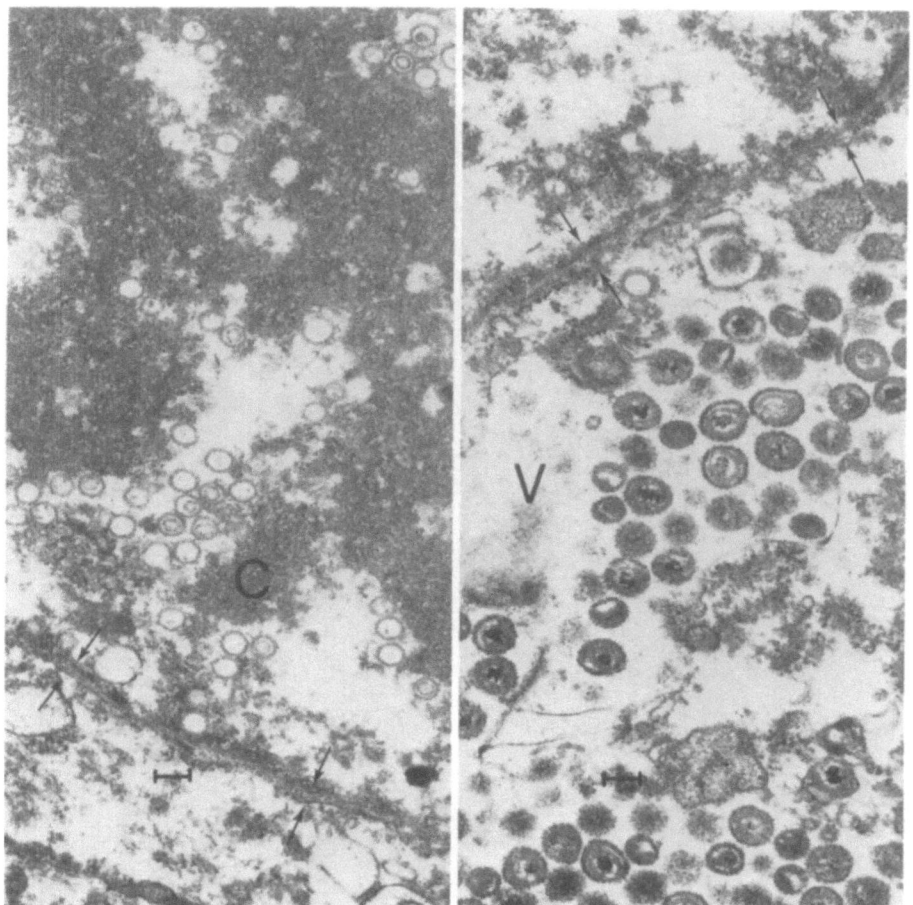

a   b

Fig. 9. Part of a cytomegalic pneumocyte representing **a** circular profiles of intranuclear nucleocapsids closely attached to the strands of the condensed chromatin grid (compare Fig. 8), and **b** mature virions within a cytoplasmic vacuole *(V)*. Perinuclear cistern marked by *arrows*. Electronmicrographs from a post-mortem specimen obtained from a 47 years old male suffering from Wegener's granulomatosis (immunosuppressive treatment) and an ultimate combined pneumocystis and cytomegalovirus pneumonia. Scale bar: 100 nm

9–10). Mature virions of this kind are accumulated in clusters (Fig. 8) that can be demonstrated quite clearly in imprint preparations as coarse, basophilic granules (Fig. 4). In PNA-stained preparations (cf. II.3) these granules show positive fluorescence probably reflecting the structures rich in carbohydrates that envelop the mature cytomegaloviruses (Figs. 5–6). Accordingly, intracytoplasmic inclusions are equally positive in histochemical reactions (PAS, Hale's iron reaction, Grocott's silver method, Alcian blue) for demonstrating carbohydrates or mucopolysaccharids (*Martin* and *Kurtz* 1966; *Ruebner* et al. 1965).

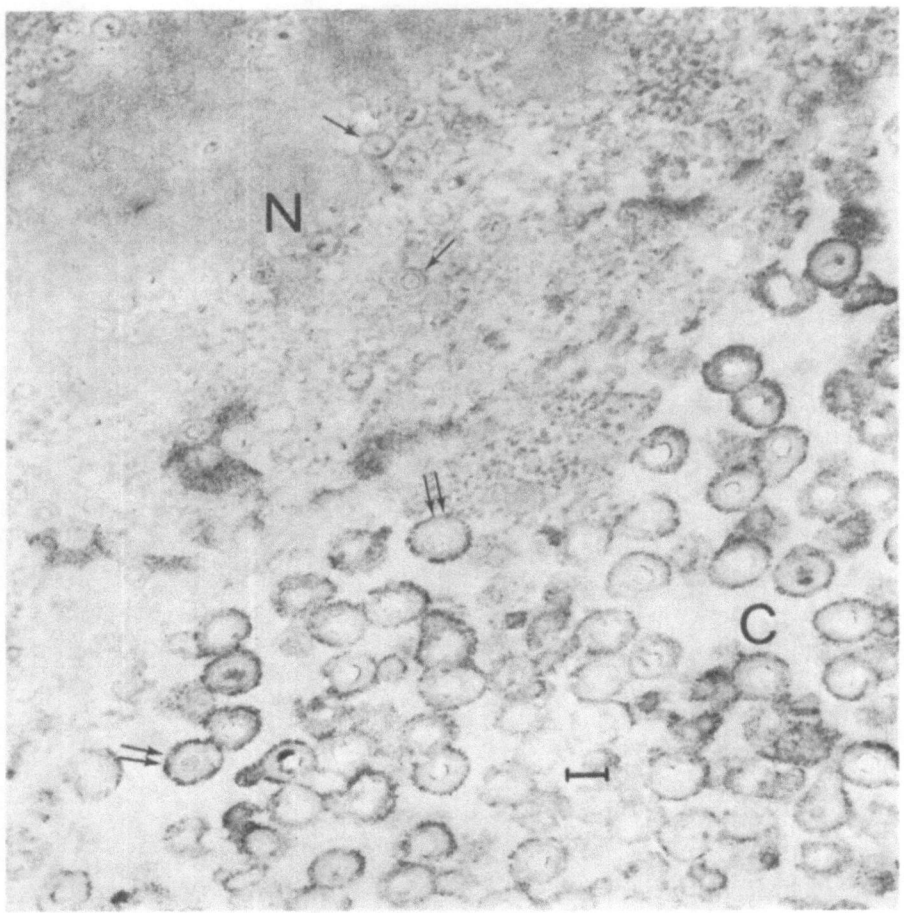

Fig. 10. Part of a cytomegalic pneumocyte (same case as Fig. 3) stained with lead citrate only. The nucleus *(N)* contains faintly contrasted nucleocapsids *(arrows)*. The mature virions *(double arrows)* clustering within the cytoplasm *(C)* are surrounded by opaque envelopes. The intense contrast of the envelope structure is due to the presence of lead binding glycoproteins corresponding to the PNA-binding sites (compare Figs. 5 and 6). Scale bar: 100 nm

The PNA technique enables us to delineate early leasions composed of pneumo-cytes which are more or less hypertrophic and obviously infected. These cuboid cells are assembled in complexes whose surface is marked by increased PNA fluorescence. Surface fluorescence, however, disappears with advancing cytomegalic transformation and development of intracytoplasmic inclusions (Fig. 5). Having lost their surface fluorescence, the completely transformed cytomegalic cells start to exfoliate from the alveolar surface; they are found in the alveolar lumen, especially of post-mortem lung tissue (Fig. 6), a localization corresponding to that of alveolar macrophages. Thus, a development of the cytomegalic cell from the alveolar macrophage might appear

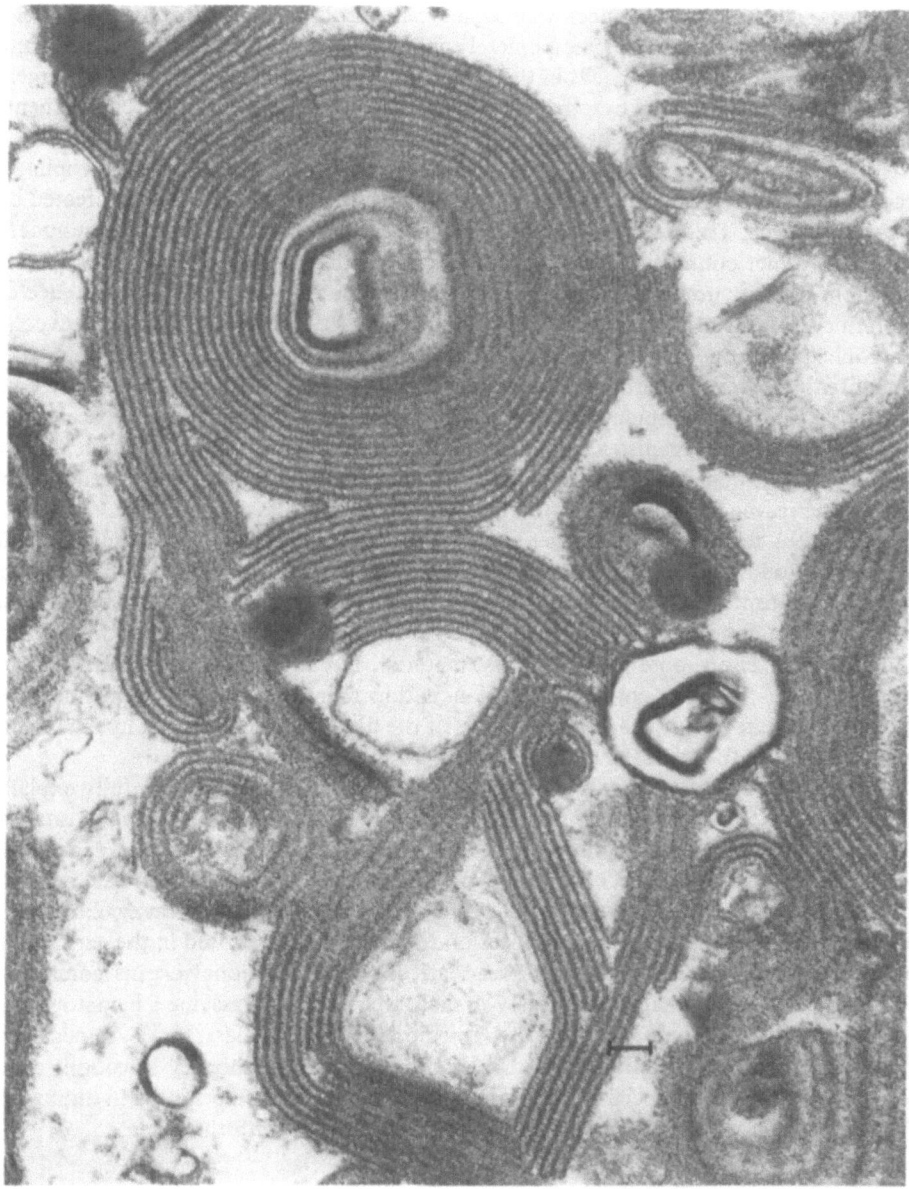

Fig. 11. Impaired macrophage clearance results in an intraalveolar accumulation of lipoproteinaceous, concentrically layered membrane residues. Post-mortem tissue obtained from a combined pneumocystis and cytomegalovirus pneumonia (same case as Fig. 9). Electronmicrograph scale bar: 100 nm

suggestive, all the more so since cytomegalic cells display a high AP activity (cf. II.1). The latter reaction, however, is completely inhibited by the addition of tartrate, and so the origin of cytomegalic cells in the lung from alveolar macrophages, can be largely excluded. In well-preserved cytomegalic cells, ultrasturctural evidence of tonofilaments will be another criterion for their truly epithelial origin (Fig. 8).

Unexpectedly, it became apparent from our material that the alveolar macrophages traceable by the TAP reaction, are extremely rare or even missing in lungs infected by cytomegalovirus. This deficiency may result from the always underlying immunodeficiency. A direct connection between pulmonary cytomegaly and the lack of alveolar macrophages, has not been proven, so far. The frequently observed concomitance of pneumocystis infection may be explained, however, by a lack of functional alveolar macrophages. In one case of combined pulmonary cytomegalovirus and pneumocystis pneumonia, electron microscopic investigation revealed some peculiar piles of concentric convoluted membraneous structures accumulating in the alveolar spaces apart from pneumocystis organisms (Fig. 11). Whatever the origin of these materials, the retention of such deposits points to a disturbed alveolar clearance due to malfunction of phagocytic scavenging activities.

The PNA technique can further serve to trace the focal occurrence of cytomegalic transformation in pneumocytes of the lung. Whenever an alveolar region shows an excess of cytomegalic cells completely exfoliated from the alveolar surface, these alveoli will be almost completely denuded of pneumocytes (Fig. 6). This strictly focal denudation is rarely observed in biopsy material, but regularly in lung tissue taken from autopsies; we may conclude that denudation represents a terminal phenomenon directly correlated with the fatal outcome of the disease. In some cases, hyaline membranes were also found in the denuded zones.

The pathways of pulmonary cytomegaly infectin in man are not yet fully explained. Experimentally, cytomegaly with interstitial pneumonia can be induced in rats and guinea pigs by intratracheal inoculation of high doses of virus (*Kuttner* and *T'Ung* 1935). However, *Brody* and *Craighead* (1974) had been able to demonstrate hematogenous infection in immunosuppressed mice. In these animals intravascular mononuclear cells with manifest virus replication had been demonstrated in the early phase of infection. In view of the widespread affection of additional organs commonly associated with pulmonary cytomegaly in man, we may safely assume a hematogenous spread of viral infection in this disease. It is possible, nevertheless, that cytomegaly of the lung, especially in adults, is an expression of primary pulmonary infection; virus-replicating mononuclear cells like those typical of hematogenic spread in animal infections, have not been observed to date in human patients with this disease.

2. Varicella Pneumonia

Although varicella virus is classified together with herpes virus, Epstein-Barr virus and cytomegalovirus in one category characterized by certain structural relationships (*Timbury* and *Edmond* 1979), the morphologic picture of pneumonia due to varicella is distinctly different from that of pulmonary cytomegaly.

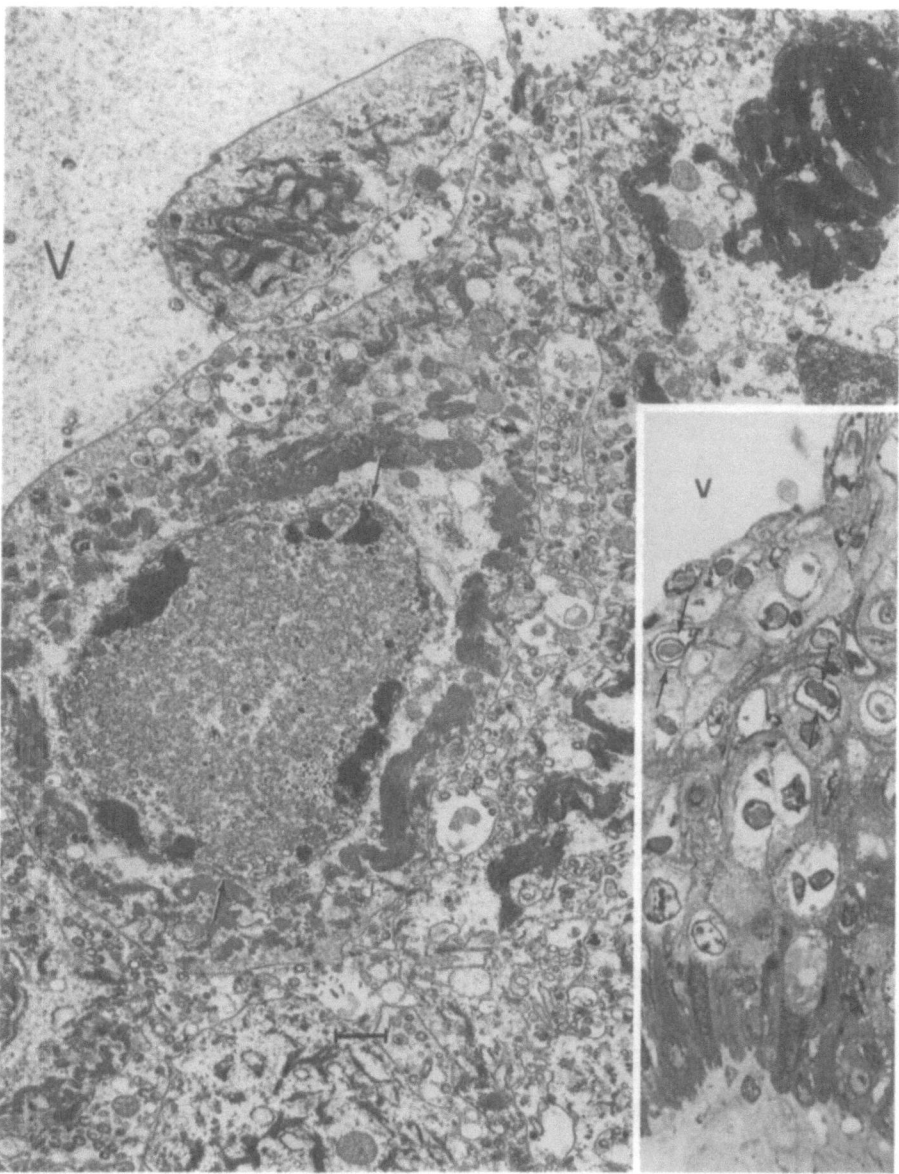

Fig. 12. Varicella blister. Electronmicrograph of a virus-replicating epidermal nucleus *(arrows)*, situated beneath the lumen of the vesicle *(V)*. In part chromatin has become marginated and condensed. The remainder nucleus consists of a homogenous, fine granular material and peripherally situated circular profiles of immature virions budding into the cytoplasm. This peculiar ultrastructural arrangement corresponds to the more homogenous looking lightmicroscopical appearance of the inclusion bodies as seen in the inset at lefthand. Post-mortem specimen obtained from a 3 years old girl, suffering from acute lymphoblastic leukaemia, prior to fatal generalized varicellosis. Scale bar: 1 μm

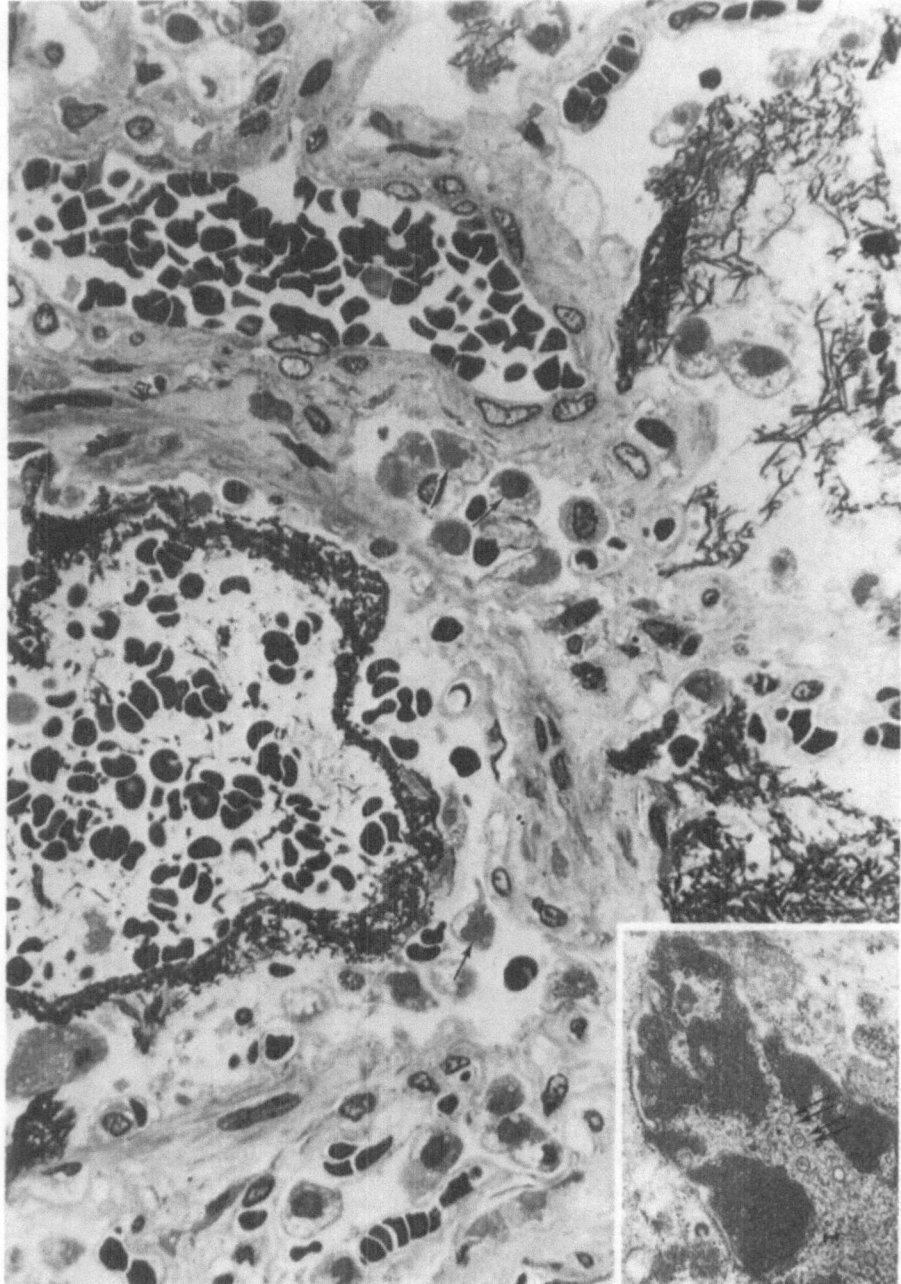

Fig. 13. Varicellosis pneumonia (same case as Fig. 12). The denuded alveoli are covered by hyaline membranes and contain a haemorrhagic exsudate. There are homogenous nuclear inclusions in the few remaining, unless desquamating pneumocytes. Semithin section from Epon-embedded post-mortem tissue, Mallory's stain. *Inset:* Electronmicrograph showing few intranuclear virions *(double arrows)* in an endothelial nucleus. Scale bar: 100 nm

Two forms of varicella pneumonia can be distinguished by clinical criteria: while the normal varicella infection of childhood takes a rather harmless dermotropic course only rarely associated with pulmonary complications, some fatal cases have been described in newborns who had acquired a transplacental infection from primary varicellosis of the mother (*Waring* et al. 1942; *Oppenheimer* 1944; *Lucchesi* et al. 1947; *Weinstein* et al. 1956; further review in *Taylor-Robinson* and *Caunt* 1972). If adults are exposed to varicella infection for the first time, primary varicella pneumonia of varying severity may develop as reported by *Frank* (1950), *Knyvett* (1966) and *Triebwasser* et al. (1967).

Pneumonic complications occur in adults at the rate of 16%, but at only 5% in children beyond the neonatal period (*Weinstein* and *Meade* 1956). In childhood, the nature and severity of such complications is mostly determined by bacterial superinfections, predominantly by Haemophilus influenzae, whereas in adults the course depends primarily on the effects of viral infection itself. Generally, varicellosis pneumonia takes a more severe course in adults than in children. Apart from the special form of fatal perinatal varicellosis pneumonia, similar infections with a fatal outcome have been observed in children after immunosuppressive therapy (*Sperk-Bard* et al. 1977).

The morphologic characteristics of varicellosis pneumonia in both children and adults are an exudative necrotizing form of inflammation with predominantly lymphomonocytic infiltration particularly in the interstitial area. Necrotizing lesions will often begin in terminal bronchioles, and necrotic epithelial cells exfoliate from the surfaces of bronchioles and alveoli. In the marginal areas of these foci we may find typical inclusions in epithelial nuclei (Fig. 13) whose structure resembles that of epidermal vesicles (Fig. 12). In varicella pneumonia of neonates, the cellularity of inflammatory exudates appears to be rather low (*Oppenheimer* 1944). Hyaline membranes may develop in zones of extensive bronchiolar and alveolar epithelial necrosis (Fig. 13).

In cases of fatal varicellosis in infancy, necrotic foci with intranuclear inclusions appear to be disseminated in other organs, especially in the liver. While viral inclusion bodies are formed predominantly in epithelial cells, electron microscopy reveals few virions in endothelial nuclei as well (*Sperk-Bard* et al. 1977; Fig. 13).

Limited notice has been taken of another late sequel to varicella pneumonia of adults. In a large series of such cases, *Knyvett* (1966) described the formation of central necrotic foci with calcifying and nodular scarring, which he was able to differentiate convincingly from similar residual foci of tuberculosis or histoplasmosis.

3. Adenovirus Pneumonia

The discovery of the adenoviruses was also initiated by the pathoanatomical description of typical inclusion bodies marking both in-vitro and in-vivo infected cells with active virus replication (*Meerbach* et al. 1968; *Güthert* et al. 1969; *Strano* 1976). The first observation of such inclusions was reported by *Goodpasture* et al. (1939). In two children dying of epidemic pneumonia, these authors found evidence of atypical necrotizing bronchopneumonia with intranuclear inclusions; their smaller size and lack of intracytoplasmic inclusions permitted the correct differentiation from cytomegalic inclusion disease. In contrast to herpes, the presumed viral agent was not transferable to rabbits. As late as 1953 *Rowe* et al. were able to isolate an "adenoid degeneration agent" from the tonsil; it was identical with the virus isolated by *Hilleman* and *Werner* (1954) from patients who (in the winter of 1952/53, Fort Leonard/Missouri) had been affected by an epidemic of acute respiratory disease or by primary atypical pneumonia (without cold agglutinins). On account of their presence in latently infected tonsils and adenoids, these viruses, subclassified into several subgroups, were termed adenoviruses (*Bell* et al. 1956).

Respiratory infection by adenoviruses has been recorded particularly often in persons living in close communities such as soldiers living in barracks (*Hilleman* and *Werner* 1954), in pediatric wards (*Chany* et al. 1958; *Teng* 1960) or in large families (*Osada* and *Hanayama* 1958). In familial occurrence, adenoviral infection would occasionally show different manifestations in the individual members of a family: While infants reacted with severe and even fatal pneumonia, adults would only get keratoconjunctivitis, common cold or febrile pharyngitis. These differences depend essentially on the age and immune reactivity of the individual patient. In cases of fatal bronchopneumonia, however, serotypes 3 and 7 were found to predominate (*Schier* 1957; *Chany* et al. 1958; *Osada* and *Manayama* 1958; *Kawai* 1959; *Teng* 1960; *Hsiung* 1963; *Wright* et al. 1964; *Becroft* 1969; further reviews in *Schier* et al. 1965). Serotypes 2, 3, 7 and 9 had been isolated from epidemic adenoviral infections (*Beale* et al. 1957).

In view of the very wide spread of adenoviral infections we have to ask whether reactivation of a latent infection might be specifically associated with pneumonic manifestations. The very frequency of epidemics of pneumonic respiratory disease in childhood, seems to speak against this interpretation. Moreover, latently infected tonsils were found to contain predominantly serotypes 1, 2 and 5 which occur rarely or exceptionally (type 1: *Deinhardt* et al. 1958) in pneumonic manifestations (*Evans* 1958). Fatal adenoviral pneumonia, as described sporadically in adults, may in fact be an exception: Adenoviral pneumonia in adults has been reported during renal transplant rejection (*Myerowitz* et al. 1975) and in several immune deficiencies (*Wigger* and *Blanc* 1966; *Roos* et al. 1972; *Chou* et al. 1973) as well as in newly recruited soldiers under stress (*Schier* et al. 1957; *Levin* et al. 1967; type 4: *Budding* et al. 1972). Our two cases (a man of 34 with secondary adenovirus pneumonia in chronic tuberculosis, and a man of 44 with adenovirus pneumonia after a traffic accident) may be classified among these sporadic pneumonias of adenoviral origin.

Independent of the patient's age, fatal adenovirus pneumonias at least, are characterized by relatively stereotypic pathoanatomical changes. Starting from the bronchioles, we see necroses which affect first the bronchial epithelium and glands, and then spread to the alveoli in bronchiolo-fugal direction. The development of necroses is preceded by proliferation and hypertrophy of bronchial epithelia and pneumocytes, the latter being transformed to cuboid complexes whose cell surfaces show at first a somewhat increased PNA fluorescence (Fig. 16). In the nuclei of these hyperplastic epithelial cells inclusion bodies are formed in parallel to advancing virus replication. Under the light microscope, these inclusions appear as homogenous basophilic masses ("smudge cells") rimmed only exceptionally by a slim dense outer nuclear membrane (Fig. 14). Occasionally such cells may take on binucleated forms by fusion. Electron microscopy reveals in these inclusions, an abundance of viruses in paracrystallinic array which have been released in the course of necrotic disintegration (Figs. 17–19).

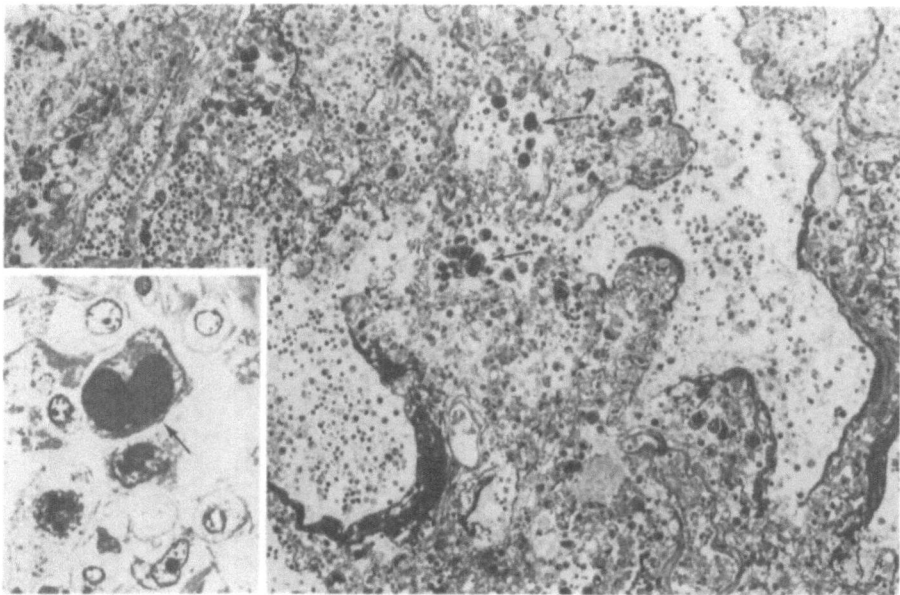

Fig. 14. Adenovirus pneumonia. Necrotizing inflammation in a peribronchial area with widespread karyorhexis and hyaline membranes. Desquamated pneumocytes *(arrows)* contain enlarged inclusion nuclei (smudge cells) filled with virions (compare Figs. 17 and 18). 34 years old male, chronic pulmonary tuberculosis, ultimate fatal adenovirus pneumonia. Semithin section from post-mortem tissue embedded in Epon, Mallory's stain

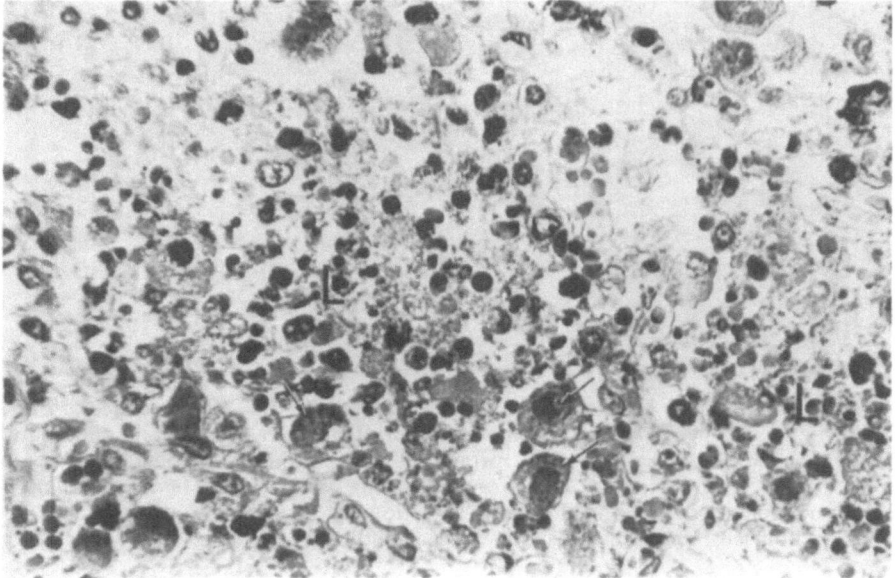

Fig. 15. Adenovirus pneumonia (same case as Fig. 14). Leukoclastic alveolar exudate; granulocytic remnants *(L)* stained (red) for naphthol AS-D chloroacetate esterase. Few desquamating pneumocytes with nuclear inclusion bodies *(arrows)* stained (blue) with Mayer's haemalum

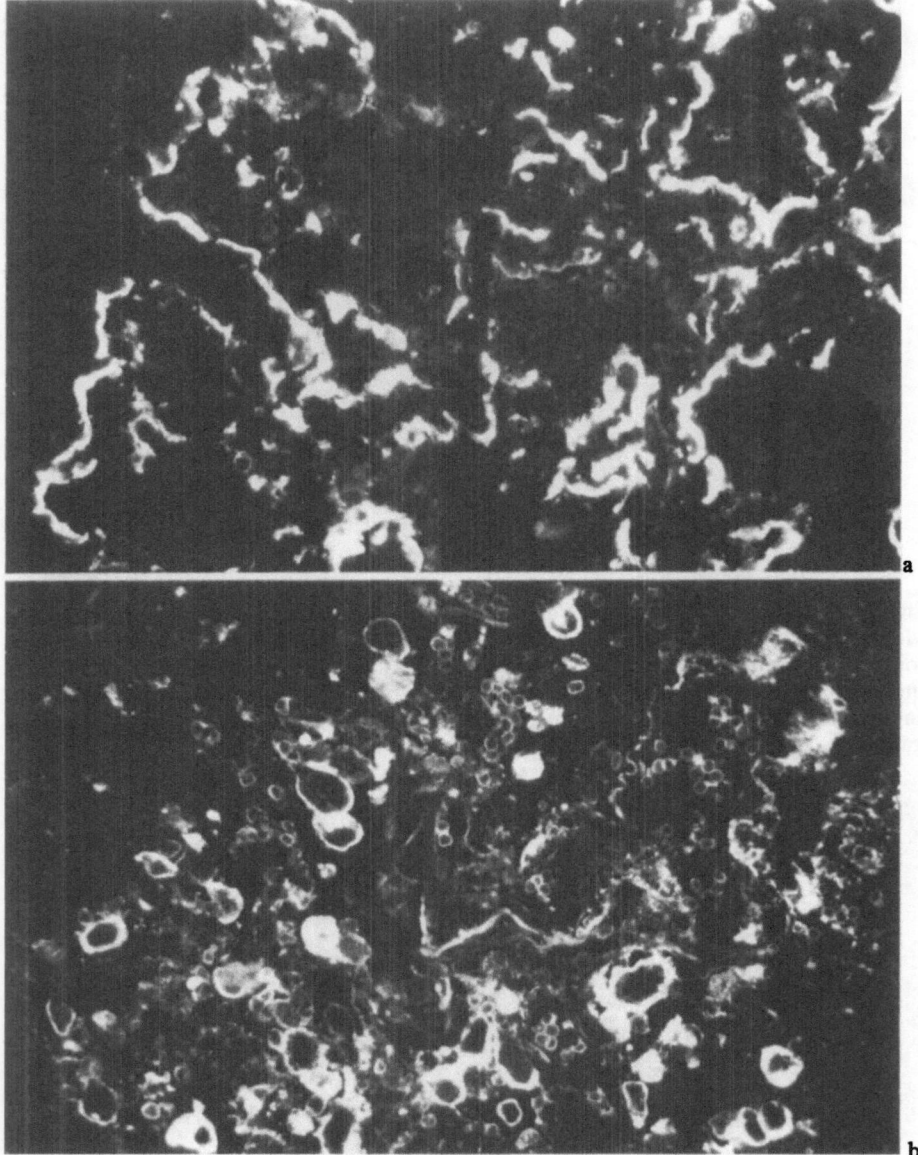

Fig. 16a, b. Adenovirus pneumonia (same case as Fig. 14). FITC-fluorescence of PNA-binding sites (after neuramidase treatment). **a** Peripheral part of a bronchopneumonic focus: enhanced PNA-binding to the surface of proliferating pneumocytes. **b** Central part of a bronchopneumonic focus: virus-replicating pneumocytes (smudge cells) become desquamated. Due to the alveolar destruction erythrocytes (fainter circular fluorescence: Thomsen-Friedenreich-antigen) appear in the alveoles

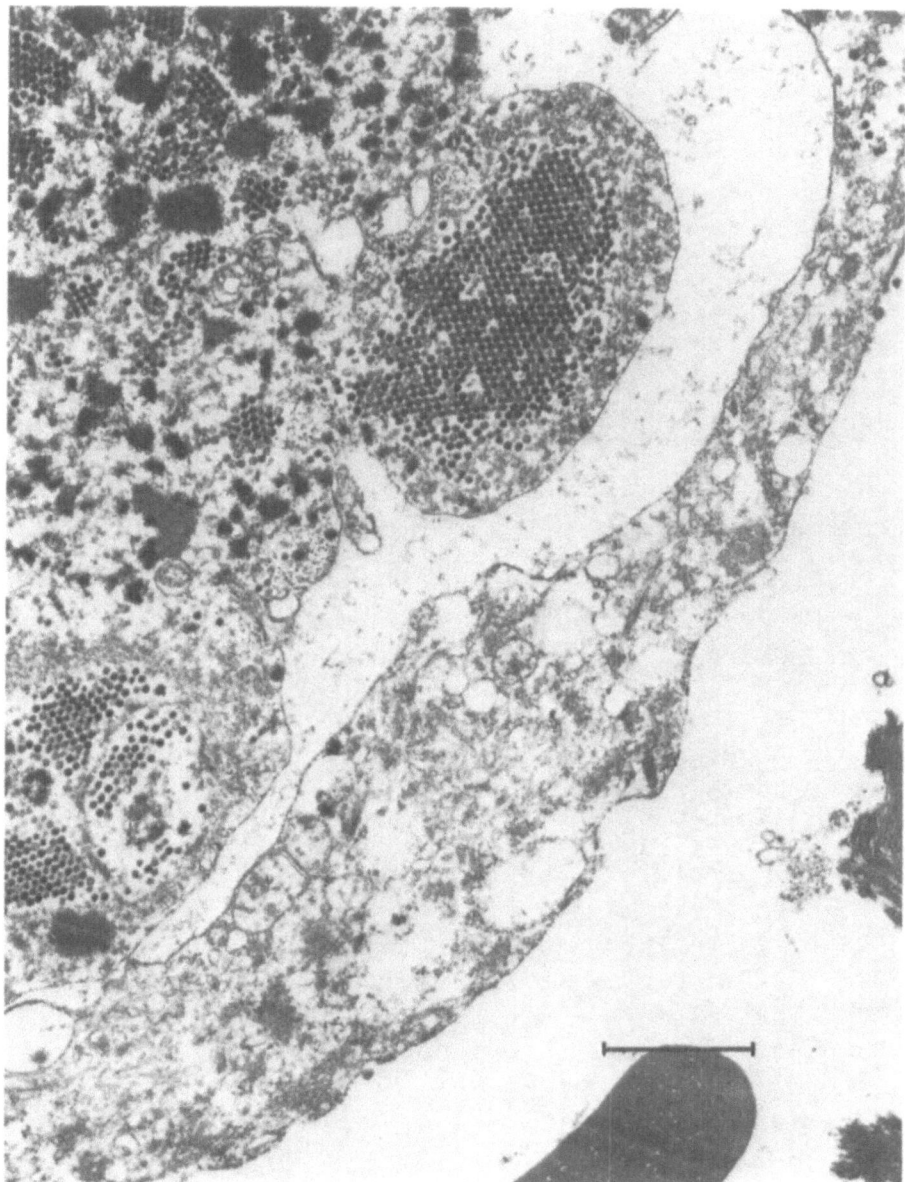

Fig. 17. Adenovirus pneumonia (same case as Fig. 14). Electronmicrograph representing part of a desquamated pneumocyte with a paracristalline arrangement of intranuclear adenovirions. Widening of the perinuclear cistern. Post-mortem material, transferred from paraffin to Epon-embedding; scale bar: 1 μm

174

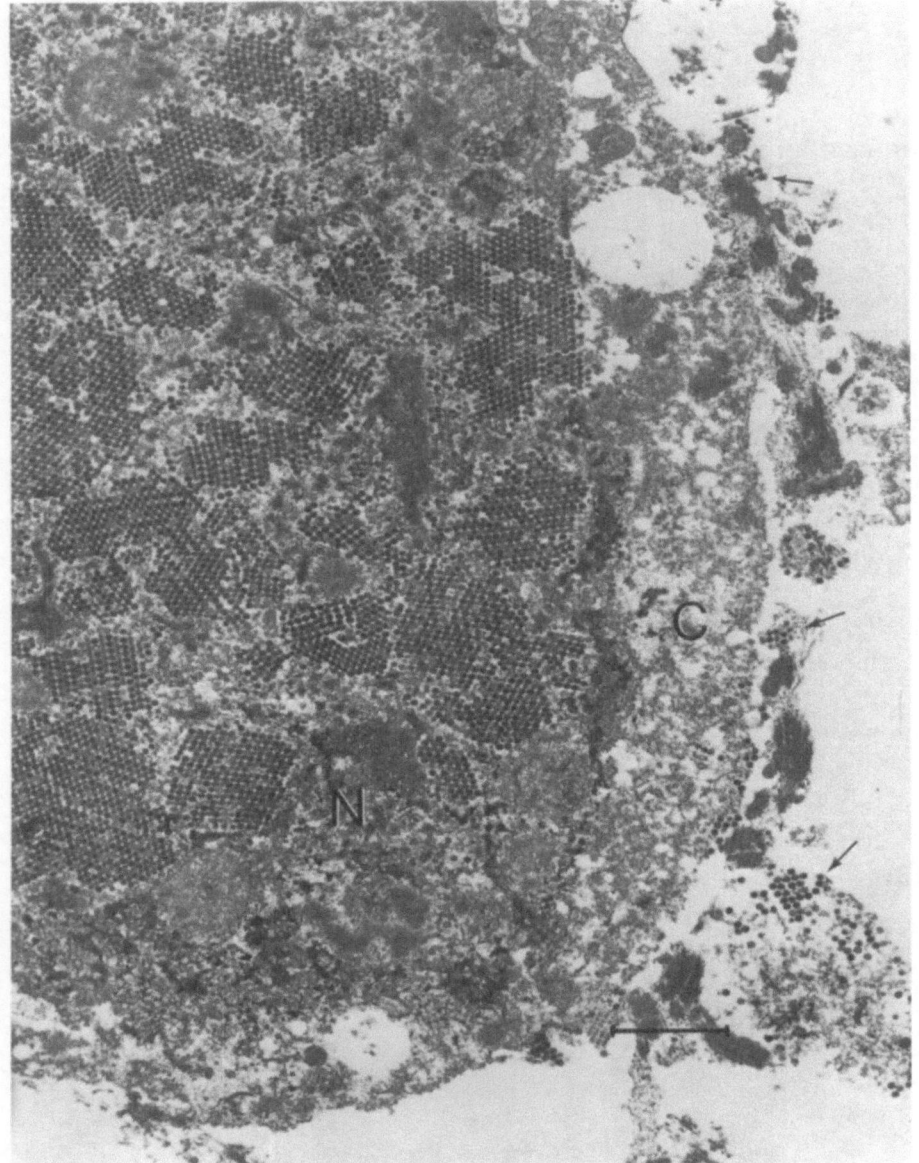

Fig. 18. Adenovirus pneumonia (same case as Fig. 14). Electronmicrograph taken from a necrobiotic pneumocyte with disintegrating cytoplasm *(C)*, shedding virions into the extracellular space *(arrows)*. Numerous paracristalling clusters of virions still remain within the nucleus *(N)*. Post-mortem material transferred from paraffin to Epon-embedding; scale bar: 1 μm

Bronchioles and alveolar lumina become filled with necrotic masses consisting of fibrin and cell detritus. Several authors have emphasized the absence of neutrophilic granulocytes from the field of inflammation (*Kawai* 1959; *Wöckel* et al. 1963). On a first look, our two cases also failed to show any evidence of intact granulocytes. Chloroacetate esterase reaction (II.2), however, demonstrated the presence of numerous enzyme positive granulocytic residues of cytoplasm between the cell detritus filling the alveoles (Fig. 16). Thus, the apparent leukocytopenia must be caused by leukocytoclastic cell destruction, a phenomenon that is well known from the Arthus reaction. We may assume that necrosis, thought to be a typical feature of adenoviral pneumonia, may be at least partly due to the proteolytic activity of released leukocytic enzyme. In this supposed local immune reaction, adenoviruses could play the role of antigens. Our electron microscopic studies have shown that viruses are not only enclosed in the nucleus (Fig. 17) where they would not be available as partners of an extracellular immune response, but that they are also abundantly released from decomposing cells, and then acquire clear extracellular visibility (Fig. 18). This behavior of the adenovirus is well contrasted to that of the cytomegalovirus. Although mature cytomegaloviruses will abound in the cytoplasm of affected cells (pneumocytes), where they accumulate to form intracytoplasmic inclusions visible even by light microscopy (*McAllister* et al. 1963; *Luse* and *Smith* 1965; *Smith* 1959), they are hardly demonstrable outside the cells, neither in vivo nor in vitro (*Ruebner* et al. 1965). Accord-

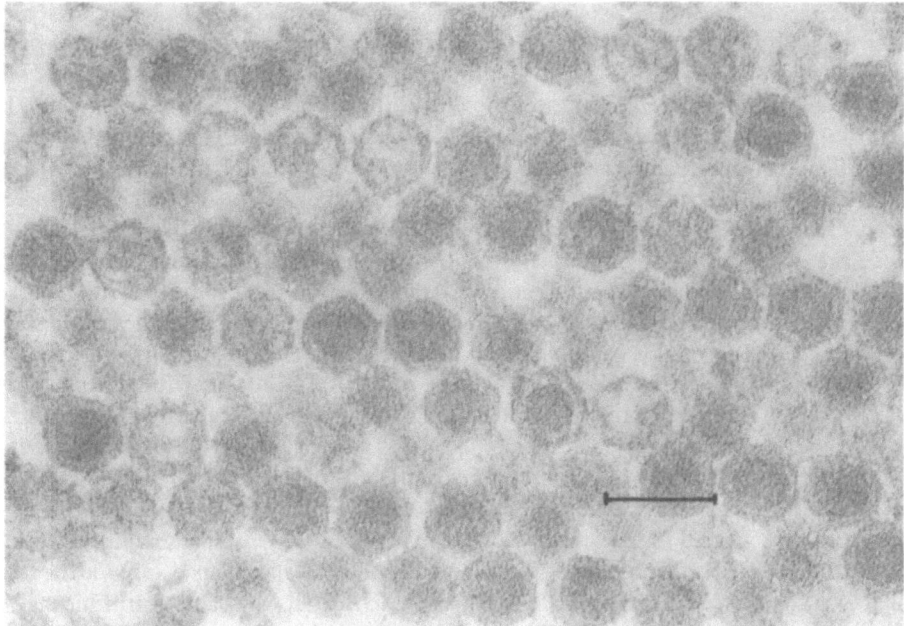

Fig. 19. Hexagonal profiles of adenovirions accumulated in a paracristalline, intranuclear cluster. Electron micrograph from post-mortem material, transferred from paraffin to Epon-embedding. Fatal adenovirus pneumonia, occurring in a 44 years old man after a polytrauma due to an accident. Scale bar: 100 nm

ingly, the phenomena of acute antigenantibody reactions are hardly ever mentioned in the context of pulmonary cytomegalic (*Geiler* 1957; *Seifert* and *Oheme* 1957; *Weller* 1971; *Dahm* 1980).

The tendency to necrosis typical of and particularly marked in adenovirus pneumonia, may also lead to vascular involvement and secondary formation of arterial and venous thrombosis with eventual infarction (*Teng* 1960): If necrotic foci involve the pleura, they provoke pleuritis (*Chany* et al. 1958). Bronchial occlusion by necrotic masses will lead to marked alveolar, interstitial and partly mediastinal emphysema, especially in children (*Becroft* 1967). The particular liability of the juvenile lung to acute emphysema has also been noted in other pulmonary virus infections (cf. IV.1).

Fatal adenovirus pneumonia may be associated with pathologic changes in other organs including perivenous encephalitis. In this context, special attention should be paid to the occurrence of inclusion bodies in adult renal tissue (*Myerowitz* et al. 1975);

IV. Pulmonary Infection by RNA Viruses

Inflammatory diseases of the lung provoked by RNA virus infection are less readily classified by morphologic criteria than infections by DNA viruses. Although the reaction patterns to paramyxovirus, orthomyxovirus, and measles virus infection are relatively characteristic and although even typical inclusion bodies may occur in some cases, their ultrastructural features give no reliable clues to a definition of the viral species involved. In fact, the exact identification of the respective virus depends on serologic followup, on demonstration by viral culture, and on the general epidemiological situation. Culture tests for respiratory syncytial viruses (RSV) have their particular difficulties: due to the specific instability of RSV, such tests in pharyngeal tissue will bring reliable results only if very rapid inoculation of the material is ensured (*Aherne* et al. 1970; *Schneweis* et al. 1966a).

If the organizational conditions are favorable, and the virus concentration is at least 10^9/ml, direct electron microscopical demonstration in negatively stained nasal secrete may succeed (*Donne* et al. 1969). A methodology for these studies was developed and used successfully by *Joncas* et al. (1969b). Here, RSV is visualized as a polymorphous, sometimes filamentous particle of some 200–500 nm with spicular protrusions on its surface, about 15 nm in length. RSV is differentiated from other "enveloped" viruses, in particular from the other myxoviruses, by the diameter of its inner helix (nucleocapsid) of 13 nm (*Joncas* et al. 1969a; *Zakstelskaya* et al. 1967), that of the influenza virus being 9 nm, and of the paramyxoviruses proper 18 nm. Finally, *Aherne* et al. (1970) successfully demonstrated RSV antigen in imprints, and *Shedden* and *Emery* (1965) had even found histochemical evidence in paraffin sections of autopsy material. *Hers* (1963) has been able to do the same for influenza A infection in imprints of lung tissue.

1. Infections by Respiratory Syncytial Viruses (RSV) and by Parainfluenza Virus

Infections by these paramyxoviruses are often epidemic in winter or spring, and are responsible for a large part of all cases of bronchitis and pneumonia in early childhood (*Adams* et al. 1961; *Beem* et al. 1960; *Jensen* et al. 1955; *Reynolds* 1967; *Schneweis* et al. 1966a; *Strano* 1976). RSV infections are in fact the cause of at least 19% (*Vivell* et al. 1962) or even 45% (*Mall* 1981) of children's hospitalizations for acute diseases of the respiratory tract. Since the outcome of such infections is benign in most cases, pathoanatomical data about the group of RSV infections are rather limited (*Adams* 1941; *Adams* et al. 1961; *Gardner* et al. 1967; *Holzel* et al. 1965; *Schedden* and *Emery* 1965; *Schneweis* et al. 1966b; *Strano* 1976; *Wöckel* and *Meerbach* 1968). Experimental results were published by *Coates* and *Shanock* (1962).

The histologic picture of fatal RSV infections of early childhood is relatively stereotypic, i.e. bronchiolitis associated with peribronchial interstitial pneumonia of higher or lower degree (*Adams* et al. 1961; *Aherne* et al. 1970; *Holzel* et al. 1965; *Reynolds* 1967; *Schneweis* et al. 1966b; *Wöckel* et al. 1968). Widely congruent patterns were described in the first papers on fatal infection of newborns by Sendai virus (parainfluenza I) (*Sano* et al. 1953). Intra-alveolar granulocytic and fibrinous exudates seem to be a sequel to bacterial superinfection; haemophilus influenzae in particular, was rather frequently isolated in RSV infections of childhood (*Holzel* et al. 1963). The cell reaction provoked by RSV infection alone is identified as a lympho-monocytic infiltration, especially by monocytes which pervade bronchiolar epithelia and eventually accumulate in the bronchial lumen together with desquamated epithelial cells and mucus (Fig. 20). Incidentally, these infiltrating blood monocytes, having just emigrated from the circulation, differ in several traits (despite their common cytogenetic origin) from the alveolar macrophages frequently found in peribronchial alveoli: infiltrating monocytes still have the typical horse-shoe shape of blood-monocytic nuclei, their acid phosphatase (AP) becomes inactivated by conventional paraffin embedding; in contrast, the nuclear profile of alveolar macrophages is round, they contain the tartrate-resistant isoenzyme of acid phosphatase (TAP) which is demonstrable even in paraffin sections by the histochemical method described in II.2.

Another histologic feature of RSV bronchiolitis is seen in partly bud-like epithelial proliferation (Fig. 21) which may lead to the facultative and often rather unobtrusive formation of multinucleated giant cells. Virus replication inside epithelial cells may also be associated with equally facultative formation of intracytoplasmic acidophilic inclusion bodies of about 3–5 μm (*Aherne* et al. 1970; *Güthert* et al. 1969; *Schneweis* et al. 1966b; *Strano* 1976). Similar phenomena with equally inconstant giant cells and inclusion bodies, have also been observed in parainfluenza infections, especially of type I (Sendai virus) and type III, and so are obviously not RSV-specific (*Aherne* et al. 1970; *Arrobio* 1964; *Delage* et al. 1976; *Buthala* and *Soret* 1964; *Jarvis* et al. 1979; *Noda* 1953). On the other hand *Sano* et al. (1953) in their first description of fatal pneumonitis in newborns caused by Sendai virus infection, had stressed the absence of (viral) inclusion bodies. In fact, *Adams* (1941) was the first to describe inclusion bodies of the types mentioned above (Fig. 22) which he found, during a viral epidemic of newborns in Minnesota, not only in bronchial and alveolar epithelia, but also in adrenal epithelia (cf. *Strano* 1976).

Inflammatory reactions occurring in this category of viral infections (parainfluenza virus, RSV) seem to affect primarily just that area of terminal bronchioles which is lined by nonciliated "Clara cells" (*Clara* 1936). This region of the bronchial system seems to be a preferential site for primary inflammatory changes in other viral infections as stated in *Kromayer's* classical description (1889) of so-called catarrhal pneumonia in measles (and pertussis). The proliferation of cuboid epithelium in and near alveolar passages and adjacent alveoli which had been observed in some very severe cases (type Friedländer 1876), may be interpreted as an excess proliferation of Clara cells involving the alveolar walls. With the advancing severity of this process, epithelial necrosis may develop in the bronchioles.

Terminal bronchiolitis — occasionally necrotic, mainly proliferative — often leads to obstruction of the respiratory pathways which ends in more or less acute, obstructive emphysema (Fig. 20a), clinically manifesting as pseudospastic bronchiolitis; the picture is well documented in clinical and roentgenological publications (*Schneweis* et al. 1966a; *Vivell* et al. 1962). The particular susceptibility of the infantile lung to acute obstructive emphysema has been explained in part by the absence of Kohn's pores, and by the imperfect capacity to resort to bypass ventilation of partly occluded acini (*Spencer* 1973). The loss of cilia from the respiratory epithelia of bronchial mucosa — observed in some cases — may also favor the retention of occlusive plugs composed of mucus and cellular detritus; the process of ciliar regeneration takes no less than 15 days (*Aherne* et al. 1970).

The occurrence of emphysema which may be extreme as well as discontinuous in individual cases can be attributed to these particular features. The findings represented in our Fig. 20a, b were observed in a left upper lobe resected from a boy of 2 months on account of a suspected (histologically unproven) diagnosis of honeycomb lung. In postoperative follow-up, a rise in titers did demonstrate RSV infection, but the clinical course was otherwise favorable.

Histologic phenomena of RSV (peri)bronchiolitis may vary in their individual manifestation. In the perinatal period, especially in premature infants, an almost asymptomatic form may take a rapid course resembling "sudden infant death" (*Hall* et al. 1979; *Hall* 1981). In some cases, *Aherne* et al. (1970) encountered more distinct necroses of bronchial epithelium with enhanced exudate spreading centrifugally to the alveoli. *Spencer* (1973) chose the term "type Becroft" for this necrotizing variant (cf. III.3). These particular features as well as the preferential occurrence of RSV bronchiolitis within the first two years of life, have been explained by conditioning immunologic factors. Generally speaking, the local immunity of a mucosa against respiratory virus infection would depend on the presence of specific antibodies of secretory IgA type (*Bellanti* 1971). Immunoglobulins of this type are lacking in the neonate, and so any exposure to RSV will lead to manifest infection; due to the high rate of infection in the general population, however, most neonates will possess maternal antibodies of IgG type from diaplacental transfer. These IgG antibodies are incapable of preventing the "take" of an infection or the primary virus replication in epithelial cells of the respiratory tract, but they will interfere with subsequent virus propagation in the infant's body. Viruses replicated in bronchial epithelia (*Chanock* and *Parrott* 1965) may induce local accumulation of antigens capable of forming immune complexes (with complement activation with pre-existing maternal IgG anti-

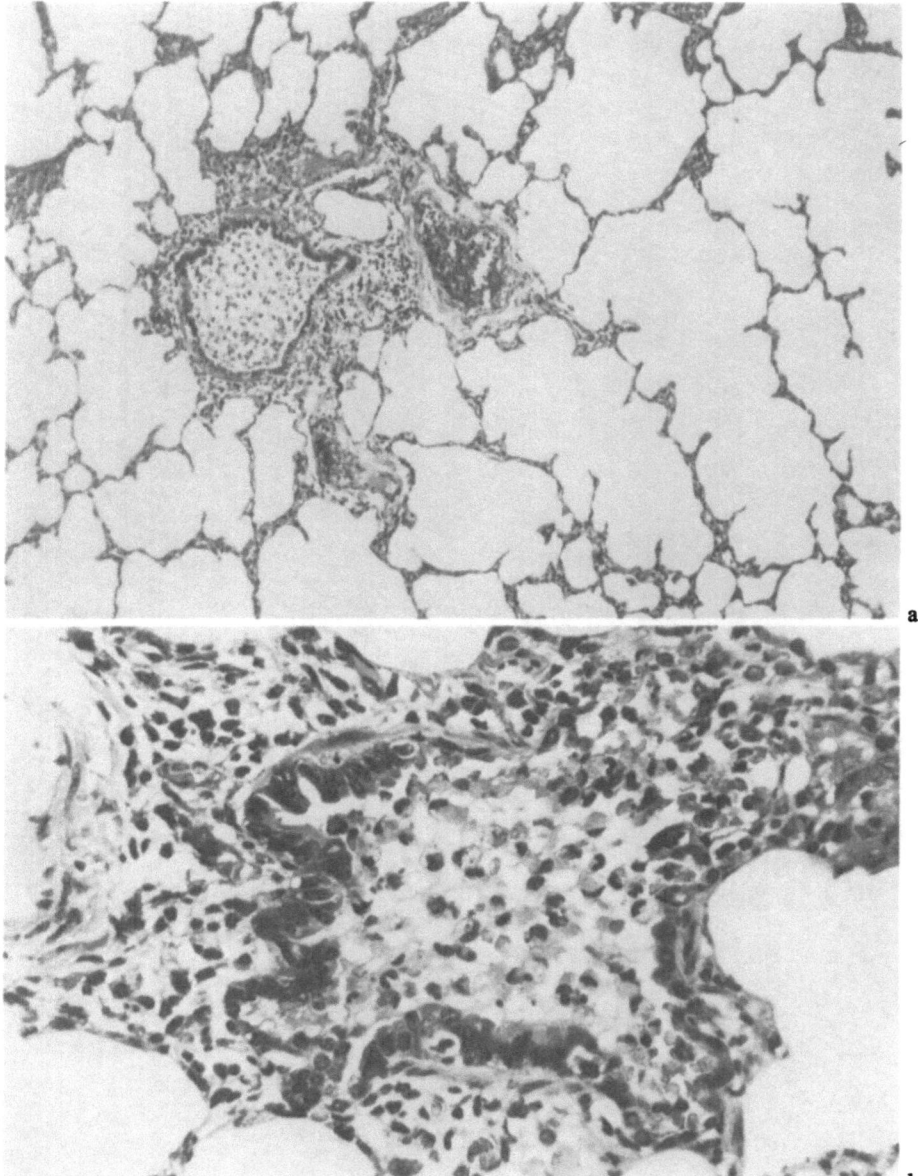

Fig. 20a, b. Obstructive RSV-bronchiolitis in a 2 months old girl. After a few days' febrile process with vomit, cough and progressive dispnoea, the left upper lobe has been resected because of a specious X-ray diagnosis of congenital lung cysts. However, on histological examination the removed lung tissue disclosed an acute emphysema (**a**) due to an obstructive acute bronchiolitis with a predominantly monocytic and lymphocytic cellular infiltrate and small erosive (**b**) or proliferative (compare Fig. 21) epithelial lesions in the bronchioles. After a benign outcome, RSV-infection was proved by a significant titer rise. Bioptical tissue, HE-stain

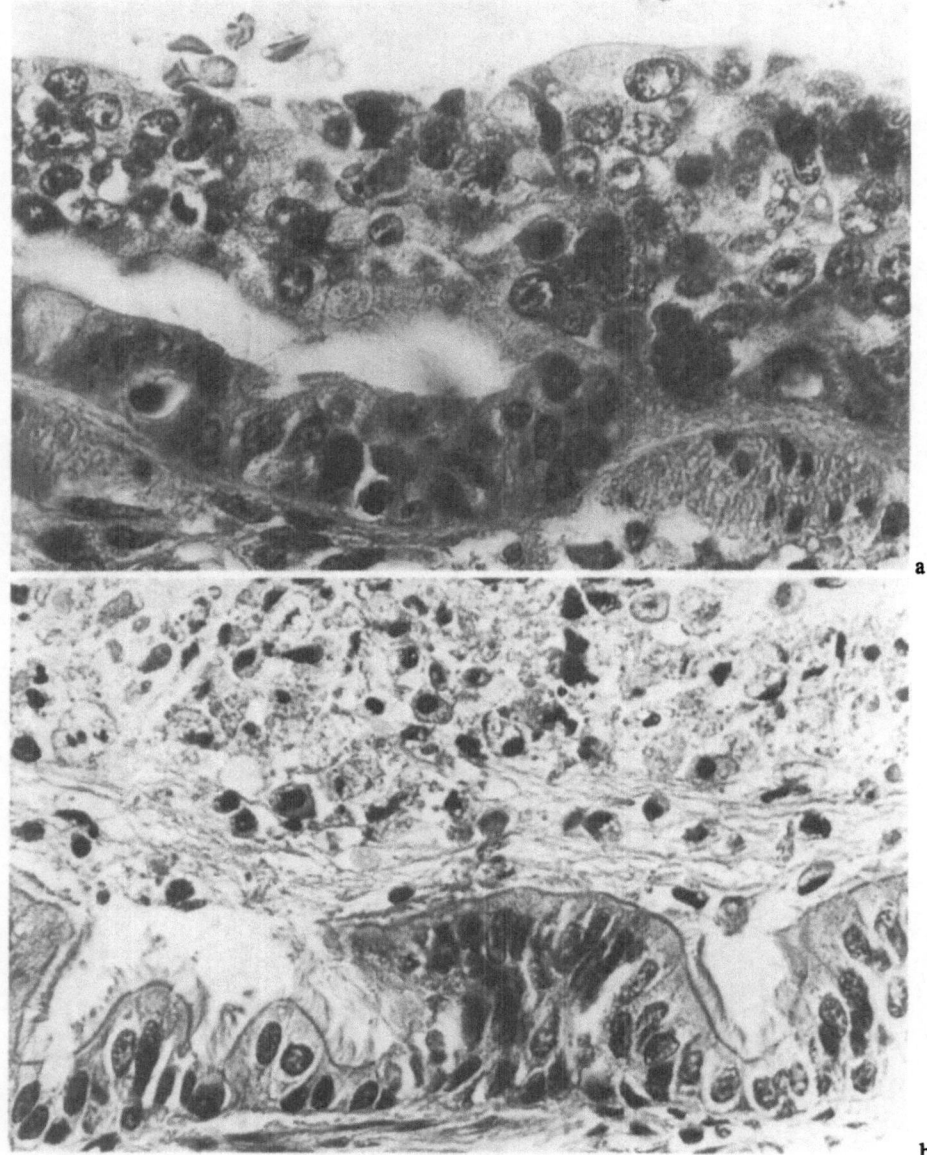

a

b

Fig. 21a, b. Obstructive RSV-bronchiolitis (same case as Fig. 20). a Marked proliferation of the bronchiolar epithelium with sketched syncytial fusion of cells. b The ciliated epithelia of larger bronchi remain intact, the bronchial lumen is obstructed with mucus and cellular debris discharging from smaller bronchioles

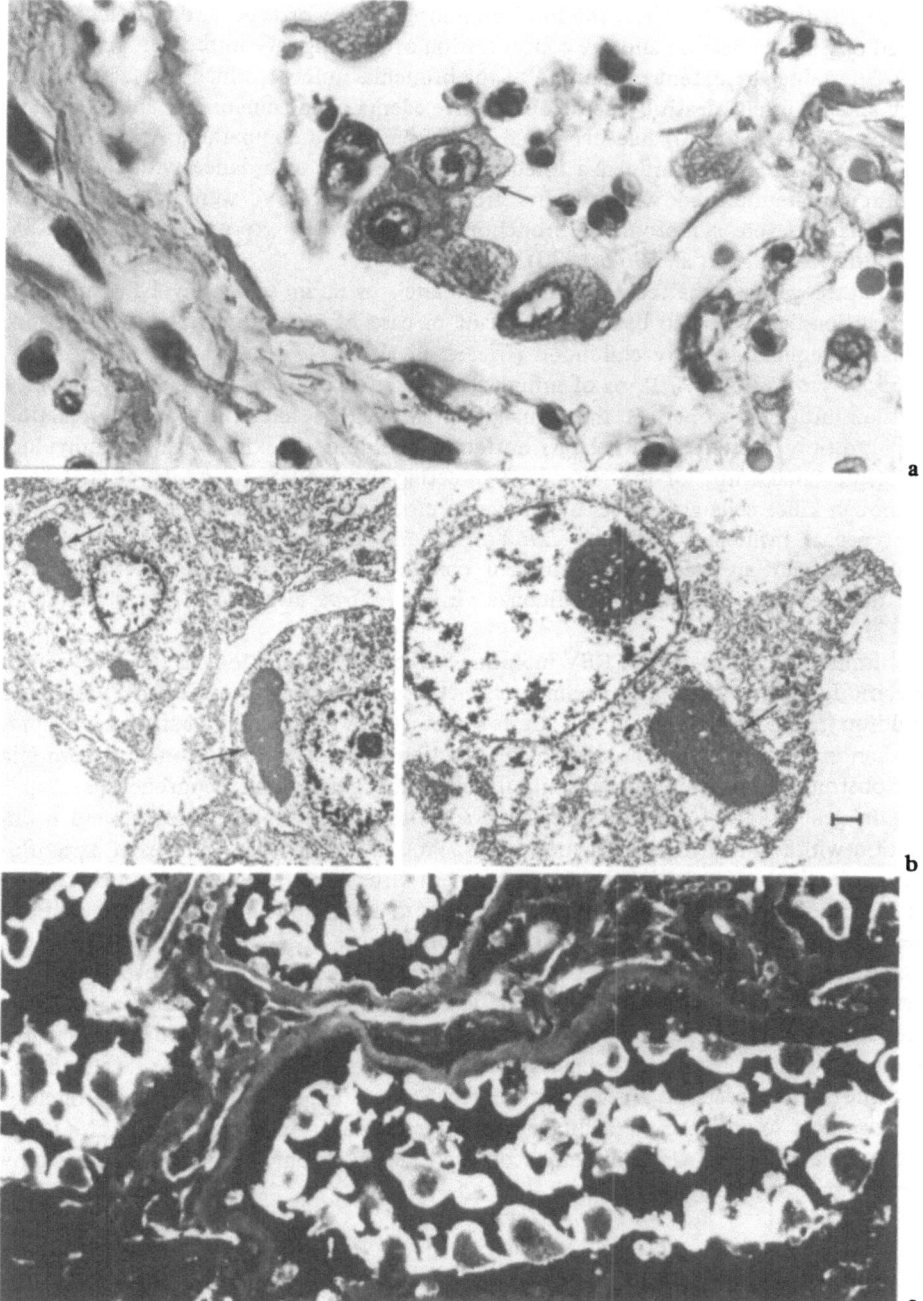

Fig. 22a–c. Presumptive paramyxovirus (not identified) bronchopneumonia with cytoplasmic inclusion bodies, type Adams (1941). a Desquamating proliferated alveolar epithelia contain acidophilic intracytoplasmic inclusion bodies *(arrows)*. HE-stain. b Electron micrograph representing inclusions *(arrows)*. Scale bars: 1 μm. c Enhanced PNA-binding to the surfaces of proliferated alveolar epithelia. Post-mortem tissue obtained from a 55 years old male suffering from Crohn's disease with secondary amyloidosis. Fatal respiratory distress after abdominal surgery

bodies (*Bellanti* 1971). Thus, the local immune reaction of type 3, depending on the speed of virus replication and the concentration of reacting IgG antibodies, can eventually determine the extent of damage to the bronchial mucosa, which may also explain very sudden infant death by acute obstructive edema of the mucosa. In animal experiments *Blandford* (1970) had been able to demonstrate a comparable Arthus-like immune response in parainfluenza infections of mice. In accordance with these facts children preimmunized with vaccine from devitalized RSV, were found to show particularly severe symptoms of bronchopneumonia when exposed to primary RSV infection (*Chanock* et al. 1968, 1970).

Pathologic immune reactions in the neonate's or infant's lung involving maternal IgG antibodies, seem to be less important in case of parainfluenza virus infection, equally frequent in early childhood (*Glezen* et al. 1971; *Jensen* 1955; *Keith* et al. 1955; *Mufson* et al. 1970), or of influenza virus infection. Due to the high variability of their antigenic properties, this virus group is much less likely to provoke a reaction with possibly present maternal IgG antibodies, seldom checking with the individual antigenic "make up" of the myxovirus infecting the neonate (*Chanock* et al. 1970). Although killer cells were recently shown to cross-react with cells infected by diverse subtypes of Influenza A viruses (*Lin Yun Lu* and *Askonas* 1981), the humoral antibodies relevant in the above-mentioned context are known to be strictly specific for the respective subtypes of influenza viruses (*Effros* et al. 1977; *Zveerink* et al. 1977).

Immunity acquired after RSV infection will persist only as long as the secretion of specific IgA lasts. Adults may become reinfected, as observed in nurses of RSV-infected children (*Hall* 1981). In reinfected adults secretory IgA formation will start more rapidly than in primary infection, and so the reactions do not include bronchopneumonia nor obstructive bronchiolitis, but only flu-like symptoms or trancheobronchitis.

In general, the formation of specific secretory IgA antibodies puts an end to infection within a few days, recognizable by a stop in virus release. In cases of parainfluenza infection, chronic forms with permanent virus excretion have been observed in patients with various pulmonary diseases (*Gross* et al. 1973) and also in apparently healthy members of a polar research team (*Muchmore* et al. 1981). In the latter, extreme cold and low air humidity seemed to impair IgA secretion. Moreover, this team living for 8.5 months in complete isolation in an antarctic base, brought incidental proof for the latent persistence of parainfluenza viruses even without manifest virus excretion — in contrast to former experience — which would then be reactivated and become again infectious several weeks later. Some other forms of chronic bronchitis are also able to enhance or facilitate viral infection; according to *Carilli* et al. (1964) more than half of all acute inflammatory episodes in chronic bronchitis are caused by viruses, predominantly by RSV.

2. Measles Pneumonia

The extremely variegated picture of measles pneumonia can only be understood by considering the different immunologic preconditions of the hosts. There are some descriptions of so-called measles pneumonias corresponding, in principle, to the patterns of mostly terminal bronchiolitis with peribronchial interstitial pneumonia and faculta-tive, partly bacterial, lobulo-alveolar pneumonia described above (*Kromayer* 1889; *Feyrter* 1925). The picture of these pneumonias in fatal measles cases is said not to differ essentially from that of pertussis pneumonia (*Giese* 1960). In fact, the very interaction between measles and whooping cough is not infrequently responsible for a fatal outcome of the disease (*Kromayer* 1889; *Feyrter* 1925; *Goodpasture* et al. 1939; *Weller* 1952). Referring to this fact *Spencer* (1973) asked whether Bordetella pertussis could not be an opportunistic germ like haemophilus influenzae, whose pathogenicity depends on primary viral infections. Thus, a pre-existing pertussis may be triggered by subsequent measles infection. Figures 23 and 24 demonstrate the case of a 17-months-old boy who, some days after presenting with a measles rash, developed recurrent symptoms of pertussis and died suddenly. His bronchioles were found to be surrounded by predominantly lymphocytic and monocytic infiltration. Neutrophilic granulocytes (Fig. 23) were found only sparsely in the intraepithelial infiltrations of the bronchial mucosa (by chloroacetate esterase reaction). All these changes had eventually provoked acute severely obstructive pulmonary emphysema. Some intraalveolar giant cell residues dated obviously from the stage of acute measles infection (Fig. 24).

On the other hand, there is *Hecht*'s description of a so-called giant cell pneumonia characterized by the presence of multinucleated giant cells derived from bronchial epithelia — frequently proliferating in several layers, to form transitional epithelial metaplasia — and from alveolar epithelia (*Hecht* 1910; *Masson* and *Pare* 1931). *Masuji* and *Minami* (1938) were the first to publish a detailed description of intracytoplasmic inclusion bodies in these giant cells, although certain intracytoplasmic inclusions had already been mentioned by *Feyrter* (1925) in the giant cells of measles pneumonia. Another description of apparently identical inclusions in pulmonary giant cells can already be found in *Dürck*'s publication of 1887. Abnormal staining properties of the nuclei (*Masson* and *Pare* 1931) or of intracytoplasmic inclusion bodies were men-tioned by *Sherman* and *Ruckle* (1958). However, many of the earlier authors may just have overlooked these intracytoplasmic or intranuclear inclusions, and so *Pinkerton* et al. (1945), in a histologic re-examination of the cases of giant cell pneumonia previously published by *Chown* (1939), *Karsner* and *Mayers* (1913), and *Denton* (1925), were able to trace typical inclusion bodies. *Pinkerton* et al. (1945) also pointed out the morphologic congruence of these giant cells with those found in canine dis-temper (*Green* and *Evans* 1939; *de Monbreun* 1937; *Sinigaglia* 1912). They further suggested that Hecht's giant cell pneumonia might be caused by measles virus which is related to distemper virus, both belonging to the category of morbilliform myxoviruses. Even Hecht himself had actually speculated about the possible relationship between the giant cell pneumonia he described, and the still unknown pathogen responsible for measles; this connection, however, had hardly been considered by any of the later authors, since most cases would come to a fatal end without ever developing measles rash, and often after a history much longer than the usual prodromal stage of measles. The cases published by *Denton* (1952) take a medium position between Hecht's giant cell pneumonia and the typical measles pneumonia without giant cells, in so far as his pneumonia type was rather poor in giant cells, but combined with a typical measles rash.

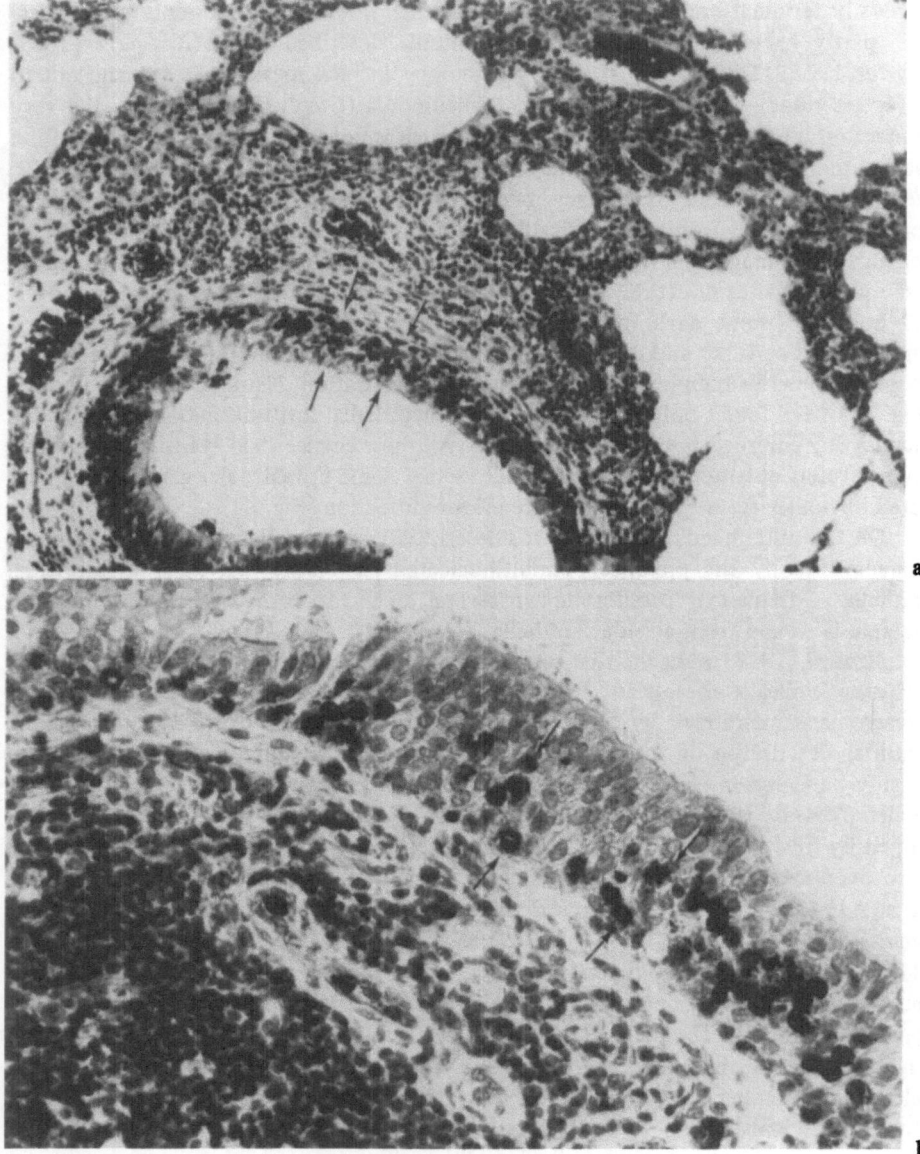

a

b

Fig. 23a, b. Fatal post-measles pertussis bronchopneumonia in a 17 months old boy suffering 3 months prior to death from pertussis. One month before death he developed symptoms of measles with a typical exanthem. **a** Peribronchial interstitial infiltrates, predominantly composed of lymphocytes, histiocytes and plasmacytes. **a, b** The bronchial epithelium is infiltrated by neutrophilic granulocytes (*arrows*) selectively stained (red) for naphthol AS-D chloroacetate esterase (method II.2)

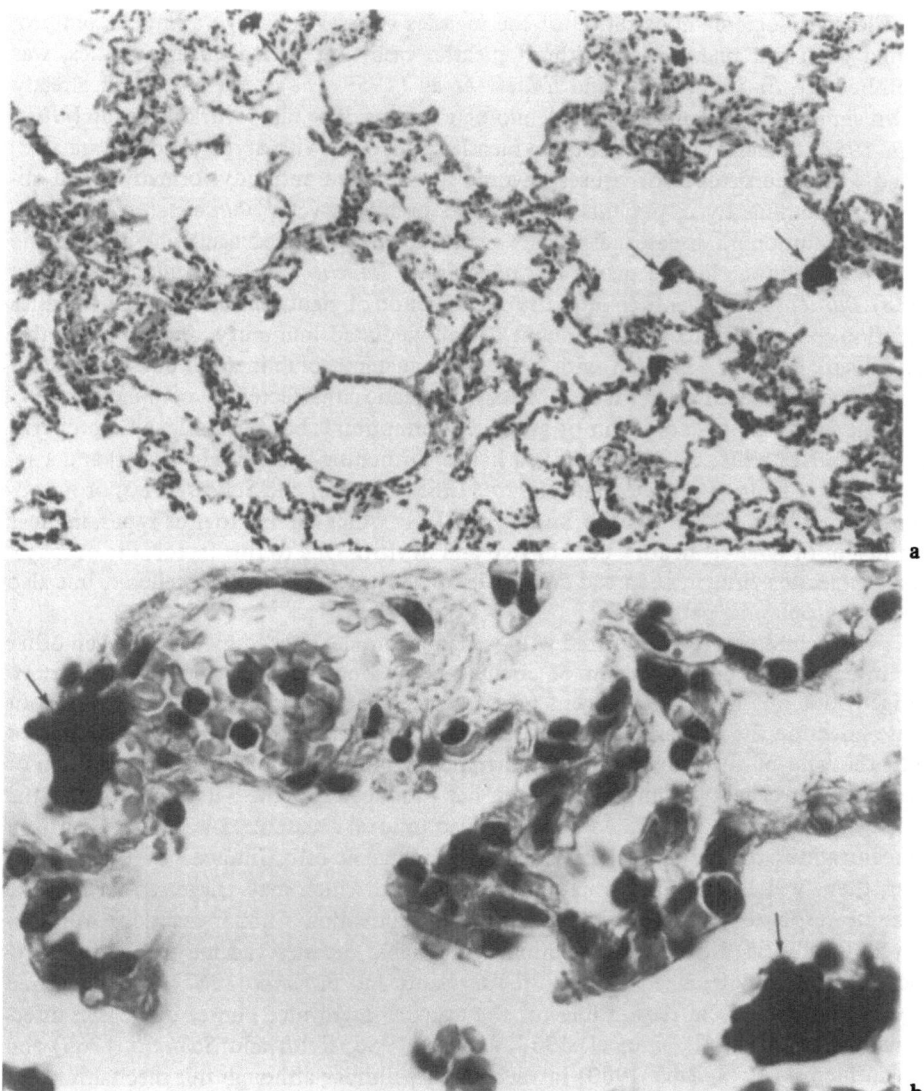

Fig. 24a, b. Fatal post-measles pertussis bronchopneumonia (same case as Fig. 23) a with marked acute obstructive alveolar emphysema. Additionally, autopsy has disclosed an interstitial emphysema. **a, b** There are few remnants of measles giant cells consisting of fused basophilic nuclear masses *(arrows)*. HE-stain

Clear virologic demonstration of the measles virus as causative agent of even protracted giant cell pneumonias without measles rash, but with inclusion bodies, was published by *Enders* (1956) and *Enders* et al. (1959); *Feyrter* (1925) had already drawn similar conclusions from epidemiologic criteria. The same working group (*Mitus* et al. 1959) had also shown that these measles infections with atypical course are associated with a persistence of viruses, favored by impaired antibody formation, and observed predominantly in patients with tumors or anemia (cf. *Fohlmeister* et al. 1979). Several conditioning diseases, especially rachitis, are mentioned again and again in the casereports about Hecht's giant cell pneumonia (*Hecht* 1910; *Masuji* and *Minami* 1938). *Burnet* (1968) wants to refer the phenomenon of giant cell pneumonia in measles infection exclusively to an impairment of cell-mediated immunity. According to this (unproven) concept, children with congenital agammagolublinemia, but with intact T-cell function would always have a history of measles unaffected by complications.

The cytologic phenomenon of giant cell formation is based on a specific property of the measles virus: On its envelope a hemagglutinating antigen (H-antigen) and a so-called fusion factor (*Cascardo* and *Kurzon* 1965; *Choppin* and *Scheid* 1980) or F-antigen are expressed. This F-antigen, known also from other paramyxovirus types, induces the fusion of virus-replicating cells in vivo and in vitro. Due to this factor, the propagation of measles virus may spread from cell to cell not only via extracellular, but also by intracytoplasmic pathways.

When children are immunized with vaccine from devitalized measles or even other paramyxoviruses, the formation of circulating antibodies is directed only against H-antigen, but not against F-antigens (*McClelland* 1980; *Merz* et al. 1980). In case of acute infection the propagation of viruses via extracellular pathways may be suppressed with the help of anti-H-immunoglobulins, thereby possibly impairing the formation of specific killer cells; but since vaccination has produced no anti-F-immunity, syncytial propagation goes on unchecked and may lead to local accumulation of high H-antigen concentrations on the surface of virus-producing giant cells. Induced by the vaccination, there will be a rapid formation of anti-H-IgG which may trigger an Arthus-like immune response of type 3 with complement activation. Similar reactions were observed locally at the site of injection with viable measles vaccine in children prevaccinated with devitalized viruses (*McNair* Scott and *Bonanno* 1967). This undesired reaction has been held responsible for the atypical aggravated course of measles infections (*Buser* 1967; *Nader* et al. 1967; *Norrby* 1966; *Rauh* and *Schmidt* 1965) and parainfluenza (*McClelland* 1980) in vaccinated children, although this mechanism was not documented in cases of giant cell pneumonia.

The particular histologic picture of measles giant cell pneumonia is now interpreted to be the result of superimposing immunologically uncontrolled F-antigen activity (possibly via T-killer cell deficiency) and proliferative bronchiolitis together with interstitial peribronchial pneumonia, both known from other myxoviral infections. As an expression of deficient T cell function, the extent of interstitial lymphocytic infiltration is probably lower in fully developed giant cell pneumonia than it is in measles pneumonia *without* giant cells. Not only the giant cells of hyperplastic bronchoepithelial complexes (Fig. 25), but also intra-alveolar giant cells (Fig. 26) are of epithelial origin. According to our own observations, neither bronchial nor alveolar giant cells contain TAP (cf. II.2), in contrast to alveolar macrophages and foreign body giant

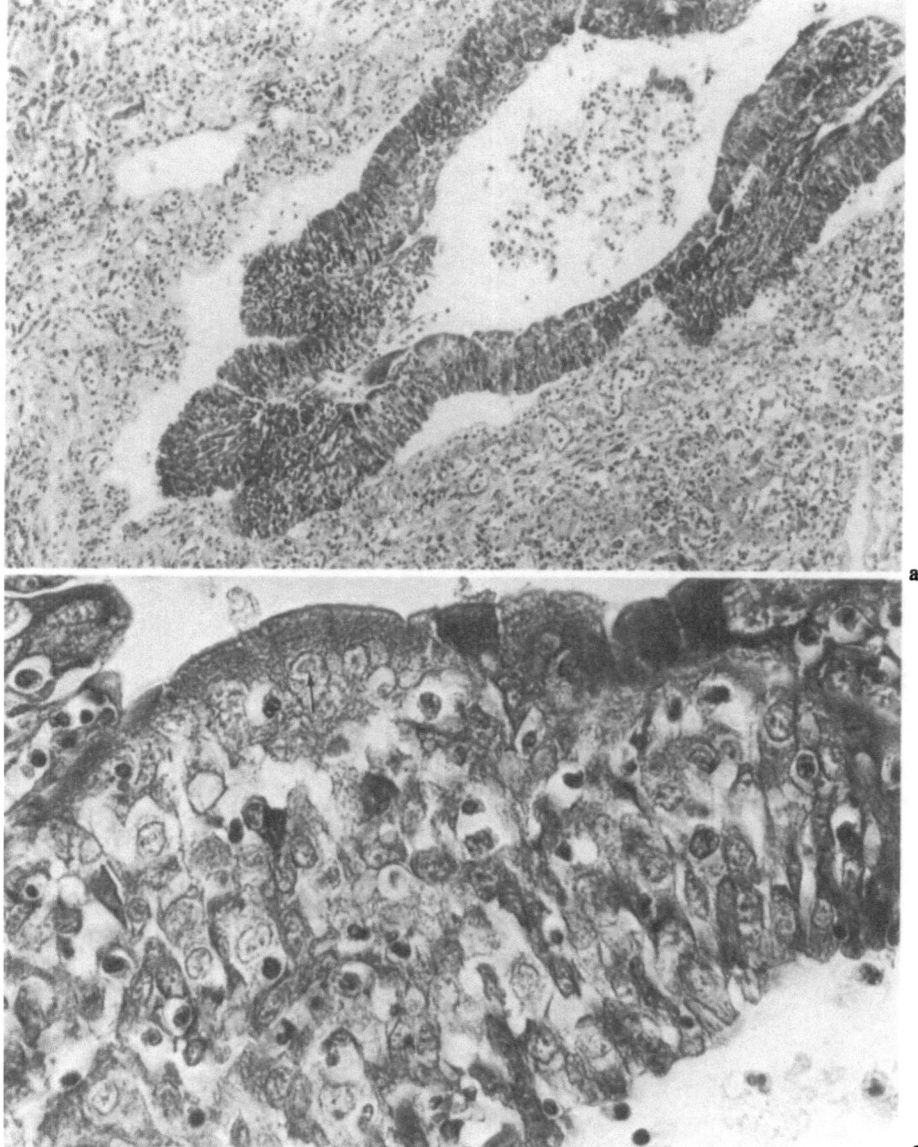

Fig. 25a, b. Fatal measles giant cell pneumonia. **a** With transitional cell-like hyperplasia of the bronchial epithelium and **b** intranuclear inclusion bodies *(arrow)* in the upper cells. HE-stain. 6 years old girl: after X-ray and cytostatic treatment because of medulloblastoma, the symptom of a diffuse pneumonia developed suddenly without any exanthem after contact with other children infected with measles

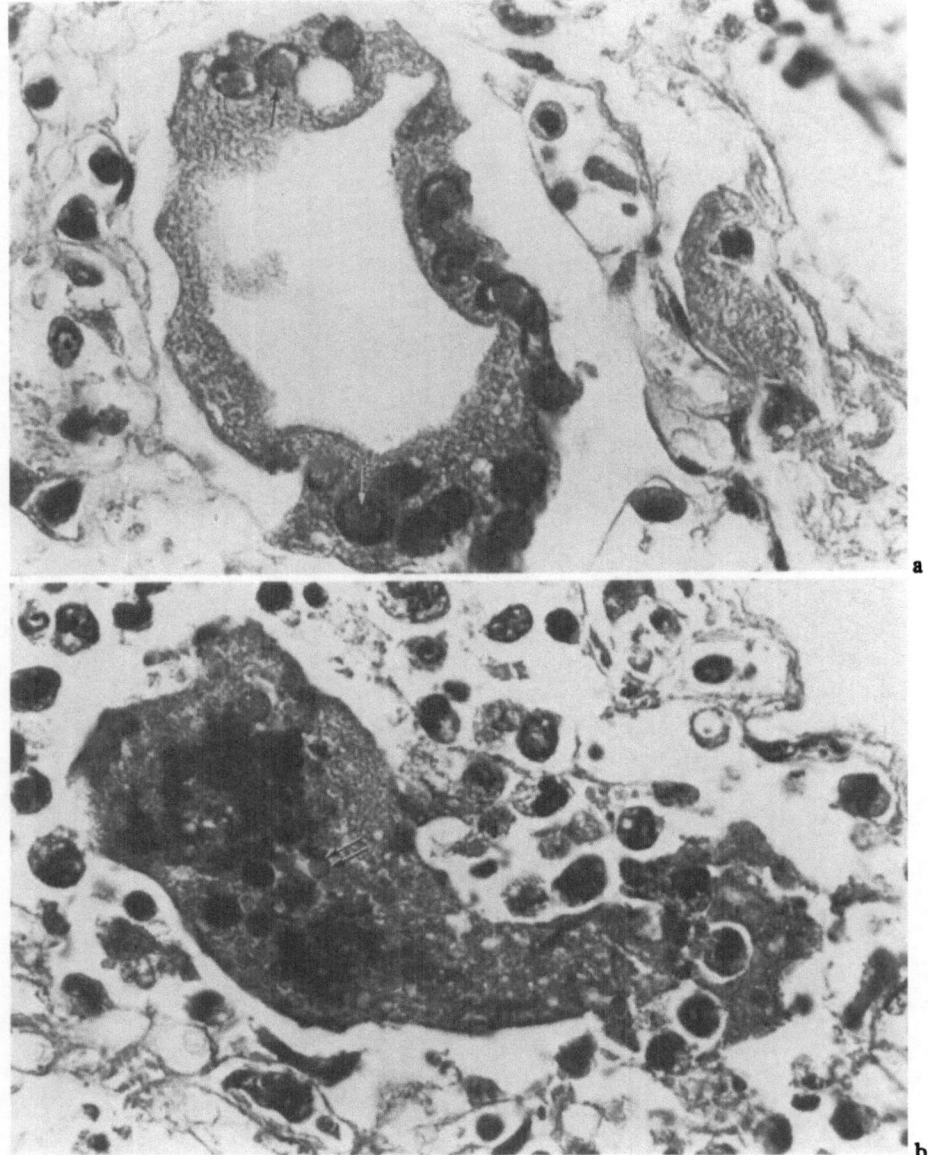

Fig. 26a, b. Measles giant cell pneumonia (same case as Fig. 25). **a** Early and **b** late developmental stages of alveolar giant cells resulting from fusion of proliferated pneumocytes. Intranuclear (**a**, *arrow*) and cytoplasmic (**b**, *double arrows*) inclusion bodies. Post-mortem tissue, HE-stain

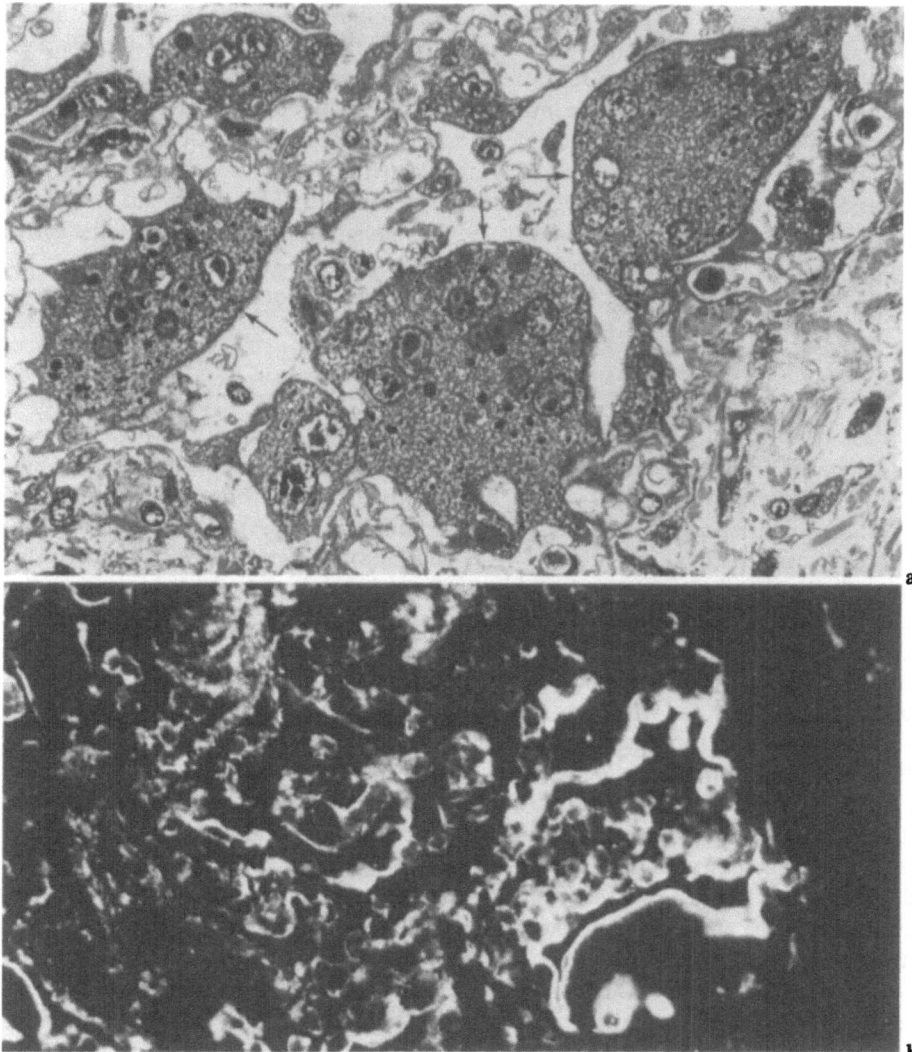

Fig. 27a, b. Measles giant cell pneumonia (same case as Fig. 25). **a** Semithin section from Epon-embedded post-mortem tissue, Mallory's stain: the luminal surfaces show condensed margins. **b** These surface structures exhibit an enhanced PNA-fluorescence (after neuraminidase treatment), comparable to the pattern found in other types of virus-induced pneumocytic proliferations

cells (e.g. in aspiration pneumonia). The lumen-oriented surface of measles giant cells, however, bears PNA receptors, mostly covered by neuraminic acid (Fig. 27). Ultra-structurally, the alveolar surface of giant cells has a microvillous configuration which may characterize and explain the light microscopic surface structure and polarity of measles giant cells which *Masson* and *Pare* (1931) have described, as a condensed rim with delicate striations.

The formation of pathognomonic inclusion bodies is correlated with the ultra-structurally proven replication of helical nucleocapsids, at least initially (*Archibald* et al. 1971; *Cohen* et al. 1955; *Sobonya* et al. 1978). *Llanos-Rhodas* and *Liu* (1965), however, had pointed out that the level of histochemically demonstrable viral antigens would decrease in intracytoplasmic inclusion bodies in parallel with their increasing size. The giant cells frequently seen in lymphoid tissue during the prodromal stage of measles — discovered 1911 by *Alagna* and named after *Warthin* (1931) and *Finkeldey* (1931, 1932) as proposed by *Hathaway* 1935 — equally seem to depend on the activity of F-antigen. They differ, however, from the epithelial giant cells of the lung by necrobiotic changes which may be dominant and by the absence of inclusion bodies.

3. Influenza

The picture of primary influenzal pneumonia without noticeable bacterial super-infection, caused by orthomyxoviruses, is distinctly different from the tissue reactions to paramyxoviruses (parainfluenza, RSV, morbilliform viruses) discussed in the previous chapters. The pathogenicity of virus subtypes manifested in various successive pandemics is known to vary considerably; their virulence depends on the varying activity of envelope antigens, that is, of the hemagglutinating HA-antigen (corresponding to the F-antigen of morbilliform viruses) and in particular, of the neuraminidase-active NA-antigen (*Laver* and *Kilbourne* 1966; *Choppin* and *Scheid* 1980). HA-antigen is responsible not only for virus adsorption, but especially for cell penetration; like the F-antigen of morbilliform paramyxoviruses, it has to be activated by cellular proteases, which may explain why its infectiousness depends, to a certain extent, on the presence of suitable target cells. Neuraminidase-active NA-glycoproteins facilitate the access of influenza viruses to those cell surfaces whose neuraminic acid-bearing structural elements are gangliosides and glycoproteins. But NA-antigen facilitates, above all, the release of new virus generations from these surfaces and a propagation of viruses in an environment rich in neuraminic acid such as the respiratory tract with its bronchial mucus.

In normal lung tissue, the PNA lectin binding method (cf. II.2) can demonstrate the predominant neuraminic acid coating of galactose(1-3)-N-acetylgalactosamine sequences which are found in high concentration in non-ciliated bronchiolar epithelia and in pneumocytes II, and which bind to PNA only after pretreatment with neuraminidase. Based on these observations, we have studied a series of 6 influenza pneumonias recorded in Hannover in the course of three A 2 epidemics (A/Hongkong 1/68 H3N2) between 1968 and 1972 (*Löblich* 1981; *Roetterink* 1981) and another case of (virologically unclassified) influenzal pneumonia, to find out whether the neuraminidase activity of influenza viruses would provoke an increase in free epithelial PNA receptors. Similar release reactions have been observed in erythrocytes during bacterial infections inducing the symptoms of the hemolytic uremic syndrome. In such processes neuraminidase released by pneumococci is particularly capable of splitting neuraminic acid from the erythrocyte surface, thereby releasing Thomsen-Friedenreich-cryptantigen with its terminal galactose(1-3)-N-acetylgalactosamine sequence which is then demonstrable with FITC-labeled PNA (*Klein* et al. 1977, 1978, 1979).

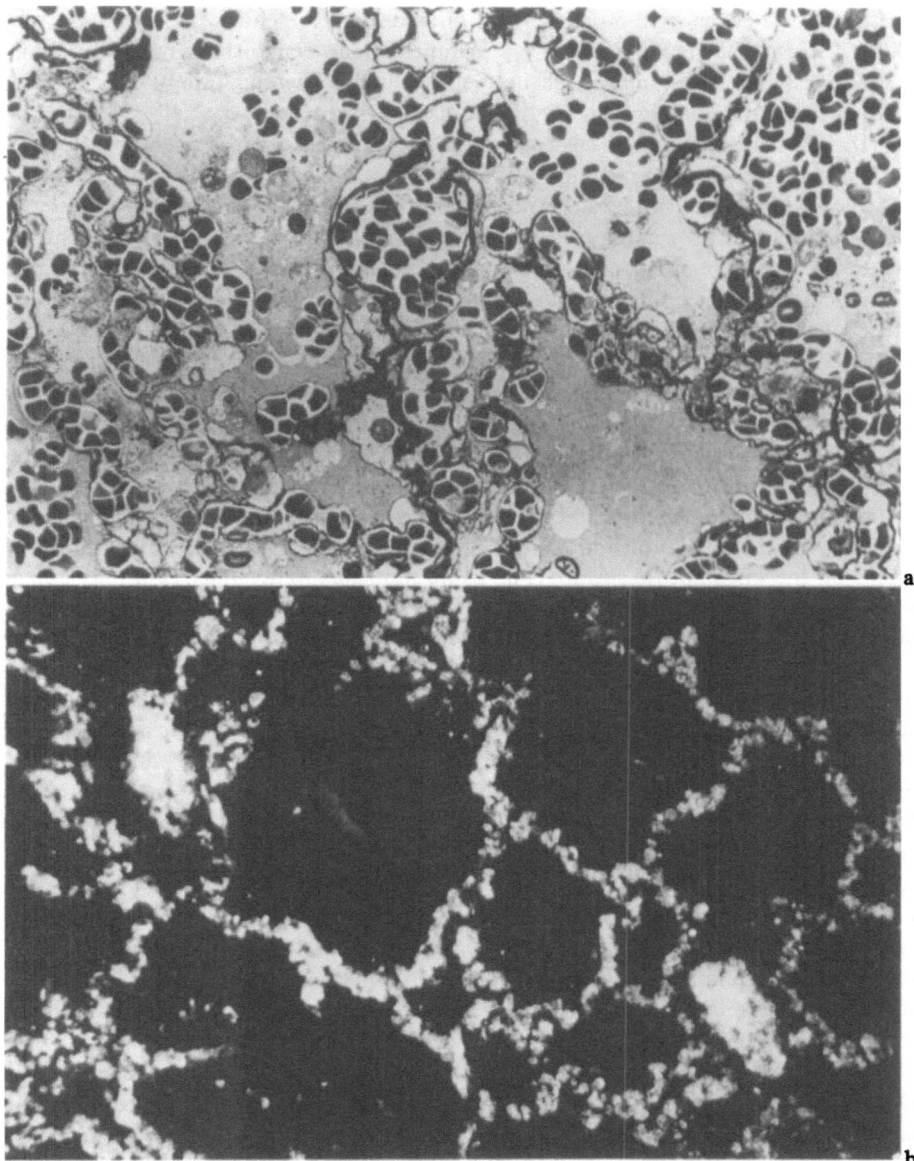

Fig. 28a, b. Fatal influenza in a 15 years old boy suddenly succumbing to a diffuse haemorrhagic pneumonia. **a** Aneurysmal dilatation of alveolar capillaries with incipient extravasation of erythrocytes. Semithin section from Epon-embedded post-mortem tissue, Movat's silver stain. **b** PNA-fluorescence (after neuraminidase treatment) discloses a complete loss of pneumocytes (compare Fig. 2 for normal). Capillaries are filled with fluorescent erythrocytes

Lung tissue taken post-mortem from influenza cases included in our study, was subjected to the PNA technique, but it was impossible to demonstrate free lectin-binding sites of pneumocytes or bronchial epithelial cells which would have been uncovered by influenza neuraminidase. Our results confirmed instead that the very substrate for the PNA test, namely the Clara cells of terminal bronchioles and the pneumocytes, had been lost by complete desquamation and necrosis.

Most of the previous histologic descriptions of influenzal pneumonia have mentioned, besides marked capillary hemostasis and frequently hemorrhagic alveolar exudate, the presence of more or less extensive epithelial necrosis and desquamation of the tracheobronchial mucosa (*Goodpasture* 1919; *Hers* and *Mulder* 1961; *Himmelweit* 1943; *Louria* et al. 1959; *Mulder* and *Verdongk* 1949; *Parker* et al. 1946; *Shope* and *Francis* 1936; *Straub* and *Mulder* 1948; *Walsh* et al. 1961). Experimentally, such findings were reported also from nasal mucosal tissue (*Francis* and *Stuart-Harris* 1930). Due to the low density of alveolar epithelia, especially in pneumocytes I, their visualization in light microscopy is very difficult, and so we lack reliable data about the structure of alveoli under the conditions of primary, fulminant influenzal pneumonia. Only hyaline membranes often mentioned in the literature, may give an indirect clue to primary lesions of the pneumocytes. By demonstration of PNA receptors normally present on the pneumocyte surface (Fig. 2) we were able to document not only extensive denudation of the bronchial mucosa, but also an almost complete loss of alveolar epithelia in all cases of primary influenza pneumonia included in the study (Fig. 28b).

An autolytic effect may be excluded by the evident intactness of lectin receptors on the surface of erythrocytes accumulating in the aneurysmatically dilated alveolar capillaries (PNA binding to the Thomsen-Friedenreich-antigen). The loss of pneumocytes may be visualized with acceptable accuracy even in epon-embedded semithin sections under light microscopy (Fig. 28a). In contrast to semithin sections or even electron microscopic preparations, our lectin technique offers the advantage of a wide survey over pulmonary tissue even at lower magnification. Hemorrhages may occur in typical cases without any cellular inflammatory reactions and without serous exudation or hyaline membranes: they can be interpreted as sequela to impaired barrier functions resulting from extensive epithelial losses. This destruction of epithelium might be aptly interpreted as an immediate cytopathogenic effect of the virus itself. Whether the process can be actually attributed to viral neuraminidase activity will have to be ascertained by experimental studies of early stages of viral infection.

In our cases, large accumulations of bacteria were often demonstrated by light microscopy within the protein-rich alveolar exudate. Such bacterial, predominantly staphylococcal superinfections have been mentioned by several authors as an important secondary pathogenetic event (*Himmelweit* 1943; *Parker* et al. 1946; *Mulder* and *Verdongk* 1949; *Martin* et al. 1959). In porcine influenza with its similar pathoanatomical features, frequent superinfections by Haemophilus influenzae suis were described by *Shope* (1936). Granulocytic infiltration which is rather inconstant in influenzal pneumonia, seems to depend on the extent of bacterial superinfection.

V. Desquamative Interstitial Pneumonia (DIP)

In 1965, *Liebow* et al. described the clinical and histologic picture of desquamative interstitial pneumonia. Histologically, DIP is manifested in diffuse interstitial infiltration of plasma cells and in follicular lymphocytic infiltration into predominantly peribronchial and subpleural tissue (Fig. 29). This chronic interstitial inflammatory reaction parallels, to some extent, the forms of peribronchitis we know from paramyxoviral infections, and therefore a viral etiology was often postulated, but never proven (*Liebow* et al. 1965; *Farr* 1970). Virus-like intranuclear inclusions were observed in some cases (*Farr* et al. 1970; *McNary* and *Gaensler* 1971; *Patchefsky* 1971). Follow-up studies have shown that DIP, though initially unconnected with interstitial fibrosis, may show a progressive picture of diffuse fibrosing alveolitis (diffuse intersitital fibrosis), during its prolonged and often fatal course turning eventually into the honeycomb phenomenon (*Scadding* and *Hinson* 1967; *Patchefsky* et al. 1975).

The significant morphologic criterion for DIP is seen in a massed accumulation of cells with abundant cytoplasm in alveoli and in terminal bronchioles, where their obstructive effect is an essential factor in the development of advanced respiratory insufficiency. The rich cytoplasm of these cells shows a fine, PAS-positive granulation, and partly weak positive reactions with Prussian blue staining. The nuclei are somewhat larger and of a looser structure than those of normal alveolar macrophages; mitoses are rare. The first authors describing these intraalveolar cells traced them from proliferating and desquamating alveolar epithelial cells.

Our own histochemical results of an open pulmonary biopsy taken from an 11-year-old girl who died later (*Schaefer* and *Müntefering* 1982) illustrate the histiocytic properties of these intraalveolar cells which would identify them as a special form of proliferating stimulated alveolar macrophages. They show, for instance, high TAP activity (Fig. 31). This isoenzyme of acid phosphatase is strictly limited to alveolar macrophages on paraffin sections of the lung, and will never occur in epithelial cells. Alveolar epithelia do in fact show distinct proliferation with occasional mitoses. They are seen in cuboid transformation with an increased number of PNA binding sites on their surface, demonstrable with FITC-labeled PNA after pretreatment with neuraminidase (Fig. 30). No transitional forms were found between TAP positive/PNA negative intraalveolar cells, and TAP negative/PNA positive alveolar epithelial cells. The reciprocal distribution of these two absolutely independent histochemical markers can thus refute the postulated epithelial origin of intraalveolar cells in DIP. In this context the term of "desquamative" interstitial pneumonia is histogenetically misleading, although it will remain as the accepted nomenclature. In electron microscopy, intraalveolar DIP cells show characteristics typical of the alveolar macrophage (*Farr* et al. 1970), but the loose chromatin structure of their rather large nuclei and the occasional occurrence of mitoses is certainly unusual. These phenomena point to a specific stimulation, possibly due to a latent viral infection. A similar cause might be triggering the striking hyperplasia of these alveolar epithelial cells. That such processes could also be elicited by an abnormal immune reaction might be discussed as an alternative, by analogy with the interpretation of diffuse fibrosing alveolitis with its closely related phenomena (*Scadding* 1974).

194

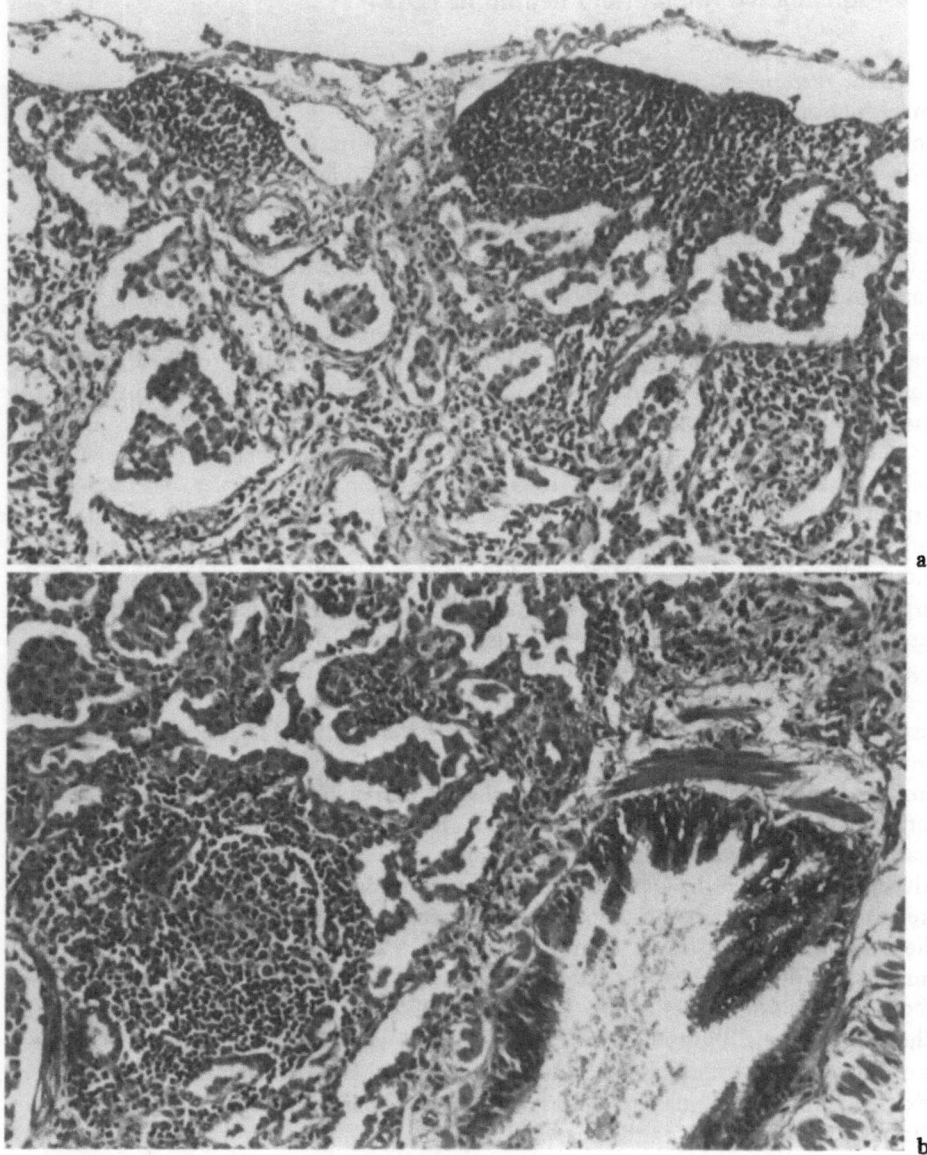

Fig. 29a, b. Desquamative interstitital pneumonia type Liebow in an 11 years old girl.
Open lung biopsy taken a few days prior to the fatal outcome. Follicular lymphoid
infiltrates beneath the pleura (a) and adjacent to a small bronchiole (b). Alveoli filled
with large "desquamated" cells. HE-stain

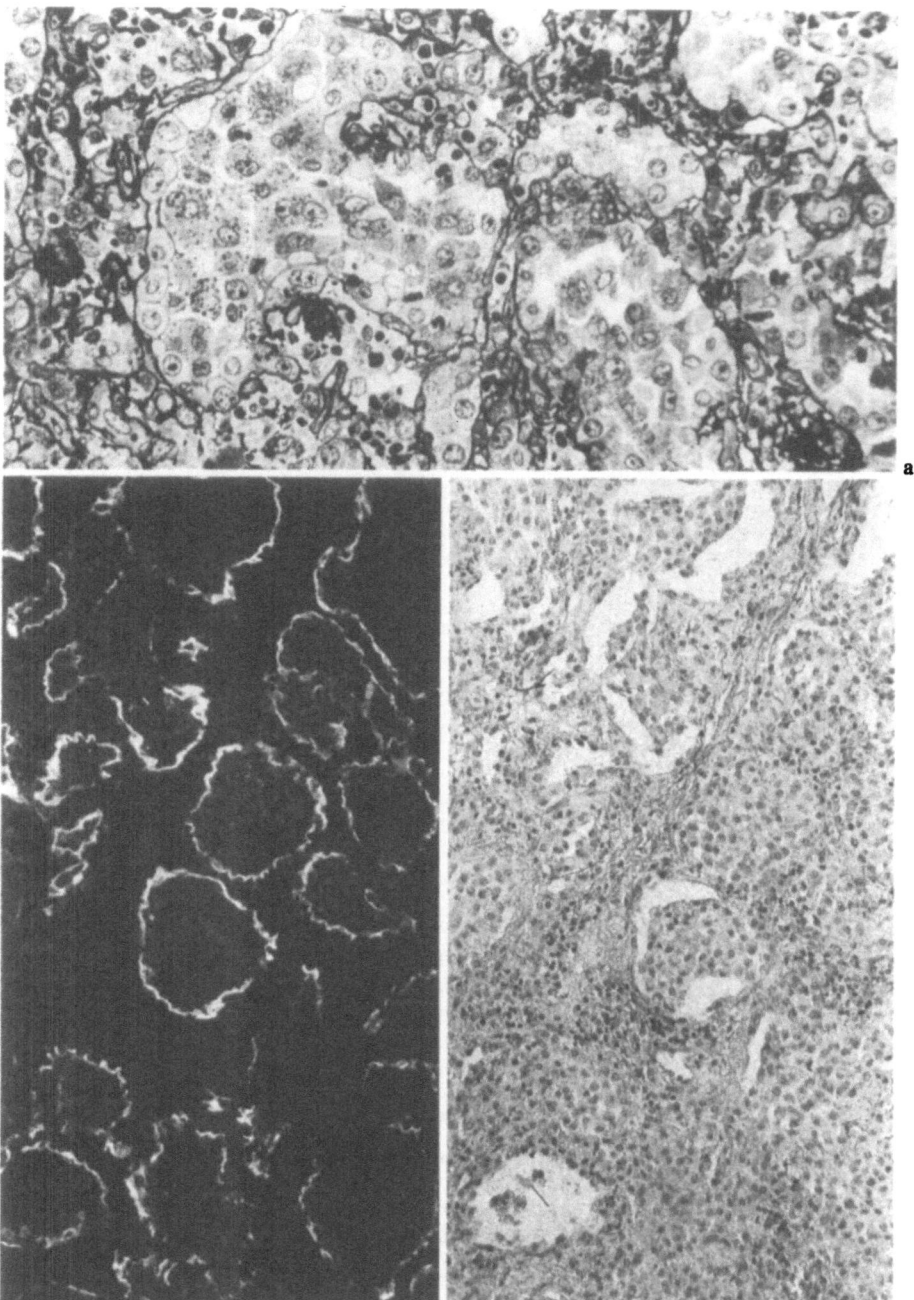

Fig. 30a—c. Desquamative interstitial pneumonia (same case as Fig. 29). a Semithin
section from Epon-embedded tissue, Movat's silver stain. Fairly broadened alveolar
septa, alveoli completely obstructed by large cells, scarcely distinguishable from hyperplastic pneumocytes. b Bright PNA-fluorescence (after neuraminidase treatment)
restricted to surfaces of pneumocytes, intraalveolar cells reacting negative. c Identical
area as b, seen in the visible light, nuclei stained with Mayer's haemalum

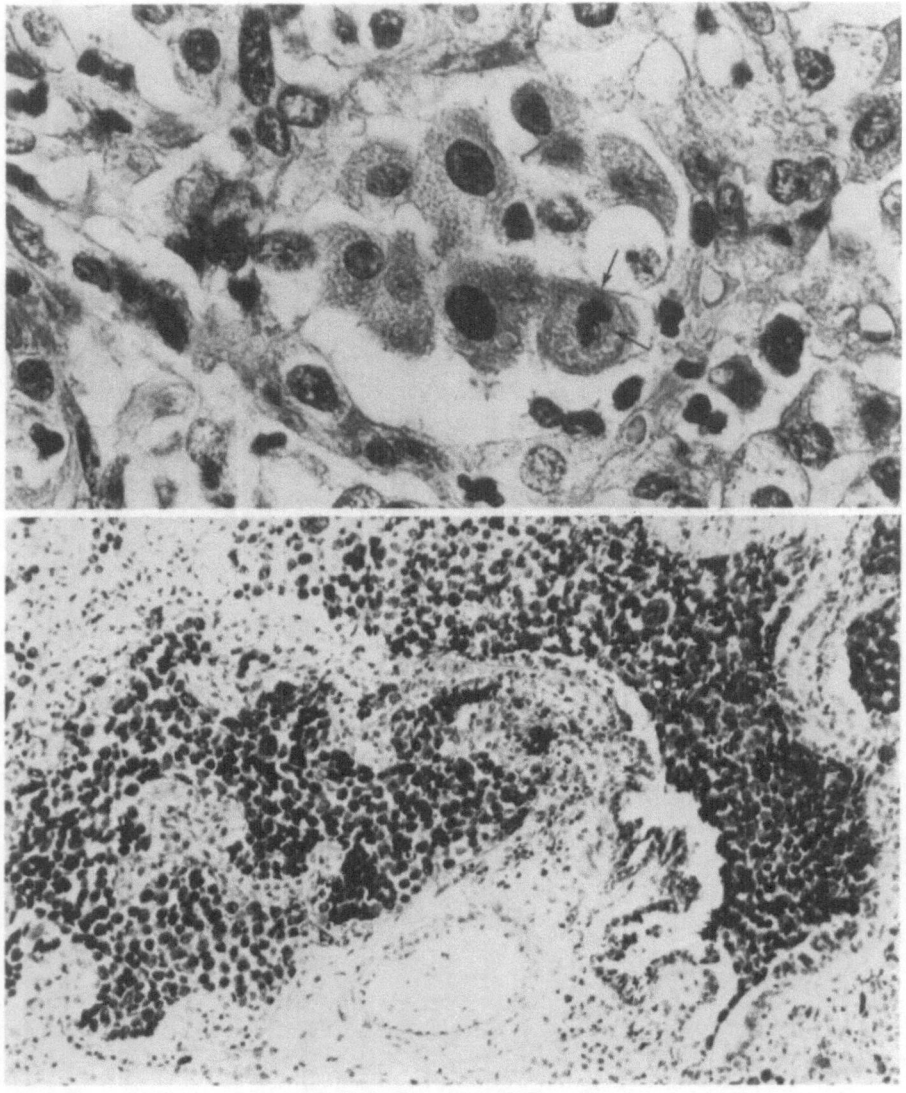

Fig. 31a, b. Desquamative interstitial pneumonia (same case as Fig. 29). **a** Mitotic intraalveolar cell (HE-stain). **b** Intraalveolar cells stained for TAP (method II.1). By their negative TAP reaction pneumocytes are clearly discriminated from the dark (red) stained intraalveolar cells, the latter corresponding to macrophages

With regard to interstitial inflammatory reactions and hyperplasia of alveolar epithelia, DIP certainly displays a number of histologic phenomena that might be typical of RNA viral infection, and so its patterns of inflammatory reactions may be of only limited etiologic specificity.

VI. Summary

The histologic and cytologic phenotypes of viral diseases of the lung appear extremely variegated, depending mainly on the type of virus involved, and on the immunologic responsiveness of the infected organism. Virus-induced pulmonary cell reactions may be analysed more thoroughly by certain histochemical techniques applicable to routinely formaldehyde-fixed and paraffin-embedded specimens.

Alveolar macrophages exhibit an intense activity of tartrateresistant acid phosphatase (TAP). With this selective staining reaction we realized that macrophages are widely missing in the lung affected by cytomegalovirus or combined cytomegalovirus and pneumocystis pneumonia. There is circumstantial evidence for alveolar clearance being disturbed due to phagocytic malfunction. It may be supposed that this precondition favors pulmonary cytomegalovirus infection, and pneumocystosis as well. – In striking contrast, TAP-staining discloses an abundant accumulation of stimulated alveolar macrophages in desquamative interstitial pneumonia (DIP). Since pneumocytes, like all other epithelial cells, are always TAP-negative, we may conclude that the intraalveolar cells characterizing DIP, that is, alveolar macrophages, are obviously *not* derived from alveolar epithelia as formerly supposed.

A unique type of leukoclastic exudate is found in fatal adenovirus pneumonia. Hitherto adenovirus pneumonia has been regarded as a form of necrotizing bronchopneumonia, more or less poor in granulocytes, or even completely agranulocytic. However, the naphthol AS-D chloroacetate esterase reaction discloses plenty of neutrophilic granulocytes in a state of advanced leukoclastic disintegration. This process can be regarded as an Arthus-like reaction that is possibly related to the rapid replication and release of virions, large amounts of these appear in extracellular spaces freely accessible to immunoglobulins or other reactive serum constituents. The release of proteolytic enzymes from granulocytes may provoke such tissue necrosis as is typically encountered in fatal adenovirus pneumonia. Under certain immunological preconditions, necrotizing inflammation (of type Becroft according to *Spencer* 1973) has also been observed e.g. in paramyxovirus pneumonia. It remains to be investigated by the naphthol AS-D chloroacetate esterase technique whether these processes are also representing a leukoclastic type of inflammation. – In general, benign paramyxovirus infections (e.g. RSV) elicit bronchiolitis with purely lympho-monocytic cellular infiltration.

In many viral diseases of the lung as well as in DIP, alveolar and (terminal) bronchiolar epithelia tend to proliferate prior to visible virus replication, or to ultimate necrobiotic events. This process is readily monitored by visualization of binding sites for peanut agglutinin (PNA). This lectin binds selectively to terminal β-D-galactose-(1-3)-N-acetylgalactosamine sequences present in surface glycoproteins of mucin-producing cells, Clara cells, and pneumocytes. In part these "PNA receptors" are covered with neuraminic acid. Most types of virus-induced epithelial proliferation are combined with an enhancement of PNA-binding. Measles giant cells will preserve to some extent, certain PNA-reactive surface structures, thereby unmasking their epithelial origin. Cytomegalic transformation ends in a complete loss of PNA surface receptors which is reciprocally correlated with the appearance of intense PNA binding to the envelope of mature cytomegalovirions accumulating within intracytoplasmic inclusion bodies. While losing their PNA-binding surface glycoproteins, the completely cytomegalo-transformed pneumocytes are seen to desquamate, leaving behind the naked alveolar walls. In cytomegalovirus pneumonia, those ultimate lesions develop in a more or less smouldering way, they remain restricted to scattered foci. However, the fatal outcome of influenza pneumonia seems to be connected with an acute alveolar denudation whose wide extent can be visualized by the PNA technique.

References

Adams JM (1941) Primary virus pneumonitis with cytoplasmic inclusion bodies. JAMA 116:925–933

Adams JM, Imagawa DT, Zike K (1961) Epidemic bronchiolitis and pneumonitis related to respiratory syncytial virus. JAMA 176:1037–1039

Aherne W, Bird T, Court SDM, Gardner PS, McQuillen J (1970) Pathological changes in virus infections of the lower respiratory tract in children. J Clin Pathol 23:7–18

Alagna G (1911) Histopathologische Veränderungen der Tonsillen und der Schleimhaut der ersten Luftwege bei Masern. Arch Laryng Rhin 25:527–530

Almeida JD (1963) A classification of virus particles based on morphology. Can Med Assoc J 89:787–798

Archibald RWR, Weller RO, Meadow SR (1971) Measles pneumonia and the nature of the inclusion-bearing giant cells: A light- and electronmicroscope study. J Pathol 103:27–34

Arrobbio J (1964) Infection with parainfluenza 3 virus: a fatal case with autopsy report. Clin Proc Child Hosp Nat Med Cent 20:298–305

Beale AJ, Doane F, Ormsby HL (1957) Studies on adenovirus infections of the eye in Toronto. Am J Opthalmol 43:26–31

Becroft DMO (1967) Histopathology of fatal adenovirus infection of the respiratory tract in young children. J Clin Pathol 20:561–569

Beem M, Wrigth FH, Hamre D, Egerer R, Oehme M (1960) Association of the chimpanzee coryza agent with acute respiratory disease in children. N Engl J Med 263:523–530

Bell JA, Dingle JH, Francis T, Hilleman MR, Huebner RJ, Payne AM-M (1956) "Adenoviruses": Group name proposed for new respiratory tract viruses. Science 124:119–120

Bellanti JA (1971) Biologic significance of the secretory yA immunoglobulins. Pediatrics 48:715–729

Blandford G (1970) Arthus reaction and pneumonia. Br Med J I:758–760

Blank H, Davis C, Collins C (1970) Electron microscopy for diagnosis of cutaneous viral infections. Br J Dermatol 83:69–80

Brody AR, Craighead JE (1974) Pathogenesis of pulmonary cytomegalovirus infection in immunosuppressed mice. J Infect Dis 129:677–689

Buescher EL (1967) Respiratory disease and the adenoviruses. Med Clin North Am 51:769–779

Burnett FM (1968) Measles as an index of immunological function. Lancet II:610—613

Buser F (1967) Side reaction to measles vaccination suggesting the Arthus phenomenon. N Engl J Med 277:250—251

Buthala BA, Soret MG (1964) Parainfluenzy type 3 virus infection in hamsters: virologic, serologic and pathologic studies. J Infect Dis 114:226—234

Carilli AD, Gohd RS, Gordon W (1964) A virologic study of chronic bronchitis. N Engl J Med 270:123—127

Cascardo H, Karzon DT (1965) Measles virus giant cell inducing factor (fusing factor). Virology 26:311—325

Chanock RM, Parrott RH (1965) Respiratory syncytial virus. In: Horsfall FL Jr, Tamm I (eds) Viral and rickettsial diseases of man. Lippincott, Philadelphia, pp 775—783

Chanock RM, Parrott RH, Kapikian AZ, Kein HW, Brandt CD (1968) Possible role of immunological factors in pathogenesis of RS virus lower respiratory tract disease. In: Pollard M (ed) Perspectives in virology, vol VI. Academic Press, New York, pp 125—139

Chanock RM, Kapikian AZ, Mills J, Kein HW, Parrott RH (1970) Influence of immunological factors in respiratory syncytial virus disease of the lower respiratory tract. Arch Environ Health 21:347—355

Chany C, Lépine P, Lelong M, Le-Tan-Vinh, Satgé O, Virat J (1958) Severe and fatal pneumonia in infants and young children associated with adenovirus infections. Am J Hyg 67:367—378

Choppin PW, Scheid A (1980) The role of viral glykoproteins in adsorption, penetration and pathogenicity of viruses. Rev Infect Dis 2:40—60

Chown B (1939) Giant cell pneumonia of infancy as a manifestation of vitamin A deficiency. Am J Dis Child 57:489—505

Coates HV, Chanock RM (1962) Experimental infection with respiratory syncytial virus in several species of animals. Am J Hyg 76:302—312

Cohen SM, Gordon J, Rapp F, Macauley JC, Bickley SM (1955) Cited by Spencer. Proc Soc Exp Biol Med 90:118

Cole R, Kuttner AG (1926) A filtrable virus present in the submaxillary glands of guinea pigs. J Exp Med 44:855—873

Cowdry EV (1934) The problems of intranuclear inclusions in virus diseases. Arch Pathol 18:527—542

Craighead JE (1971) Pulmonary cytomegalovirus infection in the adult. Am J Pathol 63:487—504

Dahm HH (1980) Zytomegalie des Neugeborenen und des Erwachsenen. Med Welt 31:64—69

Davis BJ, Ornstein L (1959) High resolution enzyme localization with a new diazo reagent, "hexazonium pararosaniline". J Histochem Cytochem 7:297

Deinhardt F, May RD, Calhoun HH, Sullivan HE (1958) The isolation of adenovirus type 1 from a fatal case of viral "pneumonitis". Arch Intern Med 102:816

Delage B, Bronchu P, Pelletier M, Jasmin G, Lapointe N (1979) Giant cell pneumonia caused by parainfluenza virus. J Pediatr 94:426—429

De Monbreun WA (1937) The histopathology of natural and experimental canine distemper. Am J Pathol 13:187—212

Denton J (1925) The pathology of fatal measles. Am J Med Sci 169:531—543

Dingle JH, Feller AE (1956) Noninfluenzal viral infections of the respiratory tract. N Engl J Med 254:465—471

Doane FW, Anderson N, Zbitnew A, Rhodes AJ (1969) Application of electron microscopy to the diagnosis of virus infections. Can Med Assoc J 100:1043—1049

Dürck H (1897) Studien über die Aetiologie und Histologie der Pneumonie im Kindesalter und die Pneumonien im Allgemeinen. Dtsch Arch Klin Med 58:368—444

Effros RB, Doherty PC, Gerhard W, Bennink J (1977) Cited by Lin Yun Lu et al. (1981). J Exp Med 145:557—568

Enders JF (1956) The present status of etiologic discovery in viral diseases. Ann Intern Med 45:331–350

Enders JF, McCarthy FK, Mitus A, Cheatham WJ (1959) Isolation of measles virus at autopsy in cases of giant-cell pneumonia without rash. N Engl J Med 261:875–881

Evans AS (1958) Latent adenovirus infections of the human respiratory tract. Am J Hyg 67:256–266

Farber S, Wolbach SB (1932) Intranuclear and cytoplasmic inclusions ("protozoan-like bodies) in the salivary glands and other organs of infants. Am J Pathol 8:123–135

Farr GH, Russell AH, Hennigar GR (1970) Desquamative interstitial pneumonia. Am J Pathol 60:347–370

Feyrter F (1925) Ueber die Masernpneumonie. Virchows Arch 255:753–794

Finkeldey W (1931) Über die Riesenzellbefunde in den Gaumenmandeln, zugleich ein Beitrag zur Histopathologie der Mandelveränderungen im Maserninkubationssta-dium. Virchows Arch [Pathol Anat] 281:311–329

Finkeldey W (1932) Riesenzellbefunde bei akuter Wurmfortsatzentzündung. Ein Bei-trag zur Histopathologie der Veränderungen des Wurmfortsatzes im Maserninkuba-tionsstadium. Virchows Arch [Pathol Anat] 284:528

Fohlmeister I, Schaefer HE, Rieger M, Galanski M (1979) Masernriesenzellpneumonie. Med Welt 30:307–312

Francis T, Stuart-Harris CH (1938) Studies on nasal histology of epidemic influenza virus infection in ferret. J Exp Med 68:789–802

Frank L (1950) Varicella pneumonitis. Report of a case with autopsy observations. Arch Pathol Lab Med 50:450–456

Friedländer (1876) Experimentaluntersuchungen über chronische Pneumonie und Lungenschwindsucht. Virchows Arch [Pathol Anat] 68:325–363

Friedman HM (1981) Cytomegalovirus: subclinical infection or disease? Am J Med 70:215–217

Gardner PS, Turk DC, Aherne WA, Bird T, Holdaway MD, Court SDM (1967) Deaths associated with respiratory tract infection in childhood. Br Med J IV:316–320

Geiler G (1957) Über die Erwachsenenform der Cytomegalie. Frankf Z Pathol 68:107–118

Gerbeaux MJ, Héber-Jouas J, Masse N, Beauchchef A (1957) Epidémie familiale de maladie à virus du groupe A.P.C. chez trois enfants (un cas mortel). Bull Soc Méd Hôp Paris 73:519

Giese W (1960) Die Atemorgane. In: Kaufmann E, Staemmler M (eds) Lehrbuch der speziellen pathologischen Anatomie, vol II/3. de Gruyter, Berlin

Glahn WC von, Pappenheimer AM (1925) Intranuclear inclusions in visceral disease. Am J Pathol 1:445–466

Glezen WP, Loda FA, Clyde WA, Senior RJ, Shaeffer CI, Conley WG, Denny FW (1971) Epidemiologic patterns of acute lower respiratory disease of children in a pediatric group practice. J Pediatr 78:397–406

Goodpasture EW (1919) The significance of vertain pulmonary lesions in relation to the etiology of influenza. Am J Med Sci 158:863–870

Goodpasture EW, Talbot FB (1921) Conerning the nature of "protozoan-like" cells in certain lesions of infancy. Am J Dis Child 21:415–425

Goodpasture EW, Auerbach SH, Swanson HS, Cottir EF (1939) Virus pneumonia of infants secondary to epidemic infections. Am J Dis Child 57:937–1011

Green RG, Evans CA (1939) Comparative study of distemper inclusions. Am J Hyg (Sect B) 29:73–87

Gross PA, Green RH, McCrea-Curnen MG (1973) Persistent infection with parainflu-enza type 3 virus in man. Am Rev Respir Dis 108:894–898

Günther M, Schaefer HE (1981) Nachweis von Viren in Speicheldrüsen europäischer und algerischer Igel – ein neuer Aspekt der Selbstbespeichelung. Dtsch Ges Säuge-tierkunde, Heidelberg

Güthert H, Meerbach W, Wöckel W (1969) Vorkommen und Bedeutung der Riesenzellen in der Lunge. 2. Mitteilung: Die mehrkernigen Riesenzellen. Zentralbl Allg Pathol 112:22−30

Hall CB (1931) Nosocomial viral respiratory infections: Perennial weeds on pediatric wards. Am J Med 70:670−676

Hall CB, Kopelman AE, Douglas RG, Geiman JM, Meagher MP (1979) Neonatal respiratory syncytial virus infection. N Engl J Med 300:393−396

Hamperl H (1956) Pneumocystis infection and cytomegaly of the lungs in the newborn and adult. Am J Pathol 32:1−13

Hathaway BM (1935) Generalized dissemination of giant cells in lymphoid tissue in prodromal stage of measles. Arch Pathol Lab Med 19:819−824

Hecht V (1910) Die Riesenzellpneumonie im Kindesalter. Eine histologisch-experimentelle Studie. Beitr Pathol Anat Allg Pathol 48:263−310

Hers JFPh (1963) Fluorescent antibody technique in respiratory viral diseases. Am Rev Dis [Suppl] 88:316−338

Hers JFPh, Mulder J (1961) Broad aspects of the pathology and pathogenesis of human influenza. Am Rev Respir Dis 83(2):84−97

Hers JFPh, Masurel N, Mulder J (1958) Bacteriology and histopathology of the respiratory tract and lungs in fatal asian influenza. Lancet II:1141−1143

Hilding A (1930) The common cold. Arch Otolaryngol 12:33−150

Hilleman MR, Werner JH (1954) Recovery of new agent from patients with acute respiratory illness. Proc Soc Exp Biol Med 85:183−188

Himmelweit F (1943) Influenza virus B isolated from fatal case of pneumonia. Lancet II:793−794

Holzel A, Parker L, Patterson WH, White LLR' Thompson KM, Tobin JOH (1963) The isolation of respiratory syncytial virus from children with acute respiratory disease. Lancet I:295−298

Holzel A, Parker L, Patterson WH, Cartmel D, White LLR, Purdy R, Thompson KM, Tobin JOH (1965) Virus isolations from throats of children admitted to hospital with respiratory and other diseases, Manchester 1962−4. Br Med J I:614−619

Hsiung CC (1963) Adenovirus pneumonia in infants and children. Pathologic studies of 40 cases. Chin Med J (Engl) 82:390−398

Ishida N (1957) Cited by Wöckel and Meerbach (1968). Ann NY Acad Sci 67:299

Jarvis WR, Middleton PJ, Gelfand EW (1979) Parainfluenza pneumonia in severe combined immunodeficiency disease. J Pediatr 94:423−524

Jensen KE, Minuse E, Ackermann WW (1955) Serologic evidence of American experience with newborn pneumonitis virus (type Sendai). J Immunol 75:71−77

Jesionek Kiolemenoglou (1904) Ueber einen Befund von protozoenartigen Gebilden in den Organen eines hereditär-luetischen Fötus. Münch Med Wochenschr 51: 1905−1907

Joncas J, Berthiaume L, Pavilanis V (1969a) The structure of the respiratory syncytial virus. Virology 38:493−496

Joncas JH, Williams R, Berthiaume L, Beaudry P, Pavilanis V (1969b) Diagnosis of viral respiratory infections by electron microscopy. Lancet I:956−959

Karsner HT, Meyers AE (1913) Giant cell pneumonia. Arch Intern Med 11:534−541

Kawai K (1959) Pathology and pathologic anatomy of adenovirus infection; based on 3 autopsy cases of infantile pneumonia. Jpn J Exp Med 29:359−368

Klein PJ, Bulla M, Newman RA, Müller P, Uhlenbruck G, Schaefer HE, Krüger G, Fischer R (1977) Thomsen-Friedenreich Antigen in haemolytic-uraemic syndrome. Lancet II:1024−1025

Klein PJ, Bulla M, Newman RA, Müller P, Uhlenbruck G, Krüger G, Schaefer HE, Lennartz KJ (1978a) Untersuchungen zur Pathogenese des hämolytisch-urämischen Syndroms. Zentralbl Allg Pathol 122:280

Klein PJ, Newman RA, Uhlenbruck G, Schaefer HE, Lennartz KJ, Fischer R (1978b) Histochemical methods for the demonstration of Thomsen-Friedenreich antigen in cell suspensions and tissue sections. Klin Wochenschr 56:761−765

Klein PJ, Bulla M, Newman RA, Radermacher EH, Müller P, Uhlenbruck G, Krüger G, Schaefer HE, Lennartz KJ, Fischer R (1979) The significance of pneumococcal neuraminidase for the development of haemolytic-uraemic syndrome. In: Bulla M (ed) Dialysis and kidney transplantation in children. Problems and particularities of intermittent longterm dialysis and acute renal failure in children. Bibliomed, Melsungen, pp 183–189

Knyvett AF (1963) The pulmonary lesions of chickenpox. Q J Med 35(N.S.):313–323

Kromayer E (1889) Ueber die sogenannte Katarrhalpneumonie nach Masern und Keuchhusten. Arch Pathol Anat 117:452–468

Kuttner AG, T'Ung T (1935) Further studies on the submaxillary gland viruses of rats and guinea pigs. J Exp Med 62:805–822

Laver WG, Kilbourne ED (1966) Identification in a recombinant influenza virus of structural proteins derived from both parents. Virology 30:493–501

Leder LD (1964) Über die selektive fermentcytochemische Darstellung von neutrophilen myeloischen Zellen und Gewebsmastzellen im Paraffinschnitt. Klin Wochenschr 42:553–555

Lelong M, Lépine P, Alison F, Le-Tan-Vinh, Satgé P, Chany Ch (1956) La pneumonie à virus du groupe A.P.C. chez le nourrisson. Isolement du virus. Les lésions anatomo-histologiques. Arch Fr Pediatr 13:1092–1096

Liebow AA, Steer A, Billingsley JG (1965) Desquamative interstitial pneumonia. Am J Med 39:369–404

Lin Yun Lu, Askonas B (1981) Cross-reactivity for different type A influenza viruses of a cloned T-killer cell line. Nature 288:164–165

Lipschütz (1921) Untersuchungen über die Ätiologie der Krankheiten der Herpesgruppe (Herpes zoster, Herpes genitalis, Herpes febrilis). Arch Dermatol Syph 136:428–482

Llanos-Rodas R, Liu C (1965) A study of measles virus infection in tissue culture cells with particular reference to the development of intranuclear inclusion bodies. J Immunol 95:840–845

Löblich H-J (1981) Personal communication

Löwenstein C (1907) Über protozoenartige Gebilde in den Organen von Kindern. Zentralblatt Allg Pathol Pathol Anat 18:518–518

Louria DB, Blumenfeld HL, Ellis JT, Kilbourne ED, Rogers DE (1959) Studies of influenza in the pandemic of 1957–1958. II. Pulmonary complications of influenza. J Clin Invest 38:213–265

Lucchesi PF, La Boccetta AC, Peale AR (1947) Varicella neonatorum. Am J Dis Child 73:44–54

Luse SA, Smith MG (1965) Electron microscope studies of cells infected with the salivary gland viruses. Ann NY Acad Sci 81:133–144

Martin AM, Kurtz SM (1966) Cytomegalic inclusion disease. An electron microscopic study of the virus at necropsy. Arch Pathol Lab Med 82:27–34

Martin CM, Kunin CM, Gottlieb LS, Fuland M (1959) Asian influenza A in Boston, 1957–1958. II. Severe staphylococcal pneumonia complicating influenza. Arch Intern Med 103:532–542

Masson P, Paré L (1931) Un cas de broncho-pneumonie à plasmodes. Contribution à l'étude du revêtement alvéolaire. Ann Anat Pathol (Paris) 8:13–35

Masugi M, Minami G (1938) Über einen Fall von Masern mit Riesenzellbildung an Luftwegen, Mund- und Rachenschleimhaut. Über die Einschlüsse an Masernriesenzellen. Beitr Pathol Anat Allg Pathol 101:483–502

McAllister RM, Straw RM, Filbert JE, Goodheart CR (1963) Human cytomegalovirus: Cytochemical observations of intracellular lesion development correlated with viral synthesis and release. Virology 19:521–531

McClelland AJ (1980) Vaccination against paramyxoviruses. Nature 284:404

McNair Scott TF, Bonanno DE (1967) Reactions to live-measles virus vaccine in children previously inoculated with killed-virus vaccine. N Engl J Med 277:248–250

McNary WF, Gaensler EA (1971) Intranuclear inclusion bodies in desquamative interstitial pneumonia: Electron microscopic observations. Ann Intern Med 74:404–407

Meerbach W, Wöckel W, Güthert H (1968) Vorkommen und Bedeutung der Riesenzellen in der Lunge. 1. Mitteilung: Die einkernigen Riesenzellen. Zentralbl Allg Pathol Pathol Anat 111:544–550

Merz DC, Scheid A, Choppin PW (1980) Importance of antibodies to the fusion glycoprotein of paramyxoviruses in the prevention of spread of infection. J Exp Med 151:275–288

Mitus A, Enders JF, Craig JM, Holloway A (1959) Persistence of measles virus and depression of antibody formation in patients with giant cell pneumonia. N Engl J Med 261:882–889

Moloney WC, McPherson K, Fliegelman L (1960) Esterase activity in leucocytes demonstrated by the use of naphthol AS-D chloroacetate substrate. J Histochem Cytochem 8:200–207

Moore RA, Gross P (1930) Giant cells in inflammation of the lung in children. Am J Dis Child 40:247–259

Mouchet R (1911) De la présence de protozoaires dans les organes des enfants. Contribution à l'étude de l'ictère des nouveau-nés. Arch Med Exp Anat Pathol (Paris) 23:115–124

Muchmore HG, Parkinson AJ, Humphries JE, Scott LV, Cooney MK, Miles JAR (1981) Persistent parainfluenza virus shedding during isolation at the south pole. Nature 289:187–189

Mufson MA, Krause HE, Mocega HE, Dawson FW (1970) Viruses, mycoplasma pneumoniae and bacteria associated with lower respiratory tract disease among infants. Am J Epidemiol 91:192–202

Mulder J, Verdongk GJ (1949) Studies on the pathogenesis of a case of influenza-A pneumonia of 3 days duration. J Pathol Bacteriol 61:55–61

Myerowitz RL, Stalder H, Oxman MN, Levin MJ, Moore M, Leith JD, Gantz NM, Pellegrini J, Hierholzer JC (1975) Fatal disseminated adenovirus infection in a renal transplant recipient. Am J Med 59:591–598

Nader PR, Horwitz M, Rouseau J (1967) Severe illness (atypical exanthem) following exposure to natural measles: II cases in children previously inoculated with killed vaccine. Presented at a meeting of the American Pediatric Society April, 29

Noda K (1953) Newborn virus pneumonitis, type Sendai. III. Report: Pathological studies on the 9 autopsy cases and the mice inoculated with the new-found virus. Yokohama Med Bull 4:281–287

Norrby E (1966) Present status of killed measles vaccines. Proc Int Conf Vaccines viral ricketsial Dis Man, Washington

Oppenheimer EH (1944) Congenital chickenprox with disseminated visceral lesions. Bull Johns Hopkins Hosp 74:240–250

Osada R, Hanayama R (1958) A fatal case of infantile pneumonia due to adenovirus; clinical findings. Jpn J Exp Med 28:293–295

Parker F, Jolliffe LS, Barnes MW, Finland M (1946) Pathologic findings in the lungs of five cases from which influenza virus was isolated. Am J Pathol 22:797–819

Patchefsky AS (1971) Desquamative interstitial pneumonia: significance of intranuclear viral-like inclusion bodies. Ann Intern Med 74:322–327

Patchefsky AS, Fraimow W, Hoch WS (1973) Desquamative interstitial pneumonia. Pathological findings and follow-up in 13 patients. Arch Intern Med 132:222–225

Pettavel CA (1911) Über eigentümliche herdförmige Degenerationen der Thyreoidea-Epithelien bei Purpura eines Neonatus. Virchows Arch [Pathol Anat] 206:1–11

Pinkerton H, Smiley WL, Anderson WAD (1945) Giant cell pneumonia with inclusions. A lesion common to Hecht's disease, distemper and measles. Am J Pathol 21:1–23

Pisano G (1910) Su di un reperto istologico raro in feto scleromatoso. Gazz Osp 31:249–250

Rauh LW, Schmidt R (1965) Measles immunization with killed virus vaccine: serum antibody titers and experience with exposure to measles epidemic. Am J Dis Child 109:232–237

Rector EJ, Rector BS (1934) Intranuclear inclusions in the salivary glands of moles. Am J Pathol 10:629–637

Reynolds EOR (1967) Bronchiolitis. In: Kendig EL (ed) Disorders of the respiratory tract in children. Saunders, Philadelphia

Ribbert H (1904) Ueber protozoenartige Zellen in der Niere eines syphilitischen Neugeborenen und in der Parotis von Kindern. Zentralbl Allg Pathol Pathol Anat 15:945–948

Roberts GBS, Bain AD (1958) The pathology of measles. J Pathol Bacteriol 76:111–118

Roetterink F (in preparation) Epidemiologisch-klinische und pathologisch-anatomische Beobachtungen für Influenzaepidemien mit A2 Hongkong/1/68. Inauguraldissertation, Hannover (and personal communication 1981)

Rowe WP, Huebner RJ, Gilmore LK, Parrott RH, Ward TG (1953) Isolation of a cytopathogenic agent from human adenoids undergoing spontaneous degeneration in tissue culture. Proc Soc Exp Biol Med 84:570–573

Ruebner BH, Hirano T, Slusser RJ, Medearis DN (1965) Human cytomegalovirus infection. Electron microscopic and histochemical changes in cultures of human fibroblasts. Am J Pathol 46:477–496

Sano T, Niitsu J, Nakagawa J, Ando T (1953) Newborn virus pneumonitis (Type Sendai) I. Report: Clinical observation of a new virus pneumonitis of the newborn. Yokohama Med Bull 4:199–216

Scadding JG (1974) Diffuse pulmonary alveolar fibrosis. Thorax 29:271–281

Scadding JG, Hinson KFW (1967) Diffuse fibrosing alveolitis (diffuse interstitial fibrosis of the lungs). Correlation of histology at biopsy with prognosis. Thorax 22:291–403

Schaefer H-E (198) Ein atypisches Verteilungsmuster der tartratresistenten sauren Phosphatase in Osteoklasten bei Ostitis deformans Paget – zur pathogenetischen und diagnostischen Bedeutung. Verh Dtsch Ges Pathol 64:569

Schaefer H-E (1981) The role of macrophages in storage disease. In: Schmalzl F, Huhn D, Schaefer H-E (eds) Disorders of the monocyte macrophage system. Pathophysiological and clinical aspects. Springer, Berlin Heidelberg New York. (Haematology and blood transfusion, vol 27, pp 121–130)

Schaefer H-E, Müntefering H (1982) Histochemische Untersuchungen zur Abkunft intraalveolarer Zellen bei der desquamativen interstitiellen Pneumonie (Liebow). Ber Pathol 97:215

Schaefer H-E, Hellriegel K-P, Fischer R (1977) Vorkommen tartrat-resistenter saurer Phosphatase in verschiedenen Zelltypen des lymphoretikulären und hämatopoetischen Zellsystems. Blut 34:393–397

Schneweis KE, Käckell MY, Nolte R, Sinapius D, Brandis H (1966a) Respiratory-syncytial-Virus-Infektionen im Kindesalter. Virologische Untersuchungen. Dtsch Med Wochenschr 91:53–55

Schneweis KE, Käckell MY, Nolte R, Sinapius D, Brandis H (1966b) Respiratory-syncytial-Virus-Infektionen im Kindesalter. Klinik und pathologische Anatomie. Dtsch Med Wochenschr 91:153–158

Seifert G, Oehme J (1957) Pathologie und Klinik der Cytomegalie. Thieme, Leipzig

Shedden WJH, Emery JL (1965) Immunofluorescent evidence of respiratory syncytial virus infection in case of giantcell bronchiolitis in children. J Pathol Bacteriol 89:343–347

Sherman FE, Ruckle G (1958) In vivo and in vitro cellular changes specific for measles. Arch Pathol Lab Med 65:587–599

Shope RE (1936) The influenzas of swine and man. The Harvey Lectures, 1935–36, p 183

Shope RE, Francis T (1936) The susceptibility of swine to the virus of human influenza. J Exp Med 64:791–801

Sinigaglia G (1912) Osservazioni sul cimurro. Clin Vet (Milano) 35:421–446

Smith MG (1959) The salivary gland viruses of man and animals (cytomegalic inclusion disease). Prog Med Virol 2:171–202

Sobonya RE, Hiller C, Pingleton W, Watanabe J (1978) Fatal measles (rubeola) pneumonia in adults. Arch Pathol Lab Med 102:366–371

Sohier R, Bensimon P, Lagabrielle B (1957) Infection à adénovirus (type 7 prime) avec atteinte pulmonaire et rénale. Bull Soc Méd Hôp Paris 73:37–42

Sohier R, Chardonnet Y, Prunieras M (1965) Adenoviruses. Status of current knowledge. Prog Med Virol 7:253–325

Spencer H (1973) Pathology of the lung (excluding pulmonary tuberculosis), 2nd edn. Pergamon Press, Oxford

Sperk-Bard E, Kaiserling E, Müller-Hermelink HK (1977) Letale Varizelleninfinektionen. Verh Dtsch Ges Pathol 61:452

Strano AJ (1976) Light microscopy of selected viral diseases (morphology of viral inclusion bodies). Pathol Annu 11:53–75

Straub M, Mulder J (1948) Epithelial lesions in the respiratory tract in human influenzal pneumonia. J Pathol Bacteriol 60:429–434

Taylor-Robinson D, Caunt AE (1972) Varicella virus. Virology monographs. Die Virusforschung in Einzeldarstellungen, Nr. 12. Springer, Wien

Teng CH (1960) Adenovirus pneumonia epidemic among Peking infants and preschool children in 1958. Chin Med J (Engl) 80:331–339

Timbury MC, Edmond E (1979) Herpesviruses. J Clin Pathol 32:859–881

Triebwasser JH, Harris RE, Bryant RE (1967) Varicella pneumonia in adults. Medicine 46:409–423

Tyrrell DAJ, Parsons R (1960) Some virus isolations from common colds. III. Cytopathic effects in tissue cultures. Lancet I:239–242

Vivell OM, Axmann M, Lips G (1962) Die Epidemie von Respirationstrakterkrankungen im Winter 1961/62. Dtsch Med Wochenschr 87:1996–2003

Walsh JJ, Dietlein LF, Low FN, Burch GE, Mogabgab WJ (1961) Bronchotracheal response in human influenza. Type A, Asian strain, as studied by light and electron microscopic examination of bronchoscopic biopsies. Arch Intern Med 108:376–388

Waring JJ, Neubuerger K, Geever EF (1942) Severe forms of chickenpox in adults, with autopsy observations in a case with associated pneumonia and encephalitis. Arch Intern Med 69:384–408

Warthin AS (1931) Occurrence of numerous large giant cells in the tonsils and pharyngeal mucosa in the prodromal stage of measles. Arch Pathol Lab Med 11:864–874

Weinstein L, Meade RH (1956) Respiratory manifestations of chickenpox. Special consideration of features of primary varicella pneumonia. Arch Intern Med 98:91–99

Weller RW (1952) Giant cell pneumonia with inclusions. Pediatrics 10:681–686

Weller TH (1971) The cytomegaloviruses: Ubiquitous agents with protean clinical manifestations. N Engl J Med 285:203–214 (I), 267–274 (II)

Wöckel W, Meerbach W (1968) Zur Morphologie der Lunge bei Viruskrankheiten im Säuglings- und Kindesalter. Dtsch Med Wochenschr 93:313–318

Wöckel W, Güthert H, Meerbach W (1963) Zur pathologischen Anatomie der Adenoviruspneumonie. Pathol Microbiol 26:768–788

Wrigth HT, Beckwith JB, Gwinn JL (1964) A fatal case of inclusion body pneumonia in an infant infected with adenovirus type 3. J Pediatr 64:628–633

Yam LT, Li CY, Lam KW (1971) Tartrate-resistant acid phosphatase isoenzyme in the reticulum cells of leukemic reticuloendotheliosis. N Engl J Med 284:357–360

Zakstelskaya LY, Almeida JD, Bradstreet CMP (1967) The morphological characterisation of respiratory syncytial virus by a simple electron microscope technique. Acta Virol (Praha) 11:420–423

Zweerink HJ, Courtneidge SA, Skehel JJ, Crompton MJ, Askonas BA (1977) Cited by Lin Yun Lu et al. (1981) Nature 267:354–356

Formal Genesis of Pulmonary Fibrosis: Experimental Investigations

W. KISSLER

I. Introduction

In 1976, *Crystal* et al. reported the histological results of open pulmonary biopsies from 29 patients with idiopathic pulmonary fibrosis. Apart from an interstitial fibrosis, which by definition is part of this disease, only two alterations could be regularly observed in all pulmonary biopsies: (a) proliferation of type II pneumocytes and (b) accumulation of cells in the alveolar lumen which proved on electron microscopy to be in some cases desquamated type II pneumocytes and in some cases alveolar macrophages. Other findings, such as an interstitial lymphocytic/plasmacytic infiltration, formation of lymph follicles, narrowing of bronchioli, proliferation of smooth muscle cells, pulmonary arteriosclerosis, focal precipitation of cholesterol crystals, and a faveolate parenchymal transformation were found only irregularly in 30%–97% of cases.

Crystal's observations were confirmed in animal experiments. On the basis of a comparative enzyme-histochemical and electron-microscopic investigation of ten different models of pulmonary fibrosis, however, it will be shown that very many of the histological alterations which are regarded as typical for idiopathic pulmonary fibrosis develop completely independently of the causative agent. They are to be seen as a reaction of the lungs to the mechanical stabilization of its alveolar septae due to fibrosis.

II. Materials and Methods

1. Animals and Maintenance

Experimental animals (mice, rats, guinea pigs, and rabbits, 319 in total, with a minimum age of 10 weeks) were kept conventionally with an artificial day/night rhythm and fed with industrially manufactured pellets.

2. Special Methods for the Individual Fibrosis Models

The animals were devided into ten groups, each of which was subjected to a different treatment procedure. The details of the method, the animals species chosen, and the number of animals in the individual groups are summarized in Table 1. The animals of all groups, together with control animals, were killed under Nembutal anesthesia at definite time intervals. With insignificant differences within the individual groups, as a rule the following timetable was chosen: Animals were killed 1 week, 2 weeks, 1 month, 2 months, 3 months, or 4 months after completion of treatment. Only individual animals were killed at later or earlier times. After the animals had been killed, part of their lungs was processed for light and electron microscopy, and part for enzyme histochemistry.

3. Electron-Microscopic Preparation

The animal lungs to be used for electron-microscopic examination were perfused in situ with 2% glutaraldehyde solution in phosphate buffer pH 7.2 via the pulmonary artery after cuneiform opening of the left ventricle. After lamellation of the lungs, postfixation was carried out in the same solution and then a further fixation in 2% osmium tetroxide. After dehydration in the ascending alcohol series, the material was embedded in Epon. Double staining with methylene blue (Merck) and basic fuchsin

Table 1. Methods used in the individual models

Group	Model	Method	Animal species (n)
1	Radiation fibrosis	3000 rads X-rays or cobalt rays applied to one or both lungs	Wistar rats (38) Rabbits (18)
2	Paraquat fibrosis	Acute intoxication: 35 mg paraquat [a] i.p./kg body weight Chronic intoxication: 5 mg paraquat [a] i.p./kg body weight; 3–6 times at intervals of 1 week	Sprague-Dawley rats (66)
3	Bleomycin fibrosis	Bleomycin [b] 5 mg/kg body weight i.p. in rats twice a week over a period of 4 weeks; 20 mg/kg body weight in mice	Mice (20) Sprague-Dawley rats (20)
4	Adjuvant fibrosis due to complete Freund's adjuvant	Complete Freund's adjuvant [c] (1 ml) injected subcutaneously into the skin of the neck on 5 consecutive days	Guinea pigs (31)
5	Adjuvant fibrosis due to incomplete Freund's adjuvant	Incomplete Freund's adjuvant [c] (1 ml) injected subcutaneously into the skin of the neck on 5 consecutive days	Guinea pigs (22)
6	Silicosis	Quartz [d] (20–25 mg) administered intratracheally in 0.4 ml physiological saline	Sprague-Dawley rats (20)
7	Anthracosilicosis	Quartz (12.5 mg) and coal dust [e] (12.5 mg) administered intratracheally in 0.5 ml physiological saline	Sprague-Dawley rats (21)
8	Cadmium sulfide pneumoconiosis	Cadmium sulfide [f] (6 × 15 mg) administered intratracheally at intervals of 1 week	Wistar rats (21)
9	Lead sulfide pneumoconoiosis	Lead sulfide [f] (6 × 15 mg) administered intratracheally at intervals of 1 week	Wistar rats (21)
10	Silicosis with adjuvant fibrosis	Complete or incomplete Freund's adjuvant (3–4 × 1 ml) injected on consecutive days into the skin of the neck; single intratracheal dose of 25 mg quartz	Guinea pigs (21)

[a] Commercial name Gramoxone, Celamerck, Ingelheim, West Germany
[b] Commercial preparation of bleomycin, H. Mack, Nachfahren, Illertissen, West Germany
[c] Ready-for-use preparation, Difco Laboratories, Detroit, Michigan
[d] Dörentrup 120   [e] NBAG Magerkohle   [f] Merck, Darmstadt, West Germany

(Chroma) according to *Morgenroth* et al. (1970) was carried out on semithin sections prepared from the tissue. Ultrathin sections which were prepared afterwards were contrast-stained with saturated uranylacetate solution and lead citrate.

4. Enzyme-Histochemical Reactions

Lamellated lungs in 0.3-cm-thick slices were investigated enzyme-histochemically in some cases without fixation and in some cases after fixation in formalin-calcium according to *Baker* (1944). The section thickness of all slices prepared in the cryostat type HR (Slee) was 6 μm at $-20°C$. The activity of the following enzymes was investigated:

1. Succinate dehydrogenase: method according to *Pette* and *Brandau* (1966), modified after *Fand* and *Wattenberg* (1963)
2. α-Glycerol phosphate oxidase: method as above
3. NADH and NADPH diaphorases: method according to *Nachlas* et al. (cited by *Pearse* 1968), modified after *Wattenberg* and *Leong* (1960)
4. Alkaline phosphatase: method after *Burstone* (cited by *Barka* and *Anderson* 1963)
5. Acid phosphatase: method according to *Barka* and *Anderson* (1963)
6. Nonspecific esterase: method according to *Davis* et al. (cited by *Barka* and *Anderson* 1963)

III. Results

There were appreciable differences in the extent of fibrosis in the individual models. An early and especially pronounced pulmonary fibrosis occurred in cadmium sulfide pneumoconiosis and in the model "silicosis with adjuvant fibrosis". On the other hand, the development of fibrosis in radiation-induced fibrosis, paraquat fibrosis, bleomycin fibrosis, and in the adjuvant models was irregular and mostly only slight in extent. In detail, the light-microscopic findings were as follows:

1. Radiation-Induced Fibrosis Model

After 2 days, a perivascular edema was seen as well as swelling and shedding of bronchial epithelial cells, on paraffin and semithin sections of the irradiated lungs. In the alveoli, there were large cells arranged in varying numbers with roundish nuclei and foamy cytoplasmic bodies. After 4 weeks, peribronchovascular lymphocytic/plasmacytic infiltrates appeared. After 2 months, there was a fluid transition of these alterations into a stage of increasing fibrosis. In the fibrotic lung areas, numerous free alveolar cells with a large cytoplasmic body could also be observed at later times, when they were often arranged in groups (Fig. 1).

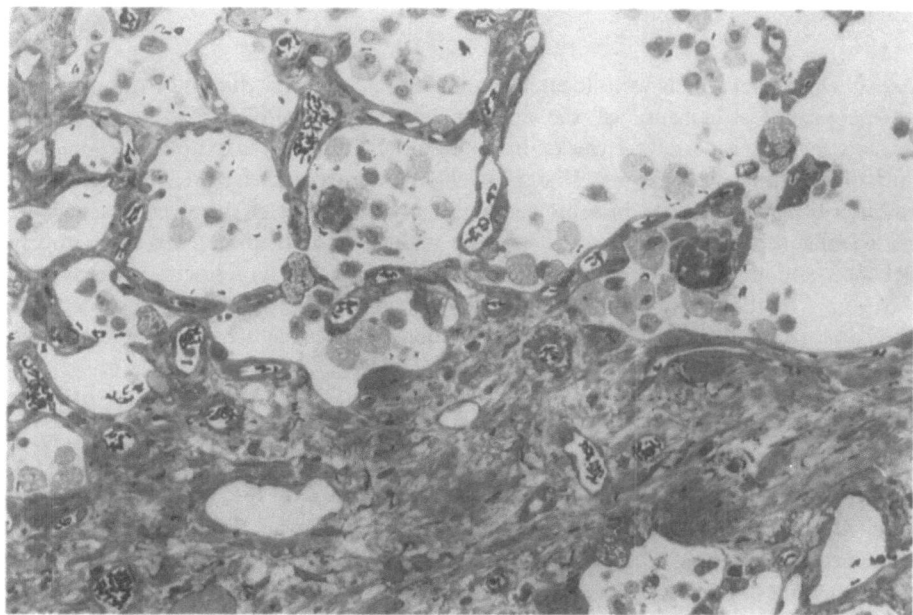

Fig. 1. Radiation-induced fibrosis of a rabbit lung 9 1/2 months after a single exposure of 3000 rads. Semithin section. In the alveoli, numerous macrophages with foamy cytoplasm. Methylene blue and basic fuchsin, × 250

2. Paraqaut Fibrosis Model

At a high dosage of paraquat (35 mg/kg body weight), there was already pronounced hyperemia after 3 h in the lungs of Sprague-Dawley rats. After 7 h, a perivascular interstitial edema had also developed. In the alveolar lumen, increasing numbers of free cells were observed in the subsequent hours: a proportion of these displayed pyknotic or karyolytic nuclei. One-third of the rats which had received this concentration of poison died spontaneously within 24 h.

On the other hand, of 21 rats which had received 5 mg paraquat/kg body weight i.p. six times over 6 weeks only one died. A slight interstitial lymphocytic/plasmacytic infiltration was seen light-microscopically in the lungs of these animals after 5 weeks. In the course of the following months, this increasingly transformed into a focal fibrosis of the alveolar septae. The alveoli in these sections were poorly inflated, and the alveolar walls were often coated with cubical cells lying side by side in rows. In the region of these foci, large cells with foamy cytoplasm were found locally in the alveoli.

3. Bleomycin Fibrosis Model

Grayish-white foci which were located mainly subpleurally in the lungs were noticed macroscopically at autopsy of the animals in which bleomycin had been applied protractedly over a period of weeks; in no case did these foci take up more than one-tenth of the lung parenchyma. Under the light microscope, the areas proved to be circumscribed fibrotic foci, in some cases with complete loss of the alveolar structure. The alveolar septae adjacent to the fibrotic regions were in some cases edematously thickened and as a whole showed a moderate degree of lymphocytic/plasmacytic infiltration. In the alveoli, abundant focally arranged cells of varying numbers with foamy cytoplasm were seen, occasionally located between slightly granular and otherwise unstructured eosinophilic material.

4. Adjuvant Fibrosis Due to Complete Freund's Adjuvant

In the 31 guinea pigs in which 1 ml complete Freund's adjuvant had been injected subcutaneously into the skin of the neck on 5 consecutive days, interstitial infiltrates of varying density consisting of lymphocytes, plasmacytes, and histiocytes appeared in the lungs in the early months.

In addition, epithelioid-cellular granulomas (Fig. 2) already developed as soon as 2 weeks after the last adjuvant administration, frequently in immediate combination

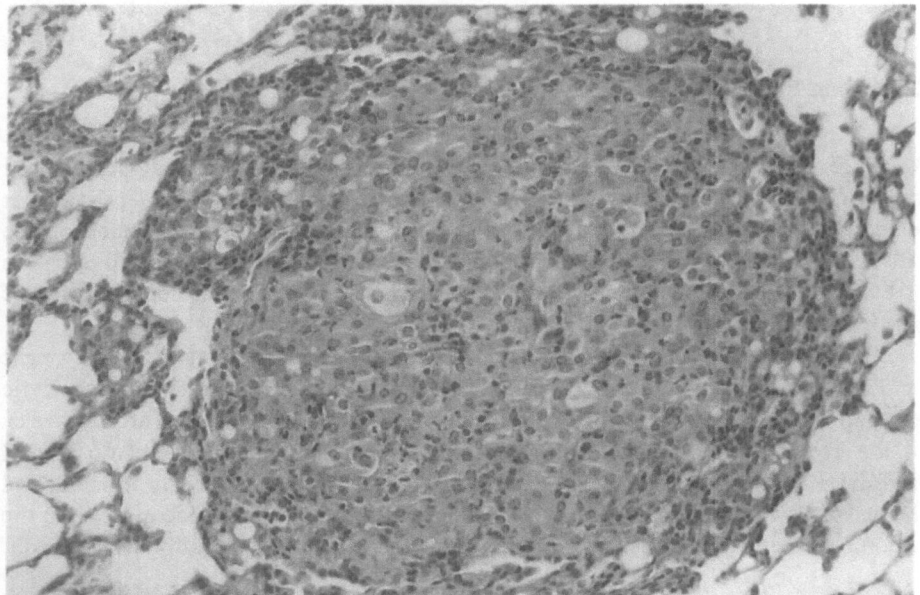

Fig. 2. Guinea pig lung 2 weeks after five subcutaneous injections of 1 ml complete Freund's adjuvant into the skin of the neck. Development of an epithelioid-cellular granuloma. H & E, × 250

with the infiltrates. Individual granulomas became confluent. Locally, there was central necrosis, in some cases with calcifications (Fig. 3).

In occasional isolated instances, a striate fibrosis developed. The neighboring alveoli were constricted partly by this fibrosis, and partly by the interstitial thickening due to the infiltrate. These constricted alveoli were lined by cubic cells, often giving rise to the appearance of "adenoid structures" (Fig. 3).

After 14 months, the epithelioid cells had disappeared and the calcifications were surrounded by fibroblasts with shell-like fibrosis. A diffuse fibrosis of the alveolar septae was found only occasionally in circumscribed lung areas after 4 months.

5. Adjuvant Fibrosis Due to Incomplete Freund's Adjuvant

After administration of incomplete Freund's adjuvant, the pathological alterations in the lung of the guinea pig were less than after administration of the complete adjuvant. However, in the early months after the treatment, focal interstitial lymphoplasmatic cellular infiltrates could also be demonstrated here. After 2 months, locally increased fibroblasts which formed delicate collagen fibers became visible between the inflammatory cells. A slight subpleural fibrous broadening of the alveolar septae remained as a final stage.

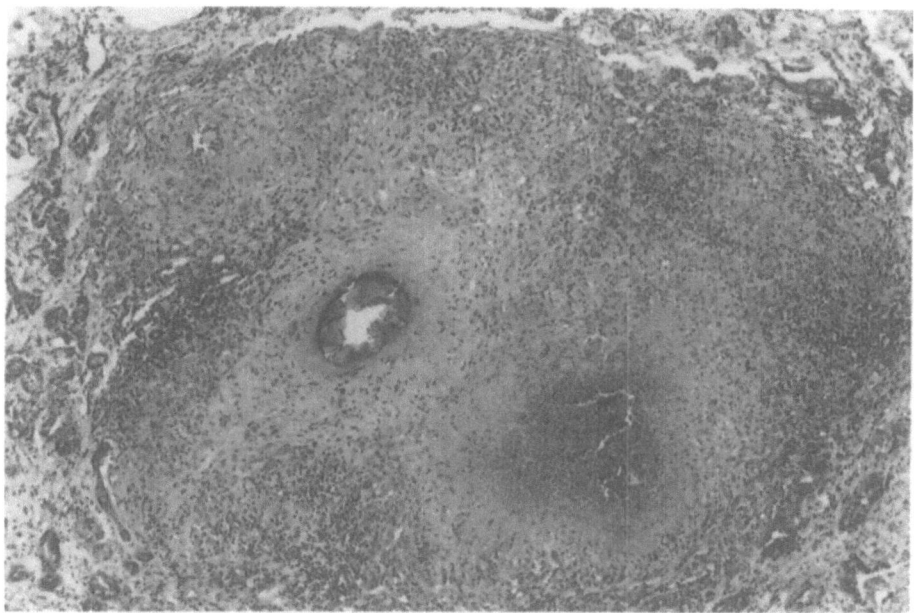

Fig. 3. Guinea pig lung 3 months after five subcutaneous injections of 1 ml complete Freund's adjuvant into the skin of the neck. Old epithelioid-cellular granuloma with central necrosis and calcification. Cubic transformation of the alveolar epithelium at the edges. H & E, × 100

6. Silicosis and Anthracosilicosis Models

A qualitative difference in the lung findings could not be observed after administration of quartz alone (Standardquarz Dörentrup 120) as compared with coal-quartz administration (NDBAG Magerkohle and Standardquarz Dörentrup 120).

From the earliest time of investigation onwards (7 days after intratracheal quartz or coal-quartz administration) increased numbers of macrophages (often arranged in groups) were found both intra-alveolarly and interstitially. After 2 weeks, the macrophages gathered into small nodules in the pulmonary interstitium. The number and extent of the nodules increased continuously up to the last time of killing; some nodules became confluent, especially in the peribronchial vascular sections. In the course of development of these foci, their cellular composition altered. After 2 1/2 months, the phagocytes resembled epithelioid cells (Fig. 4). After 4 1/2 months, the nodules were formed of fibroblasts, and occasionally formation of delicate collagenous fibers could be discerned between them. From the 6th week onward, increased numbers of cells with foamy cytoplasm became visible in the alveoli (Fig. 5). They occurred preferentially in the alveoli adjacent to the nodules. After 4 1/2 months, the alveoli were filled focally with unstructured eosinophilic material, in which spike-like gaps occasionally became visible (Fig. 5). It was striking that type II pneumocytes often proliferated in rows at the edge of the nodules (Fig. 6).

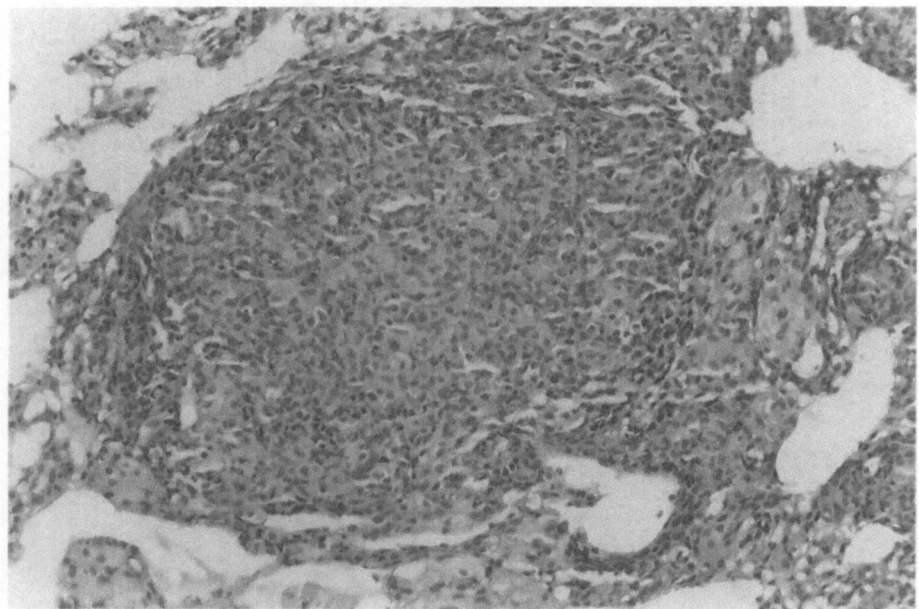

Fig. 4. Rat lung 2 1/2 months after a single administration of 25 mg quartz. Silicosis nodules. Cells with partly epithelioid-cellular character. H & E, × 250

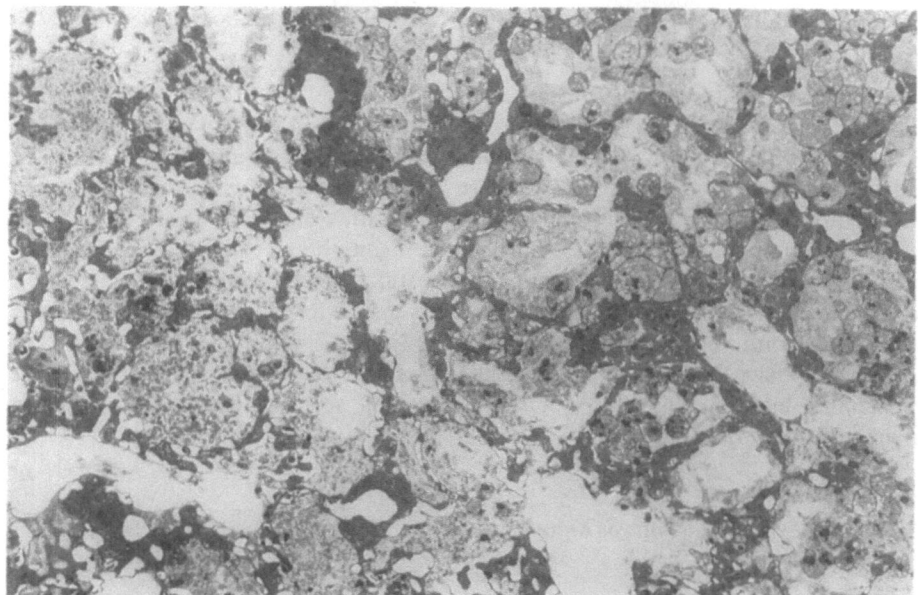

Fig. 5. Rat lung 4 1/2 months after administration of a coal-quartz dust mixture. In the alveoli, cells with foamy cytoplasm between surfactant material. Semithin section. Basic fuchsin with methylene blue, × 250

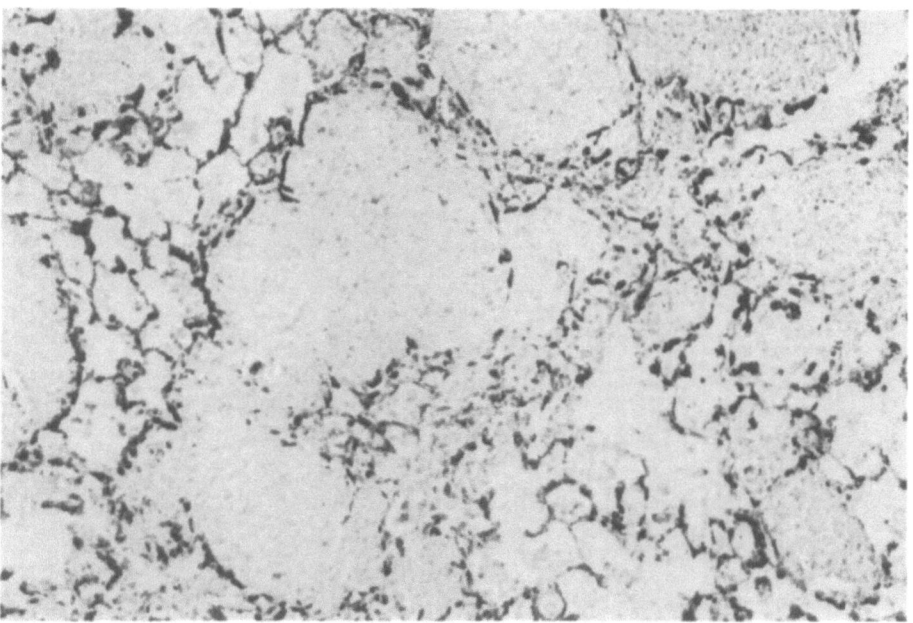

Fig. 6. Rat lung 2 1/2 months after intratracheal administration of 20 mg quartz. Non-specific esterease reaction. Complete enzyme-free silicosis nodules. At the edges of the nodules, enzyme-rich proliferated type II pneumocytes arranged in bands. × 100

7. Cadmium Sulfide Pneumoconiosis Model

In the lungs of Wistar rats in which 15 mg cadmium sulfide had been administered intratracheally six times at weekly intervals, pulmonary fibrosis of varying intensity could already be observed from 2 1/2 weeks after the last administration (Fig. 7). Many of the alveolar septae thickened with connective tissue, which were free from inflammatory infiltrates, were coated by continuous rows of cubic cells (Fig. 8).

The cadmium sulfide particles, which could readily be recognized by their bright yellow color in the histological section, were still mainly intra-alveolar after 2 1/2 weeks, and later an even greater percentage was interstitial. In the alveoli, numerous macrophages with foamy cytoplasm were seen from the beginning: the majority of these macrophages had phagocytosed cadmium sulfide particles (Fig. 8). Abundant fine-granular but otherwise unstructured eosinophilic material was found in varying amounts between the phagocytes.

8. Lead Sulfide Pneumoconiosis Model

The scars in the lungs after intratracheal administration of lead sulfide were slight. Moderately numerous connective tissue nodules occurred at an early stage in all lung regions. In the course of the month, a progressive enlargement of the nodules could not be observed but they appeared poorer in cells after 2 1/2 and 6 months than at earlier times. Whereas the intra-alveolar lead sulfide particles were still abundant initially, they were concentrated almost exclusively in these nodules after 6 months. The

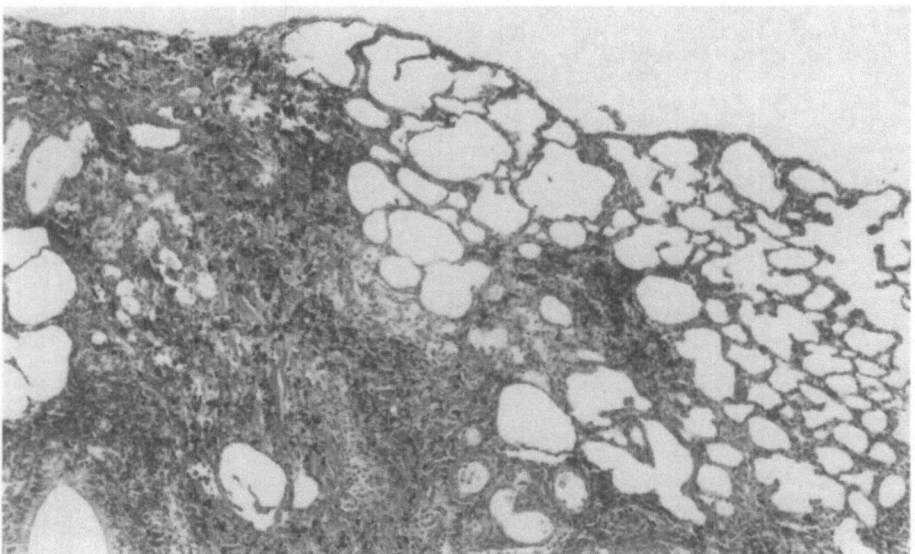

Fig. 7. Rat lung 6 months after six administrations of 15 mg cadmium sulfide. Severe fibrosis in the region of positive cadmium sulfide particles. H & E, × 100

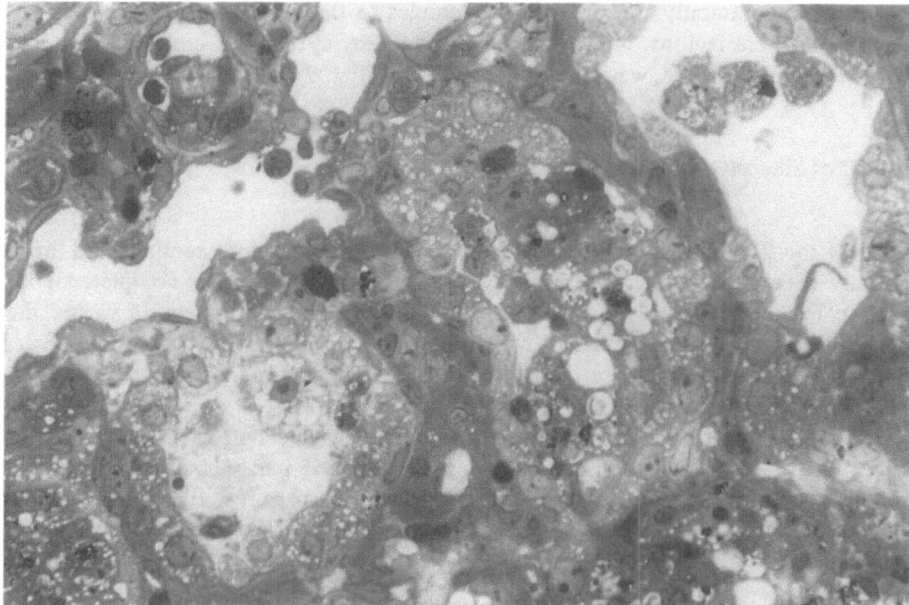

Fig. 8. Rat lung 2 months after six administrations of 15 mg cadmium sulfide. Semi-thin section. Proliferated type II pneumocytes with foamy cytoplasm arranged in rows coat fibrotic alveolar septae. In the alveoli, macrophages which have phagocytosed cadmium sulfide. × 250

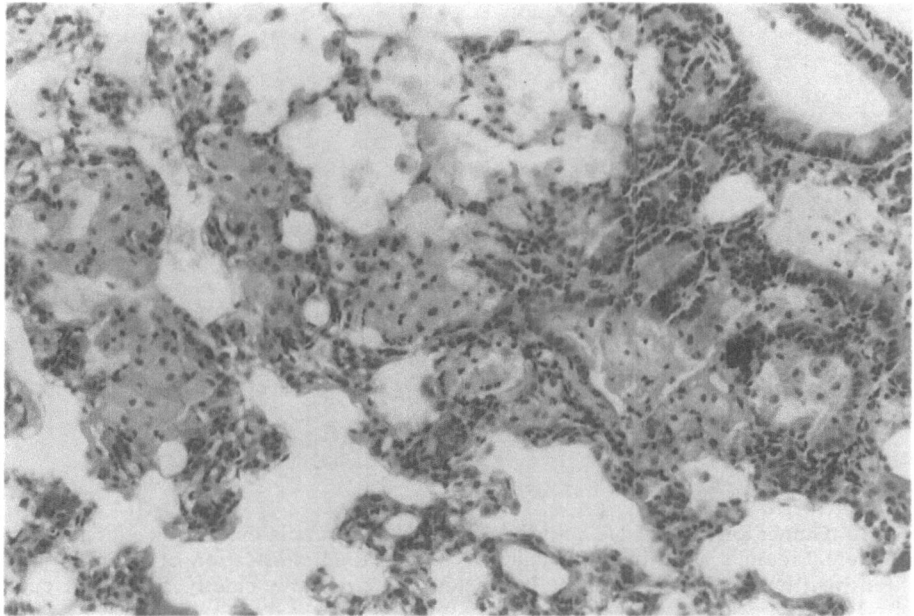

Fig. 9. Rat lung 2 months after six administrations of 15 mg lead sulfide. Focal accumulation of macrophages with foamy cytoplasm. H & E, × 100

fibrosis not uncommonly spread from the nodules to the neighboring alveolar septae. Especially in these regions, numerous cells with foamy cytoplasm, some of which had phagocytosed lead sulfide, were found in the alveoli (Fig. 9).

9. Model of Silicosis with Adjuvant Fibrosis

Several of the 21 guinea pigs initially given a single dose of quartz administered intratracheally (Standardquarz Dörentrup 120) and injected with either complete or incomplete Freund's adjuvant into the skin of the neck died spontaneously within the first month. In the other animals in which increased number of free cells could be demonstrated early in their alveoli, highly cellular, locally confluent interstitial nodules developed after the 5th week.

After 4 1/2 months, the nodules were poorer in cells and rich in fibers. Numerous nodules had fused to form calluses. The calloused tissue was partly hyalinized (Fig. 10). Adenoid structures of various sizes were found in these scar areas. These were largely coated with cubic cells, but at other points also with tall cylindrical epithelium (Fig. 11).

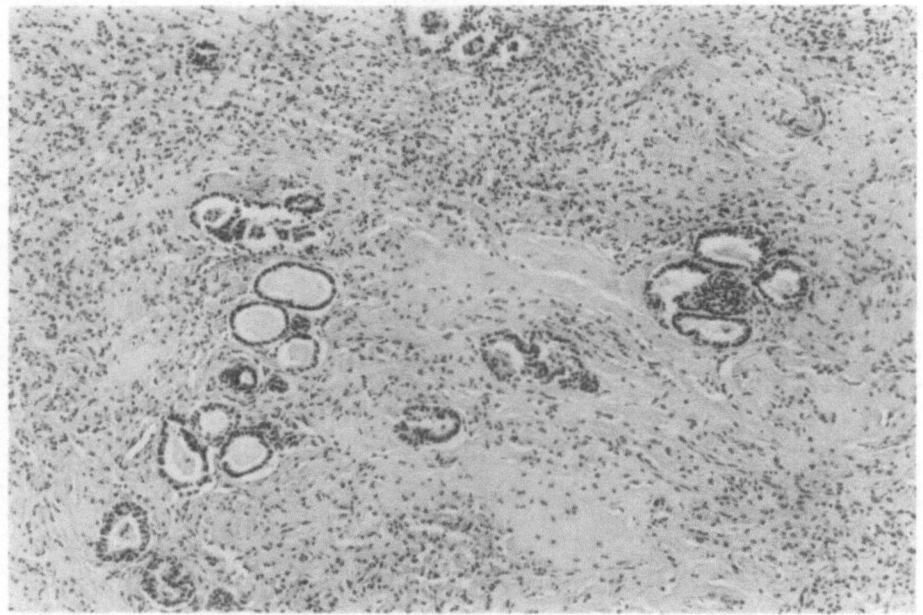

Fig. 10. Guinea pig lung 4 1/2 months after multiple subcutaneous injections of 1 ml complete Freund's adjuvant and single intratracheal administration of 25 mg quartz. Extensive fibrosis. In the fibrous tissue, adenoid structures chiefly formed of cubic cells. H & E, × 100

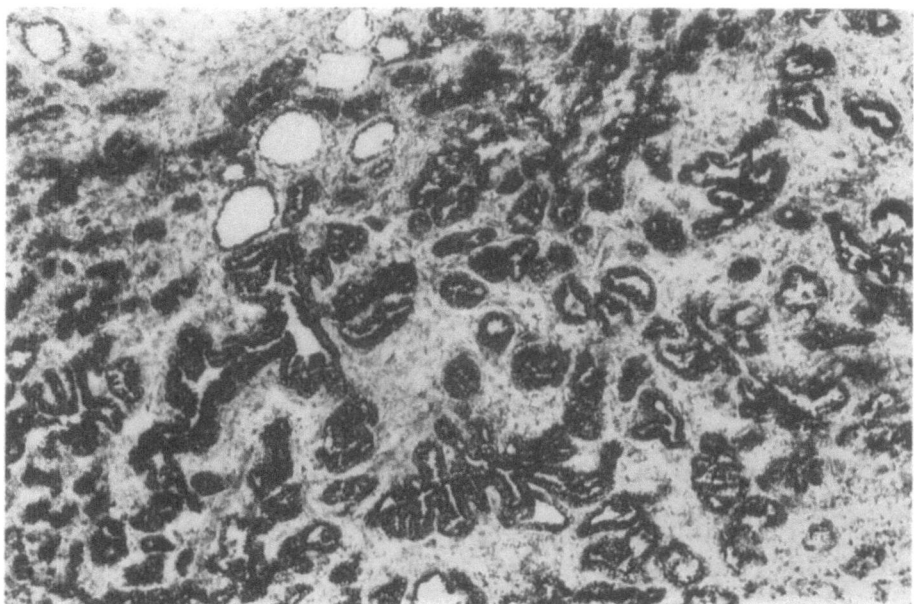

Fig. 11. Guinea pig lung 4 1/2 months after multiple subcutaneous injections of 1 ml Freund's adjuvant and single intratracheal administration of 25 mg quartz. NADPH-diaphorase reaction. Strong reaction of the enzyme in some cases in cubic cells, in some cases in cylindrical cells which form the adenoid structures in the region of an interstitial fibrosis. × 100

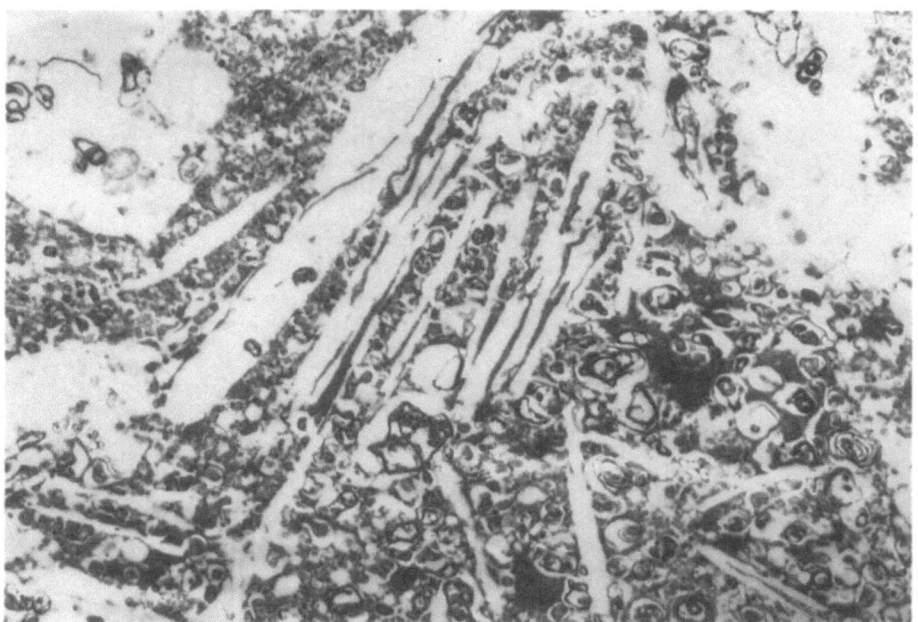

Fig. 12. Rat lung 4 1/2 months after intratracheal administration of a coal—quartz dust mixture. Spike-like gaps between lamellar structures in the alveolar lumen (probably dissolved cholesterol crystals). × 4000

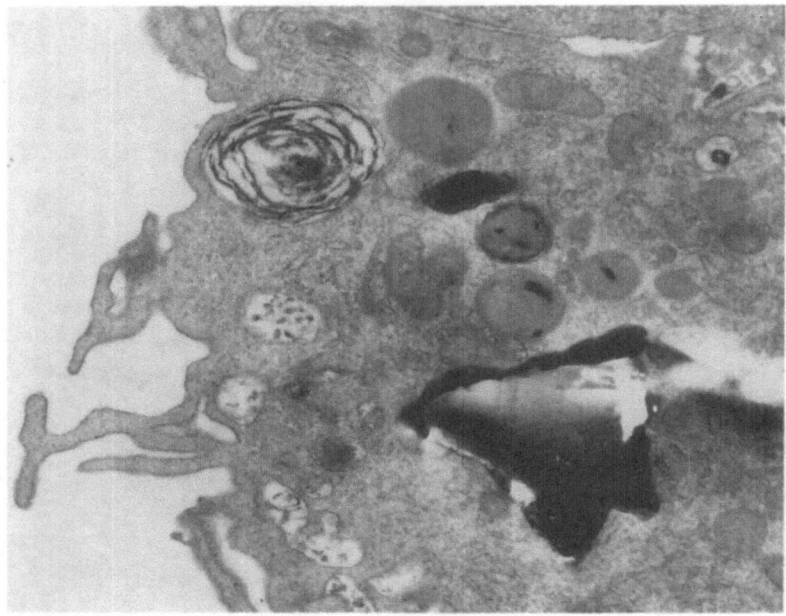

Fig. 13. Rat lung 2 weeks after intratracheal administration of a coal–quartz dust mixture. Part of an alveolar macrophage which has phagocytosed lamellar bodies and coal dust. × 10 000

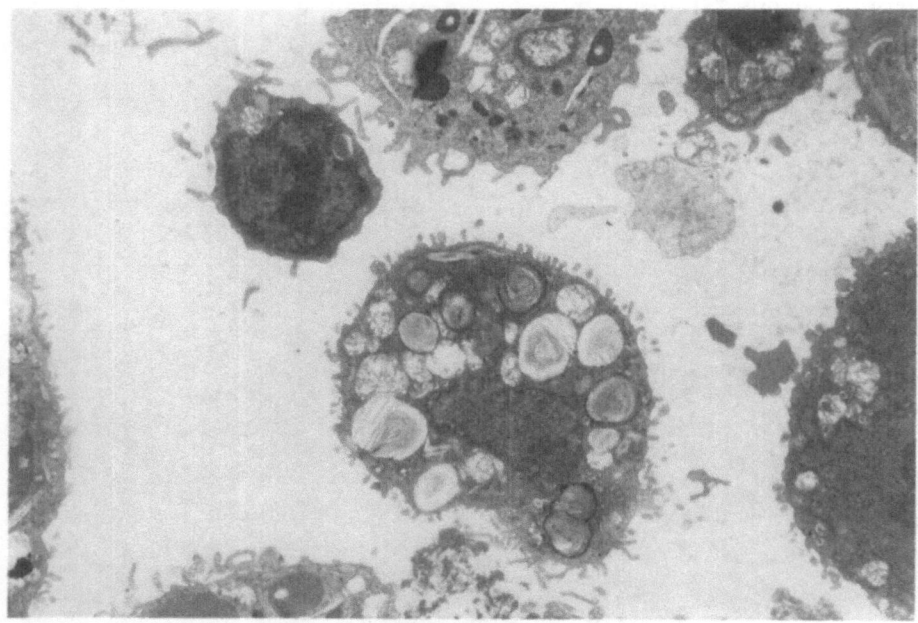

Fig. 14. Rat lung 3 months and 1 week after six injections of 5 mg paraquat/kg body weight. Desquamated type II pneumocyte with characteristic lamellar bodies and microvilli between macrophages in the alveolus. × 4000

10. Electron-Microscopic Findings

The eosinophilic material in the alveoli demonstrated under the light microscope in the fibrosis stage of the models bleomycin fibrosis, silicosis and anthracosilicosis, and cadmium sulfide pneumoconiosis proved to be a mixture of osmiophilic lamellar bodies and fine lattice-like structures (tubular myelin) under the electron microscope. Numerous free lamellar bodies also became visible in the alveolar lumen in the other models, radiation-induced fibrosis, paraquat fibrosis, the adjuvant models, and lead sulfide pneumoconiosis, in which this material had not been noticed light-microscopically. Spear-like gaps occasionally became visible between the lamellar bodies in the pneumoconiosis models: needle-shaped crystals had evidently been dissolved out of the gaps during fixation (Fig. 12). The osmiophilic lamellar bodies were not uncommonly found in the cytoplasm of the free alveolar cells and were often found together with dust particles in the pneumoconiosis models (Fig. 13).

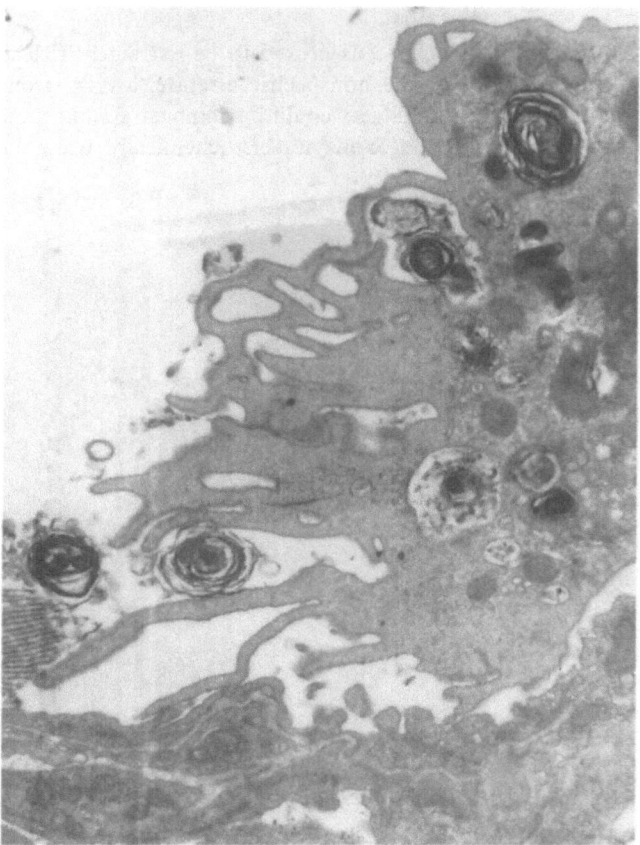

Fig. 15. Rat lung 2 weeks after intratracheal administration of a coal—quartz dust mixture. Phagocytosis of lamellar bodies by an alveolar macrophage. × 10 000

After electron-microscopic investigations alone, it could not always be definitely decided whether the free cells were desquamated type II pneumocytes or alveolar macrophages. Only individual cells could be identified unequivocally as desquamated type II pneumocytes, since they displayed microvilli on their surface which are characteristic for this cell type, and their cytoplasm contained lamellar bodies which were especially densely packed (Fig. 14). On the other hand, in other cells a lamellar body phagocytosis could be demonstrated (Fig. 15), which indicated a macrophagic nature.

The cubic cells occurring in larger numbers in paraquat fibrosis, adjuvant fibrosis with complete Freund's adjuvant, and in the pneumoconiosis models (silicosis, anthracosilicosis, cadmium sulfide pneumoconiosis, and lead sulfide pneumoconiosis) that often coated the fibrotic alveolar septae in rows proved electron-microscopically to be type II pneumocytes, which often display especially abundant osmiophilic lamellar bodies in their cytoplasm (Fig. 16).

11. Enzyme-Histochemical Findings

Almost all intra-alveolarly situated free alveolar cells proved to be extremely rich in enzymes. Apart from a moderate activity of the nonspecific esterase, a very strong reaction of all oxidoreductases and acid phosphatases could be demonstrated in these cells. They were identified as alveolar macrophages enzyme-histochemically, using the

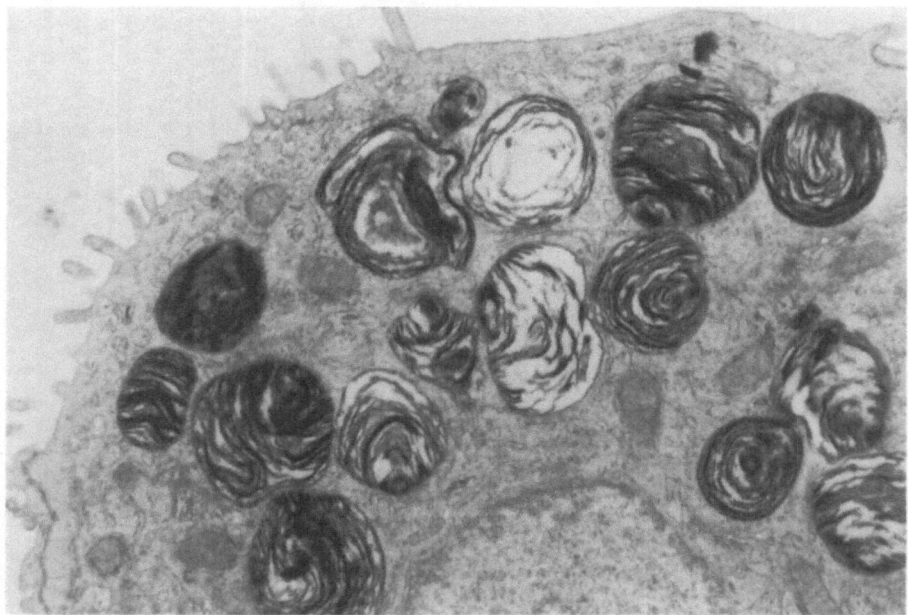

Fig. 16. Electron micrograph of rat lung 2 weeks after intratracheal administration of a coal—quartz dust mixture. Type II pneumocytes with increased and enlarged lamellar bodies. × 10 000

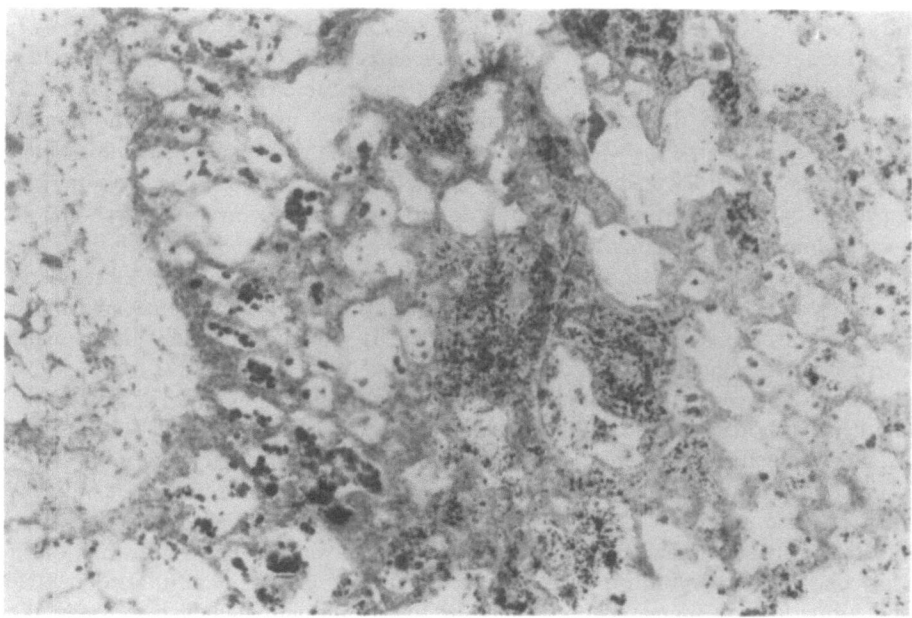

Fig. 17. Rat lung 4 weeks after six administrations of 15 mg cadmium sulfide. Acid phosphatase reaction. Intense reaction of the enzyme in intra-alveolarly situated macrophages. × 100

the acid phosphatases (Fig. 17). The alkaline phosphatase activity was the only one lacking in the majority of the free cells. However, the latter reaction was vigorous in the type II pneumocytes. Both a vigorous reaction of the oxidoreductases and of the nonspecific esterase could be demonstrated in the cubic cells which coated the fibrotic alveolar septae in rows in the various models (Figs. 6, 11). On the other hand, they displayed only a very weak acid phosphatase reaction. The enzyme constellation of the cells which had proliferated in rows entirely corresponded to that of type II pneumocytes as demonstrated in control animals.

III. Discussion

1. Common Findings in all Fibrosis Models

The results obtained essentially confirm the observation by numerous researchers who had investigated only one or two of the fibrosis models and documented them well morphologically (review studies: *Eger* and *Gregl* 1965; *Maisin* 1970; *Pickrell* et al. 1975; *Smith* et al. 1974; *Malmquist* et al. 1973; *Cegla* et al. 1975; *Fleischmann* et al. 1971; *Adamson* and *Bowden* 1974; *Sicic* et al. 1978; *Morgenroth* 1972; *Steiner* et al.

1960; *Weller* 1977; *Rosmanith* and *Breining* 1975; *Rosmanith* et al. 1976, 1977; *Kissler* et al. 1979). The present comparative enzyme-histochemical and electron-microscopic investigation of ten models makes the tissue characteristics common to the various forms of fibrosis and pneumoconiosis more evident. In all the models investigated, proliferated type II pneumocytes arranged in rows could be demonstrated in the fibrotic lung areas and at the edges of the scars in the pneumoconiosis models, irrespective of the extent of the fibrosis developing. This observation is familiar in human pulmonary fibrosis as cubic transformation of the alveolar epithelium. Like-wise, large intra-alveolarly situated cells with foamy cytoplasm were observed regularly in these areas. They proved enzyme-histochemically and electron-microscopically to be alveolar macrophages, with desquamated type II pneumocytes only occasionally occurring between them.

In addition, a further very frequent finding was a focal accumulation of free osmiophilic lamellar bodies and lattice-like osmiophilic structures in the alveoli. This observation could be made only where the type II pneumocytes occurred in larger numbers.

The similar findings described appear all the more remarkable since not only the extent, but also the cause of the scar development in the individual models was different. Despite the dissimilar cause of the fibrosis, there was a cubic transformation of the alveolar epithelium uniformly in all models with increasing interstitital connective tissue formation, an increased occurrence of free osmiophilic lamellar bodies, and a local macrophage accumulation in the alveoli. Therefore, these tissue alterations must be regarded as the consequence of *any* kind of lung scarring.

The question thus arises of why the secondary alterations develop and whether they are regressive alterations as a consequence of mechanical stabilization of the pulmonary parenchyma with modified blood circulation, or whether they involve a progressive reaction of healthy lung regions to the impairment of ventilation resulting from the pulmonary fibrosis. The function of type II pneumocytes must be discussed in order to answer these questions.

2. Type II Pneumocyte Proliferation as a Reaction to Underventilation of the Lungs

In 1954, *Macklin* was the first to suggest that the type II pneumocyte forms the sur-face-active substance of the lungs, the surfactant. This substance, which coats the alveoli as a film, reduces the surface tension at the air-liquid boundary of the lungs and thus prevents collapse of the air spaces. Today, it is known that the surfactant material is a mixture of different chemical compounds. The main constituent is dipalmitoyl phosphatidylcholine (dipalmitoyllecithin) (*King* and *Clements* 1972; *Kikkawa* et al. 1975; *Sanders* and *Longmore* 1975; *Rooney* et al. 1975), which is alleged to be loosely linked to a surfactant apoprotein (*Hallmann* and *Gluck* 1974). Phosphatidylglycerol is regarded as a further important component (*Rooney* et al. 1974; *Sanders* and *Long-more* 1975), of which it is assumed that it can modify the action of the surfactant (*Hallmann* and *Gluck* 1976). Finally, lipids, cholesterol, and proteins are present in the surfactant (*Goerke* 1974).

There is no longer any doubt that the main constituent of the surfactant is formed by type II pneumocytes, because *Gil* and *Reiss* (1973) and *Rooney* et al. (1975) demonstrated that the lamellar bodies of type II pneumocytes predominantly consist of dipalmitoyl phosphatidylcholine; *Hatasa* and *Nakumura* (1965) were able to show that these lamellar bodies are secreted into the alveolar lumen in the same way as a merocrine secretion. *Chevalier* and *Collet* (1972) and *Massaro* and *Massaro* (1972) succeeded in demonstrating with autoradiographic methods that the synthesis of the surfactant takes place in the endoplasmic reticulum of type II pneumocytes and that this material is then channeled via the Golgi apparatus into the lamellar bodies, so that it can finally be secreted. The lamellar bodies do not spread over lattice-like structures (the tubular myelin) as an intermediate to the fine surface film before they reach the alveolar lumen (*Kuhn* 1972; *Gil* and *Reiss* 1973; *Gil* and *Weibel* 1969, 1970).

Briefly, it can now be regarded as proved that type II pneumocytes have the function of preventing underventilation of the pulmonary parenchyma via surfactant formation.

This enables the question posed initially, of why a type II pneumocyte proliferation and a focal macrophages accumulation occurred uniformly irrespective of the causal genesis of the pulmonary fibrosis in the middle and late stages of scar formation, to be answered with regard to the type II pneumocyte proliferation.

In the models investigated, it was not functionally inferior type II pneumocytes which proliferated, but rather cells with an increased activity, as indicated by increased surfactant formation. Therefore the cubic transformation of the alveolar epithelium can only be interpreted in terms of a progressive reaction of healthy cells. This serves to counteract a regional hypoventilation by means of increased surfactant formation.

However, it remains unclear how the type II pneumocytes receive the information for increased surfactant formation. It is unknown at present whether biochemical, humoral, or nervous mechanisms control the secretion of the lamellar bodies (*Goerke* 1974).

According to the present studies, a mechanical component might play a role in this regulatory mechanism to the extent that the type II pneumocyte proliferation could be observed chiefly on alveolar septae which were mechanically stabilized by the fibrosis.

A further argument for the development of the concept that the cubic transformation of the alveolar epithelium constitutes a reaction to a disturbance of ventilation is the fact that focal type II proliferation was also demonstrated by other authors, some of whose studies comprised not only the same models as in the present study, e.g., bleomycin damage to the lungs (*Aso* et al. 1976), cadmium sulfide pneumonitis (*Thurlbeck* and *Foley* 1963), paraquat fibrosis (*Vijeyaratnam* and *Corrin* 1971; *Kimbrough* and *Linder* 1973), and experimental radiation-induced fibrosis (*Maisin* 1970), but also other lung lesions, e.g., those due to hypoventilation of the pulmonary parenchyma, in oxygen damage (*Kapanci* et al. 1969), and in carbon dioxide damage (*Schaefer* et al. 1964). Only *Maisin* (1970) and *Schaefer* et al. (1964) have discussed the pneumocyte proliferation as a progressive pulmonary reaction to hypoventilation.

On the other hand, the possibility that the proliferation of type II pneumocytes might constitute a meaningful reaction of the pulmonary parenchyma to a local disturbance of ventilation has not yet been considered in human pulmonary fibrosis, although *Hamman* and *Rich* (1944) described an enlargement of alveolar cells and this cubic transformation of the alveolar epithelium (as described in the Introduction) can be regarded as characteristic for idiopathic pulmonary fibrosis (*Crystal* et al. 1976).

It is possible that such a reaction mechanism has so far not been considered in man, because here other metaplastic epithelial cells, such as bronchial epithelium and squamous epithelial cells, are occasionally to be found besides proliferated type II pneumocytes on the fibrotic alveolar septae (*Carrington* 1968). In our own study, a similar finding was seen in the combination model "silicosis with adjuvant fibrosis" in which the intensely fibrously thickened alveolar septae were partly coated by type II pneumocytes arranged in rows, and partly by tall zylindrical epithelium. One has the impression that initially proliferated type II pneumocytes are gradually replaced by proliferating bronchial epithelium, a process which probably also occurs in human idiopathic pulmonary fibrosis.

3. Macrophage Accumulation as a Reaction to Increased Surfactant Formation

The second part of the question posed initially, why a focal accumulation of alveolar macrophages occurred uniformly in all models (in agreement with the tissue reaction in idiopathic pulmonary fibrosis in man), has remained unanswered so far. Since collagenases are available to macrophages (*Wahl* et al. 1975; *Horwitz* et al. 1976), *Crystal* et al. (1978) believed that the alveolar macrophages may possibly have the task of breaking down collagenous fibers in pulmonary fibrosis. According to this concept, the macrophages would have to be localized in the pulmonary interstitium, but in fact they were found chiefly intra-alveolarly. It is therefore probable that on the contrary the accumulation of macrophages is connected with their capacity for phagocytosis. This hypothesis could be proved electron-microscopically in our own study. Furthermore, it could be shown that their increased occurrence was at least partly an immediate consequence of the focal overproduction of surfactant by proliferated type II pneumocytes.

Phagocytosed lamellar bodies were seen in a large number of macrophages. It was even possible to observe the process of phagocytosis electron-microscopically.

In the pneumoconiosis models, the macrophage accumulation was also essentially due to the administered foreign particles of quartz, coal, cadmium sulfide, and lead sulfide which they had phagocytosed. However, it must be emphasized that phagocytosed lamellar bodies were also not uncommonly seen besides phagocytosed dust particles in the cytoplasm of the alveolar macrophages.

The overproduction of lamellar bodies by proliferated pneumocytes must thus be regarded as at least one of several causes of the accumulation of macrophages in the fibrosis models investigated. In contrast to properly ventilated lungs, in which these lamellar bodies spread rapidly after their secretion under the influence of the movement of the alveolar walls and with breakdown of their characteristic structure, the lamellar bodies remained like foreign bodies in the regions in which a movement-limiting stabilization of the alveoli had occurred due to the fibrosis, so that it was necessary that they be transported away by macrophages.

According to the concept developed, the accumulation of macrophages in hypoventilated lung areas as a consequence of reactive overproduction of surfactant is largely independent of the causal genesis of the fibrosis. However, this does not exclude the possibility that further macrophages additionally migrate into the alveoli to phagocytose foreign particles, such as quartz, coal, cadmium, or lead sulfide, or to ingest disrupting pneumocytes.

The initial question as to the cause of the uniform lung reaction to an etiologically different pulmonary fibrosis can thus be answered as follows:

In pulmonary fibrosis, one can and must distinguish between the scarring which can be attributed directly to the causative agent and alterations of the lung parenchyma (such as the cubic transformation of the alveolar epithelium and the local macrophage accumulation) which are also characteristic for pulmonary fibrosis, but are to be regarded essentially as a reaction of the lung tissue to the mechanical stabilization of the alveolar walls due to the scarring.

4. Classical Interstitial Pneumonia, Desquamative Interstitial Pneumonia and Alveolar Proteinosis

In 1968, *Liebow* distinguished "desquamative interstitial pneumonia" from other forms of interstitial pneumonia, especially from "common or classical interstitial pneumonia." Desquamative interstitial pneumonia is, according to his definition, a lung disease which ends in pulmonary fibrosis in the late stages, but is characterized in early stages by especially abundant desquamated type II pneumocytes.

It will be shown here that through the comparative examination of the ten fibrosis models of the lungs, a further conclusion can be drawn, in addition to the development of the concept that a sharp distinction must be made in pulmonary fibrosis between causal and formal genesis of the tissue reaction: There are close relations between the three lung diseases, common or classical interstitial pneumonia, desquamative interstitial pneumonia, and alveolar proteinosis.

Apart from alveolar macrophages, desquamated and in some cases necrobiotic type II pneumocytes occurred in the alveoli in the individual models. *Scadding* and *Hinson* (1967) and *Crystal* et al. (1976) made the same observation in idiopathic pulmonary fibrosis in man. This also gave them cause to assume that desquamative interstitial pneumonia and common interstitial pneumonia are varieties of one and the same disease.

This view is supported by the present study. However, the occasional occurrence of desquamated, necrobiotic type II pneumocytes in the alveoli in the middle and late phases of pulmonary fibrosis, in which the pneumocytes proliferate in large numbers as described, can be by no means surprising. With an alveolar cell lifetime of 28 days (*Bertalanffy* and *Leblond* 1953), such a finding had to be expected, since there is no route of shedding for moribund type II pneumocytes other than that into the alveoli. However, it must be assumed that the type II pneumocytes have an even shorter lifetime in the full syndrome of desquamative interstitial pneumonia with a still unelucidated etiology, as they are to be found in larger numbers in the alveolar lumen.

It is remarkable that the character of the intra-alveolar cells in desquamative interstitial pneumonia is still controversial today. Only *Shortland* et al. (1969) and *Gould* et al. (1971) regarded these cells exclusively as type II pneumocytes. *Rhodes* (1973) assumes that about half of the cells are type II pneumocytes, but the other half are alveolar macrophages. On the other hand, *Leroy* (1969), *Brewer* et al. (1969), *Farr* et al. (1970), *Corrin* and *Price* (1972) and *Patchefsky* et al. (1973) have identified these cells as alveolar macrophages.

According to our own observations, the divergence of these opinions may be due to the fact that even under the electron microscope, desquamated necrobiotic type II pneumocytes cannot always be distinguished clearly from alveolar macrophages which have phagocytosed lamellar bodies. However, this differentiation could be effected readily by enzyme histochemistry in the present study, since in contrast to type II pneumocytes, the macrophages have a very strong acid phosphatase reaction. In particular, this result underscores the significance of enzyme-histochemical methods for the exploration of idiopathic pulmonary fibrosis.

Apart from the relation to desquamative interstitial pneumonia, transitions to alveolar proteinosis became clear especially in the pneumoconiosis model. Alveolar proteinosis is a lung disease of which the etiology is still unclarified. It was described for the first time in 1958 by *Rosen* et al. and is characterized by a recurrent or progressive accumulation of phospholipid-containing material in the alveoli with absence of pathological interstitial lung findings; electron-microscopically, this material proves to be surfactant.

In the present study, the overproduction of surfactant in the pneumoconiosis models was often so severe that it went beyond a reaction to the hypoventilation. It appears as if the process of enhanced surfactant production, which is to be regarded in the first instance as meaningful, occasionally gets out of control and becomes pathologically elevated. This causes development of the clinical picture of alveolar proteinosis.

There are thus close relations between a type II pneumocyte proliferation in the region of fibrotic alveolar septae with reactive overproduction of surfactant, a desquamative interstitial pneumonia, and an alveolar proteinosis. According to the present investigations, there may be fluid transitions between these clinical pictures. They are the manifestation of a lung reaction which can vary in intensity, and which can occasionally be pathologically raised.

V. Summary

Using conventionally kept mice, rats, guinea pigs, and rabbits, ten models of pulmonary fibrosis (radiation-induced fibrosis, paraquat fibrosis, bleomycin fibrosis, lung scarring resulting from multiple administration of complete or incomplete Freund's adjuvant, silicosis, anthracosilicosis, cadmium sulfide and lead sulfide pneumoconiosis, and the combination model of silicosis with adjuvant fibrosis) were investigated comparatively by means of enzyme histochemistry and light and electron microscopy.

A cubic transformation of the alveolar epithelium could be observed consistently in all models in the region of diffuse fibrosis or at the edge of the scars in pneumoconiosis. This is also characteristic for idiopathic pulmonary fibrosis in man. The type II pneumocytes proliferated in this case were not functionally inferior but had raised activity, as was demonstrated by an excess surfactant formation by these cells. Their proliferation was hence interpreted as an attempt of the lungs to compensate for the hypoventilation of the pulmonary parenchyma in the region of the fibrosis by increased surfactant formation. The secreted lamellar bodies normally spread out under the influence of movement of the alveolar walls, forming the surface film of the lungs. In pulmonary fibrosis, they pile up like foreign material, as a consequence of the mechanical stabilization of the alveolar septae. In this way, they bring about an accumulation of alveolar macrophages (which phagocytose the surfactant material) in this region. Here, there are close relations between the fibrosis models and the desquamative interstitial pneumonia as well as alveolar proteinosis in man.

The cubic transformation of the alveolar epithelium and the accumulation of macrophages in underventilated lung areas are thus to be evaluated as consequences of the mechanical stabilization of the lung parenchyma. In pulmonary fibrosis, one therefore can and must distinguish between scarring, which is directly attributable to the causal agent, and alterations of the lung parenchyma, which are also characteristic for pulmonary fibrosis but only occur as a reaction of the lung tissue to the mechanical stabilization of the alveolar walls due to scarring.

References

Adamson IYR, Bowden DH (1974) The pathogenesis of bleomycin-induced pulmonary fibrosis in mice. Am J Pathol 77:185–198

Aso Y, Yonada K, Kikkawa Y (1976) Morphological and biochemical study of pulmonary changes induced by bleomycin in mice. Lab Invest 35:558–568

Baker JR (1944) The structure and chemical composition of the Golgi element. Q J Microsc Sci 85:1–72

Barka T, Anderson PJ (1963) Histochemistry. Theory, practice and bibliography. Harper & Row, New York Evanston London

Bertalanffy FD, Leblond CP (1953) The continuous renewal of the two types of alveolar cells in the lung of the rat. Anat Rec 115:515–536

Brewer DB, Heath D, Asquith P (1969) Electron microscopy of desquamative interstitial pneumonia. J Pathol 97:317–323

Carrington CB (1968) Organizing interstitial pneumonia. Definition of the lesion and attempts to devise an experimental model. Yale J Biol Med 40:352–363

Cegla UH, Kreidl RF, Kronberger H, Weber H (1975) Tierexperimentelles Modell einer Lungenfibrose bei der Ratte mittels Paraquatinjektion. Pneumonologie 152:65–74

Chevalier G, Collet AJ (1972) In vivo incorporation of cholin-^{3}H, leucin-^{3}H and galactose-^{3}H in alveolar type II pneumocytes in relation to surfactant synthesis. A quantitative radioautographic study in mouse by electron microscopy. Anat Rec 174:289–310

Corrin B, Price AB (1972) Electron microscopic studies in desquamative interstitial pneumonia associated with asbestos. Thorax 27:324–331

Crystal RG, Fulmer JD, Roberts WC, Moss ML, Line BR, Reynolds HY (1976) Idiopathic pulmonary fibrosis: Clinical, histologic, radiographic, physiologic, scintigraphic, cytologic, and biochemical aspects. Ann Intern Med 85:769–788

Crystal RG, Fulmer JD, Baum BR, Bernado J, Bradley KH, Bruel SD et al. (1978) Cells, collagen, and idopathic pulmonary fibrosis. Lung 155:199–224

Eger W, Gregl A (1965) Die Strahlenpneumonitis. Hippokrates, Stuttgart

Fand SB, Wattenberg LW (1963) A histochemical study of oxydative enzymes in the pituitary gland. Lab Invest 12:454–459

Farr GH, Harley RA, Henningar GR (1970) Desquamative interstitial pneumonia: an electron microscopic study. Am J Pathol 60:347–354

Fleischmann, RW, Baker JR, Thompson GA, Schaeppi UH, Illievski VR, Cooney DA, Davis RD (1971) Bleomycin-induced interstitial pneumonia in dogs. Thorax 26: 675–682

Gil J, Reiss OK (1973) Isolation and characterization of lamellar bodies and tubular myelin from rat lung homogenates. J Cell Biol 58:152–171

Gil J, Weibel ER (1969/1970) Improvements in demonstration of lining layer of lung alveoli by electron microscopy. Respir Physiol 8:13–36

Goerke J (1974) Lung surfactant. Biochim Biophys Acta 344:241–261

Gould VE, Gleason TH, Winterscheid LC (1971) Desquamative interstitial pneumonia. Chest 59:349–352

Hallmann M, Gluck L (1974) Phosphatidyl glycerol in lung surfactant: I. Synthesis in rat lung microsomes. Biochem Biophys Res 60:1–7

Hallmann M, Gluck L (1976) Phosphatidyl glycerol in lung surfactant. III. Possible modifier of surfactant function. J Lipid Res 17:257–262

Hamman L, Rich AR (1944) Acute diffuse interstitial fibrosis of the lungs. Bull Johns Hopkins Hosp 74:177–212

Hatasa K, Nakamura T (1965) Electron microscopic observations of lungs alveolar epithelial cells of normal young mice with special reference to formation and secretion of osmiophilic lamellar bodies. Z Zellforsch 68:266–277

Horwitz AL, Kelman JA, Crystal RG (1976) Activation of alveolar macrophage collagenase by a neutral protease secreted by the same cell. Nature 264:772–774

Kapanci Y, Weibel ER, Kaplan HP, Robinson FR (1969) Pathogenesis and reversiblity of the pulmonary lesions of oxygen toxicity in monkeys. II. Ultrastructural and morphometric studies. Lab Invest 20:101–118

Kikkawa Y, Yoneda K, Smith F, Packard B, Suzuki K (9175) The type II epithelial cells of the lung. II. Chemical composition and phospholipid synthesis. Lab Invest 32:295–302

Kimbrough RD, Linder RE (1973) The ultrastructure of the paraquat lung lesion in the rat. Environ Res 6:265–273

King RJ, Clements JA (1972) Surface active materials from dog lung. II. Composition and physiological correlations. Am J Physiol 223:715–726

Kissler W, Rosmanith J, Breining H, Niehusmann G (1979) Enzymhistochemie und Elektronenmikroskopie der experimentellen Cadmiumsulfid- und Bleisulfidpneumokoniose. Silikosebericht Nordrhein-Westfalen 12:229–233

Kuhn C (1972) A comparison of freeze-substitution with other methods of perservation of the pulmonary alveolar lining layer. Am J Anat 133:495–508

Leroy EP (1969) The blood-air barrier in desquamative interstitial pneumonia (DIP). Virchows Arch [Pathol Anat] 348:117–130

Liebow AA (1968) New concepts and entities in pulmonary disease. In: Liebow AA, Smith DE (eds) The lung. Williams & Wilkins, Baltimore, p 323

Macklin CC (1954) The pulmonary alveolar mucoid film and the pneumocytes. Lancet 266:1099–1104

Maisin JR (1970) The ultrastructure of lung of mice exposed to a supra-lethal dose of ionizing radiation on the thorax. Radiat Res 44:545–646

Malmquist E, Grossmann G, Ivemark B, Robertson B (1973) Pulmonary phospholipids and surface properties of alveolar wash in experimental paraquat poisoning. Scand J Respir Dis 54:206–214

Massaro GD, Massaro D (1972) Granular pneumocytes. Electron microscopic radioautographic evidence of intracellular protein transport. Am Rev Respir Dis 105: 927–931

Morgenroth K (1972) Experimentelle Lungenfibrose als immunologische Spätreaktion. Veroeff Morphol Pathol 89

Morgenroth K, Schröder C, Themann H (1970) Doppelfärbung von Semidünnschnitten mit basischen Farbstoffen. Mikroskopie 20:260–263

Patchefsky AS, Israel HL, Hoch WS, Gordon G (1973) Desquamative interstitial pneumonia. Relationship to interstitial fibrosis. Thorax 28:688–693

Pearse AGE (1968) Histochemistry, theoretical and applied. Churchill, London

Pette D, Brandau H (1966) Enzymhistogramme und Enzymaktivitätsmuster der Rattenleber. Enzymol Biol Clin 6:79−122

Pickrell J, Dorothy A, Harris V, Hahn FF, Belasich JJ, Jones RK (1975) Biological alterations resulting from chronic lung irradiation. II. Connective tissue alterations following inhalation of [144]Ce-labeled fused clay aerosols in beagle dogs. Radiat Res 63:299−309

Rhodes ML (1973) Desquamative interstitial pneumonia. New ultrastructural findings. Am Rev Respir Dis 108:950−954

Rooney SA, Canavan PM, Motoyama EK (1974) The identification of phosphatidyl-glycerol in rat, rabbit monkey and human lung. Biochim Biophys Acta 360:56−67

Rooney SA, Page-Roberts BA, Motoyama EK (1975) Role of lamellar inclusions in surfactant production: Studies on phospholipid composition and biosynthesis in rat and rabbit lung subcellular fractions. J Lipid Res 16:418−425

Rosen SH, Castleman B, Liebow AA (1958) Pulmonary alveolar proteinosis. N Engl J Med 258:1123−1142

Rosmanith J, Breining H (1975) Beschleunigung der Entstehung von experimentellen Lungenfibrosen durch Urethan nach intratrachealer Applikation von Cadmium-sulfid und Kohlenstaub. Beitr Silikose Forsch (Pneumokoniose) 27:12−20

Rosmanith J, Breining H, Prajsnar D (1976) Dosis- und zeitabhängige Lungenfibrosen nach Cadmiumsulfid im Tierversuch. In: Bolt W, Buchter A, Rebentisch E, Worth G (eds) Bericht über die 16. Jahrestagung der Deutschen Gesellschaft für Arbeits-medizin e.V. Genter, Stuttgart, p 251

Rosmanith J, Breining H, Prajsnar D (1977) Dosis- und zeitabhängige Lungenfibrosen nach Bleisulfid im Tierversuch. Staub Reinhalt Luft 37:433−437

Sanders RL, Longmore WJ (1975) Phosphatidylglycerol in rat lung. II. Comparison of occurrence, composition and metabolism in surfactant and residual lung fractions. Biochemistry 14:835−840

Scadding JG, Hinson KFW (1967) Diffuse fibrosing alveolitis (diffuse interstitial fibro-sis of the lungs). Correlation of histology and biopsy with prognosis. Thorax 22:291−304

Schaefer EK, Avery ME, Bensch K (1964) Time course of changes in surface tension and morphology of alveolar epithelial cells in CO_2-induced hyaline membrane dis-ease. J Clin Invest 43:2080−2093

Shortland JR, Drake CS, Crane WAJ (1969) Electron microscopy of desquamative interstitial pneumonia. Thorax 24:192−208

Sicic JB, Mimnaugh EG, Gram TE (1978) Development of quantifiable parameters of bleomycin toxicity in the mouse lung. In: Carter SK, Crooke ST, Umezawa H (eds) Bleomycin: Current status and new developments. Academic Press, New York San Francisco, London, p 293

Smith P, Heath D, Kay JM (1974) The pathogenesis and structure of paraquat-induced pulmonary fibrosis in rats. J Pathol 114:57−67

Steiner JW, Langer B, Schatz DL (1960) The local and systemic effects of Freund's adjuvant and its fractions. Arch Pathol 70:424−434

Thurlbeck WM, Foley FD (1963) Experimental pulmonary emphysema: The effect of intratracheal injection of cadmium chloride solution in guinea pigs. Am J Pathol 42:431−441

Vijeyaratnam GS, Corrin B (1971) Experimental paraquat poisoning: A histological and electron-optical study of the changes in the lung. J Pathol 103:123−129

Wahl LM, Wahl SM, Mergenhagen SE, Martin GR (1975) Collagenase production by lymphokine-activated macrophages. Science 187:261−263

Wattenberg LW, Leong JL (1960) Effects of coenzyme Q 10 and menadione on succinic dehydrogenase activity as measured by tetrazolium salt reduction. J Histochem Cytochem 8:296−303

Weller W (1977) Anthrako-Silikose. Griebsch, Hamm (Tierexperimentelle Forschung)

The Ultrastructure of Preneoplastic Changes
in the Bronchial Mucosa

K.-M. MÜLLER and G. MÜLLER

Reactions of the bronchial mucosa to acute and chronic injuries are manifested either in transitory regenerative activities, or in more permanent changes such as loss of epithelial differentiation or the onset of intraepithelial neoplastic transformation. Reparative processes are expressed as basal cell hyperplasia, goblet cell hyperplasia, and metaplastic substitution of highly differentiated respiratory epithelium by squamous epithelium.

Dealt with here are those epithelial changes that differ from regenerative structural alterations by manifesting cellular and nuclear atypia of varying severity, and which are thus classified as preneoplastic changes. The histogenetic correlations of these preneoplastic changes with overtly malignant pulmonary neoplasia are discussed.

I. Materials and Methods

Morphological studies were carried out on biopsy specimens from 26 patients of the Münster University Clinic, Department of Thoracic, Cardiac, and Vascular Surgery. During routine diagnostic fiber bronchoscopy, biopsies were taken from the bronchial mucosa, mostly in cases of suspected bronchial carcinoma. Squamous carcinomas and preneoplastic lesions were verified histologically in 11 patients, small-cell carcinomas in five, and a large-cell carcinoma in one patient. Samples for the identification of potential preneoplastic changes were taken from areas adjacent to and distant from the tumor and from the contralateral lung. Two cases involving lobectomy for carcinoma offered the opportunity for extensive workup of the whole bronchial system.

For light microscopy, tissue specimens were fixed in 4% i.p. formalin, embedded in paraffin, and processed in the usual fashion, using H & E, PAS, and EvG stains, respectively. Slides were examined with a Zeiss photomicroscope.

Material destined for electron microscopy was fixed, immediately after excision, for 2 h at 0°C in 3% glutaraldehyde buffered with phosphate to pH 7.4. It was then washed for 24 h in the same buffer at 4°C. The samples were postfixed in 1.3% buffered osmium for 1 h, dehydrated in graded ethanols, and embedded in Epon 812 via propylenoxide.

Semithin sections were stained with toluidine blue for orientation by light-microscopic examination. Ultrathin sections subsequently cut with a Porter-Blum ultramicrotome were mounted on copper grids and contrast stained with uranyl acetate and lead nitrate. These sections were examined with a Siemens electron microscope IA at 60 kV using a double condenser.

II. Normal Bronchial Mucosa: Ultrastructural Characteristics

Normal bronchial epithelium is composed of respiratory epithelium lying on a basement membrane. Its main components are superficial ciliated epithelial cells with some isolated goblet cells, and basal cells in the deeper layers of the mucosa. In larger bronchi, the respiratory epithelium shows three to four nuclear strata. The epithelial thickness decreases towards the smaller peripheral branches, until there is only a single epithelial layer in the terminal bronchioles (Fig. 1) (*Hayek* 1970; *Hartung* 1979).

Electron microscopy helps to distinguish several cell types.

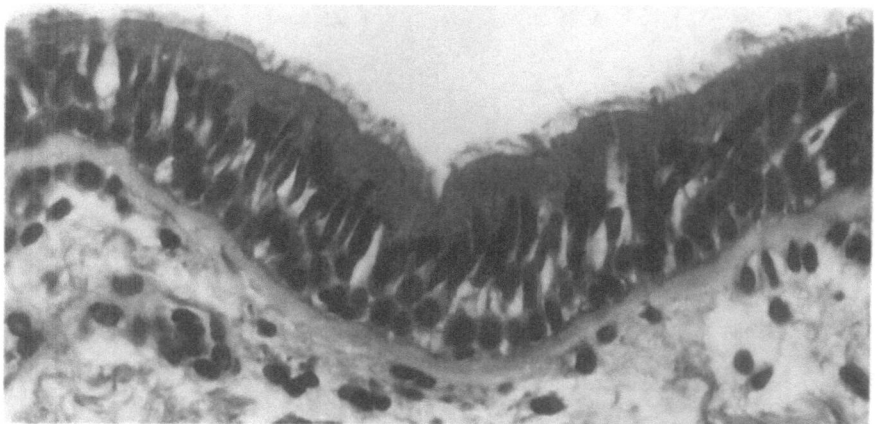

Fig. 1. Regular structure of bronchial mucosa. H & E, × 560

1. Ciliated Cells

Cylindrical ciliated cells bear up to 200 kinocilia of typical structure, firmly anchored in kinopodia on the cell's lumen-oriented surface. Between these cells we see a superficial network of terminal bars; intercellular spaces are narrow. The nucleus lodes in the basal part, and numerous mitochondria are seen in the apical part of the cell (Figs. 1, 2a).

2. Mucus-Producing Cells

Histochemical as well as electron-microscopical findings permit us to distinguish cells at several phases of secretion, up to the fully developed goblet cell (Fig. 2a). The ratio of goblet to ciliated cells is usually 1:4. *Trump* et al. (1978) introduced the term "small mucous granule cells" (SMG cells) for mucus-producing cells that are characterized ultrastructurally by the presence of small mucous granules between their Golgi field and the surface. They are thought to be capable of division (*Schulz* 1959; *Rhodin* 1956; *Gieseking* 1968, 1971, 1973).

3. Brush Cells

Brush cells are relatively rare cells of bronchial mucosa, characterized electron microscopically by superficial microvilli and finger-like cytoplasmic protrusions. Their nature and function are unclear (*Watson* and *Brinkman* 1964; *David* 1978).

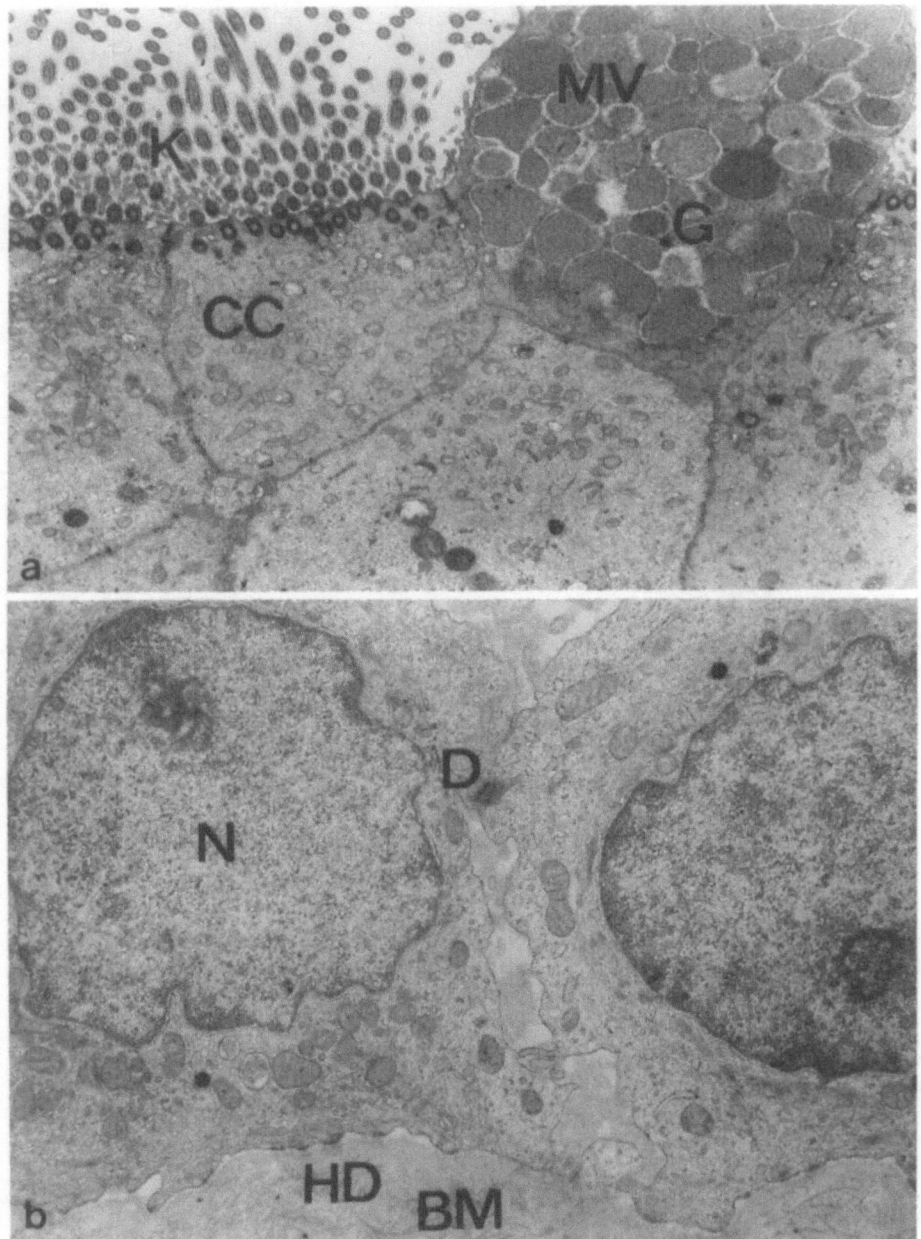

Fig. 2. a Surface layer of regular bronchial epithelium. *CC*, ciliated cell; *K*, kinocilia; *G*, goblet cell just before secretion; *MV*, mucous vacuoles. × 7500. **b** Basal cells in regular bronchial epithelium. *N*, nucleus; *D*, desmosome; *HD*, hemidesmosome; *BM*, basement membrane. × 17 000

4. Neurosecretory Cells

Neurosecretory cells are identified in light microscopy by means of silver impregnation only. They are capable of mitosis, basally oriented, and found more frequently in segmental bronchi and in the glands of the bronchial wall. Their characteristic feature on electron microscopy is the presence of neurosecretory granules of 600–1700 Å (*Bensch* et al. 1968; *Feyrter* 1969; *Terzakis* et al. 1972; *Heitz* 1977; *Pearse* and *Polak* 1974).

5. Basal Cells

Basal cells are polygonal or triangular cells localized immediately above the basement membrane. They do not usually rise to the epithelial surface. Their electron-dense cytoplasm contains tonofilaments in perinuclear array; Golgi complex and endoplasmic reticulum are poorly developed. The high mitotic capacity of basal cells is an expression of their role as stem cells for ciliated, goblet, and brush cells (Fig. 2b) (*Rhodin* 1966; *Lesch* and *Oehlert* 1966; *Gieseking* 1968; *McDowell* et al. 1978).

6. Clara Cells

Clara cells are found in the bronchiolar region. They are capable of mitosis and possess microvilli at the free surface and electron-dense granules in the apical part which rises above the general mucosal level (*Clara* 1937; *Cutz* and *Conen* 1970; *Basset* et al. 1971; *Greenberg* et al. 1975).

III. Pathological Changes in the Bronchial Mucosa

1. Epithelial Hyperplasia

In pathological states with altered proportions of cell types, we may distinguish basal cell hyperplasia from goblet cell hyperplasia and various other forms of metaplasia.

a) Basal Cell Hyperplasia

In basal cell hyperplasia, the most frequent deviation from the mucosal norm, we see the surface epithelium widened to over 50 μm (normal 30–50 μm) by an intense proliferation of basal cells. The light-microscopic appearance of basal cell isomorphism and nuclear uniformity is confirmed by electron microscopy, which shows normally differentiated cell types in a homogeneous population.

238

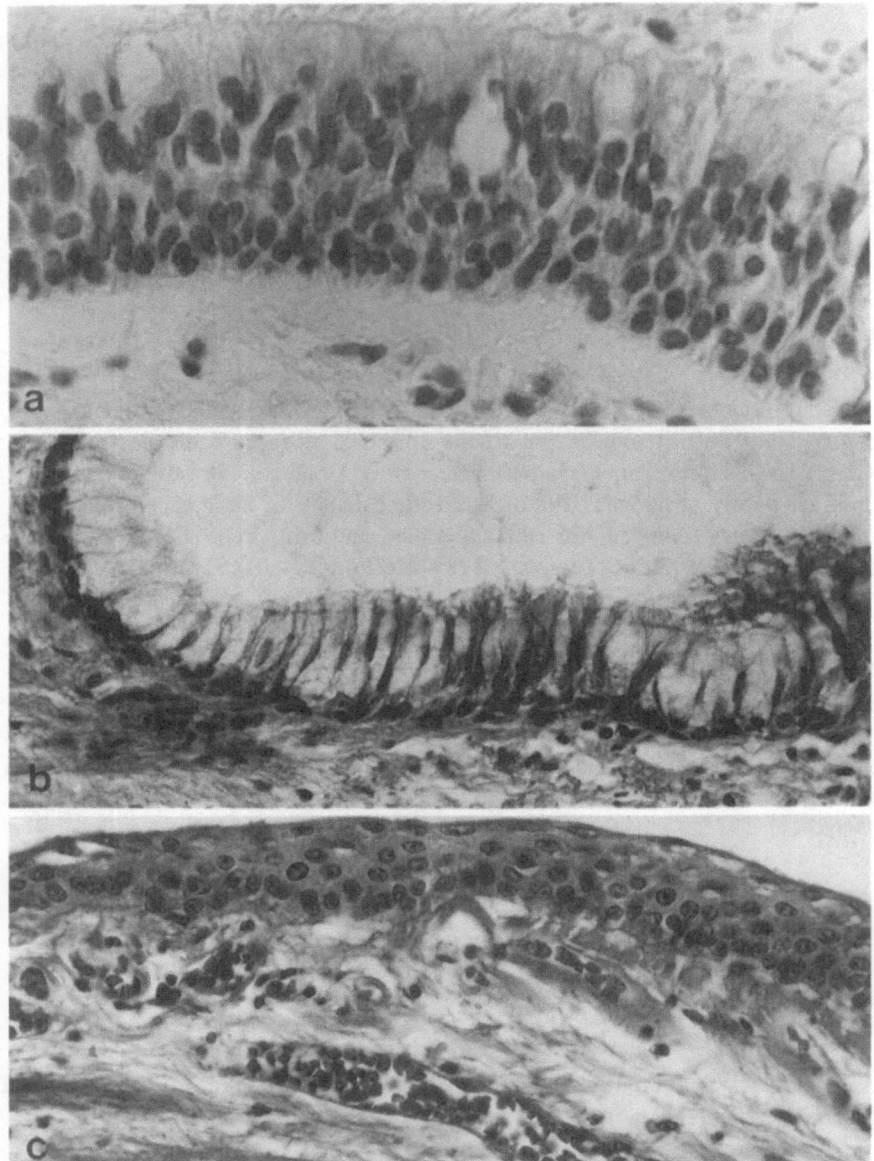

Fig. 3. a Mild basal cell hyperplasia. FE-H & E, × 600. **b** Goblet cell hyperplasia in a smaller bronchus. H & E, × 350. **c** Squamous cell metaplasia or epidermoid metaplasia. H & E, × 360

b) Goblet Cell Hyperplasia

In this slightly abnormal state of the mucosa, we find a shift of the goblet cell to ciliated cell ratio in favor of the goblet cell. Quantitation of goblet cell hyperplasia is readily possible by light-microscopical and histochemical investigation. Mucus-producing cells are arranged above a layer of regular basal cells (Fig. 3b). Goblet cell and basal cell hyperplasia are sometimes observed side by side.

Electron microscopy of goblet cell hyperplasia reveals an increased number of mucus-producing cells in various stages of the secretory cycle. In deviations from the norm, we may see some early stages of secretory cells with prosecretory granules at the lumen-oriented epithelial surface. Even the cytoplasm of ciliated cells may be dispersed by secretory droplets. Basal cells appear normal, but intercellular spaces are slightly wider.

2. Epithelial Metaplasia

Corresponding to the metaplastic changes defined in the mucosa of other organs, we may distinguish transitory metaplasia or stratification from squamous cell or epidermoid metaplasia in the bronchial mucosa.

a) Stratification

Microscopically, stratification is characterized by gradual flattening of predominantly round, cuboidal, or polygonal cells, leading to the stratified appearance of the upper layers. Ciliated cells are no longer seen. Ultrastructurally, the superficial cells, connected by terminal bars, possess microvilli interspersed with vesicular structures. The presence of small secretory droplets and larger secretory granules in cells of the middle epithelial layers is seen as a sign of mucus production (Fig. 4). A few desmosomes serve to secure intercellular contacts over slightly widened intercellular spaces.

b) Epidermoid Metaplasia

This alteration of the bronchial mucosa is characterized by the structural modification of surface epithelia to an epidermis-like array of cell layers. Unlike the pattern of normal epithelium, the picture shows predominant horizontal polarity of cells. Ciliated and typical goblet cells are absent (Fig. 3c). In contrast to stratification, light microscopy reveals intercellular bridges and occasional signs of keratinization. Electron microscopically, epidermoid metaplasia is defined by an increasing number of intracytoplamic tonofilaments in the middle layers, and an equally increased number of desmosomes. "Membrane-coating granules" are interpreted as early indicators of keratinization. In surface epithelia furnished with coarse microvilli and vesicular structures, we see occasional secretory granules like those seen in transitional metaplasia. Wider intracytoplasmic spaces interwoven with cytoplasmic protrusions are characteristic features of the middle and basal regions of the epithelium.

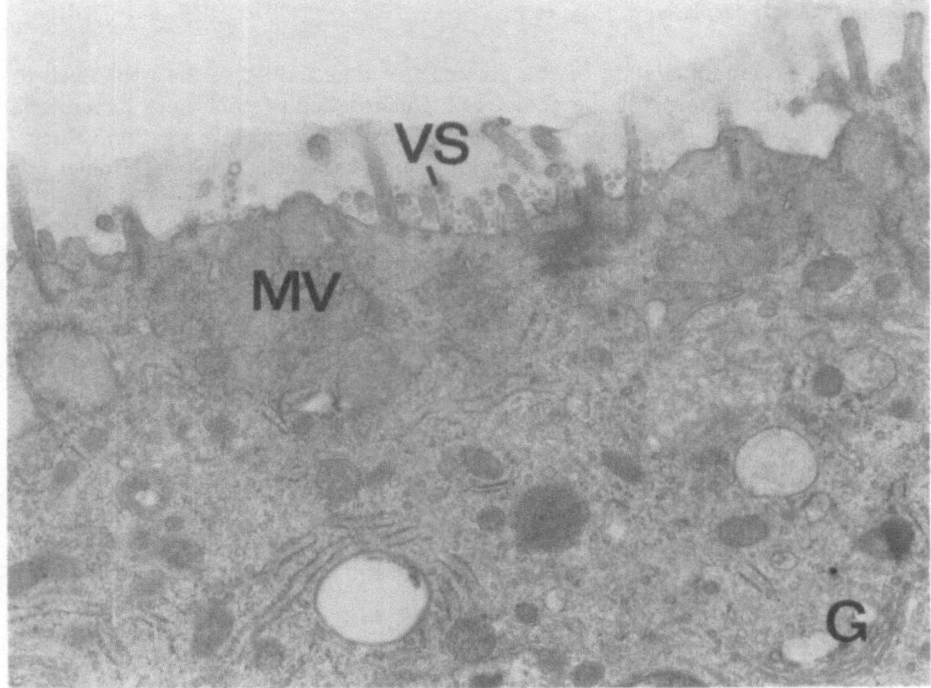

Fig. 4. Surface section from stratification. Small droplet-like vesicels bubbling up and bursting into the lumen. Note the mucous vacuoles beneath the plasma membrane and the secretory droplets of various sizes within the cytoplasm. *MV*, mucous vacuole; *G*, Golgi complex; *VS*, vesicular structure. × 19 300

3. Micropapillomatosis

Occurring mainly in metaplastic areas of the mucosa, micropapillomatosis is characterized by highly vascular portions of subepithelial stroma. The typical picture shows hernia-like protrusions of vascularized stromal papillae extending towards the surface epithelium, with or without corresponding bulges of the epithelial surface (Fig. 5a, b). Epithelial changes around these micropapillomas are similar to those found in transitional or epidermoid metaplasia. Cellular and nuclear atypia may develop to a considerable degree, eventually requiring classification as dysplasia or even as carcinoma in situ (see below).

4. Dysplasia and Carcinoma In Situ

As with preneoplastic lesions in the larynx, epithelial changes of the bronchial mucosa present various grades of atypia down to massive intraepithelial malignant transformation. Cellular and nuclear polymorphism, nuclear hyperchromasia, abnormal distribu-

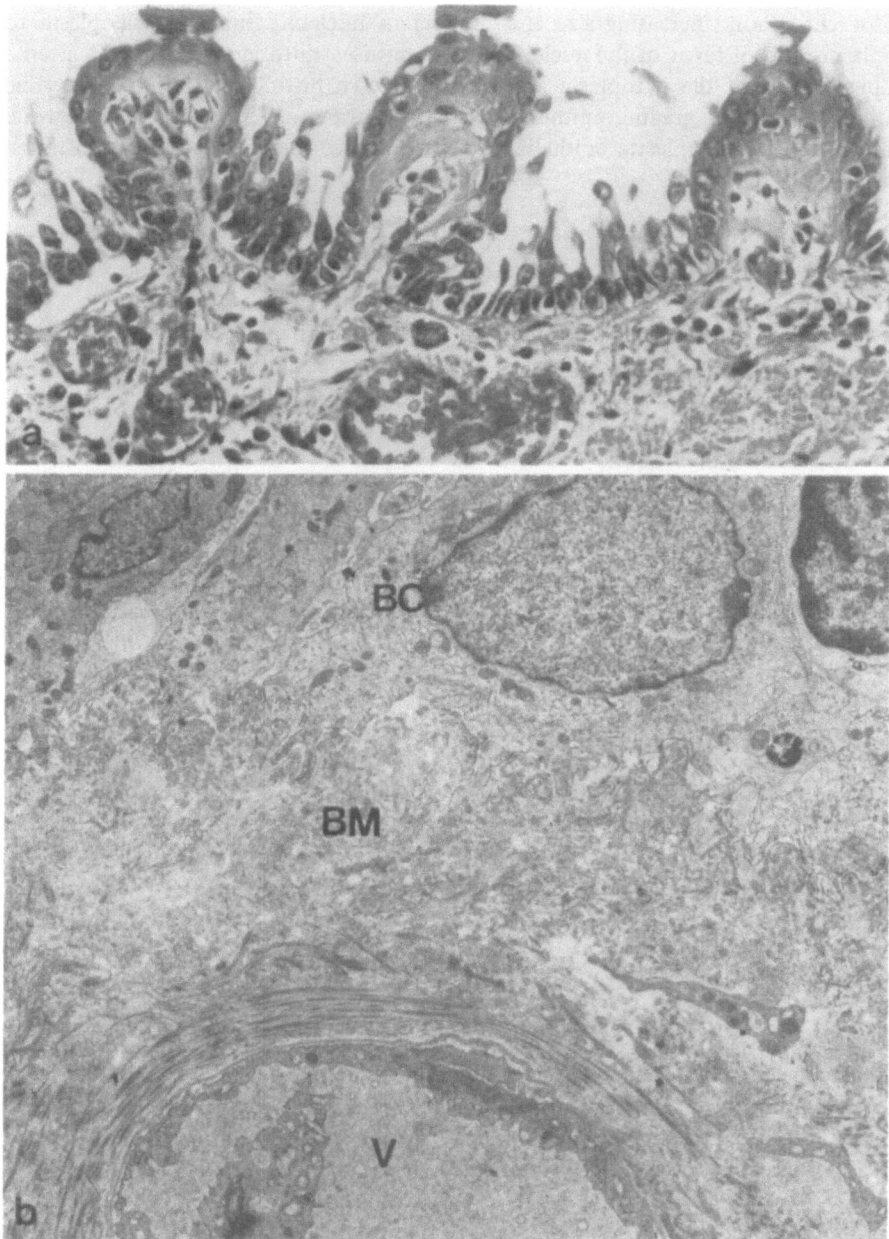

Fig. 5. a Microphotograph of micropapillomatosis in bronchial mucosa. Hernia-like, vascularized stromal papillae. H & E, × 400. **b** Section from micropapillomatosis with mild atypias (dysplasia I) seen in basal epithelial layers with basement membrane and subepithelial stroma. *BC,* basal cell; *BM,* basement membrane, *V,* vessel. × 6200

tion of chromatin, increasing size and number of nucleoli, shifting nucleoplasm to cytoplasm ratio in favor of the nuclei, frequent mitoses, mitotic atypia, and an altered staining pattern of the cytoplasm are the well-known histological criteria of atypia. Another variable for grading epithelial dysplasia is the more or less severe structural disintegration of metaplastic epithelia corresponding to the enhanced differentiation of cells.

a) Light Microscopy of Epithelial Dysplasia

From the above criteria of atypia and with the distinguishable steps of structural disintegration, three grades of dysplasia — mild, moderate, and severe — are defined as the sequence leading to carcinoma in situ.

α) Mild Dysplasia (Grade I)

Microscopically, dysplasia I is characterized by the replacement of normal mucosa, in circumscribed areas, by an orderly, stratified epithelium containing a certain number of atypical cells. Deeper strata contain more basal cells with hyperchromatic nuclei of varying form and size, and some isolated mitoses.

β) Moderate Dysplasia (Grade II)

The lesion occurs in circumscribed areas, indicated by atypia within metaplastic portions and by increased structural irregularity of cell array in the basal and middle layers of the epithelium. The lower two-thirds of the epithelium shows cellular and nuclear atypias and increased mitotic activity (Fig. 6a).

γ) Severe Dysplasia (Grade III)

In dysplasia III, metaplastic areas consist predominantly of atypical epithelium; the homogeneity of their texture is greatly disturbed. Pleomorphic nuclei with hyperchromasia, clumping of chromatin, and shifted nucleoplasm to cytoplasm ratio are seen even in the upper layers of epithelium. The size and shape of epithelial cells vary considerably; increasing mitotic activity reflects a strong proliferative trend (Fig. 6b).

δ) Carcinoma In Situ

Carcinoma in situ, found as a rule in circumscribed areas of the mucosa, shows a multilayered, highly atypical tissue, replacing the normal respiratory epithelium. Stratification is inhomogeneous, lacking the criteria of differentiation and maturity in general. Stratification, polarity, and maturation of cells are abolished in all epithelial layers up

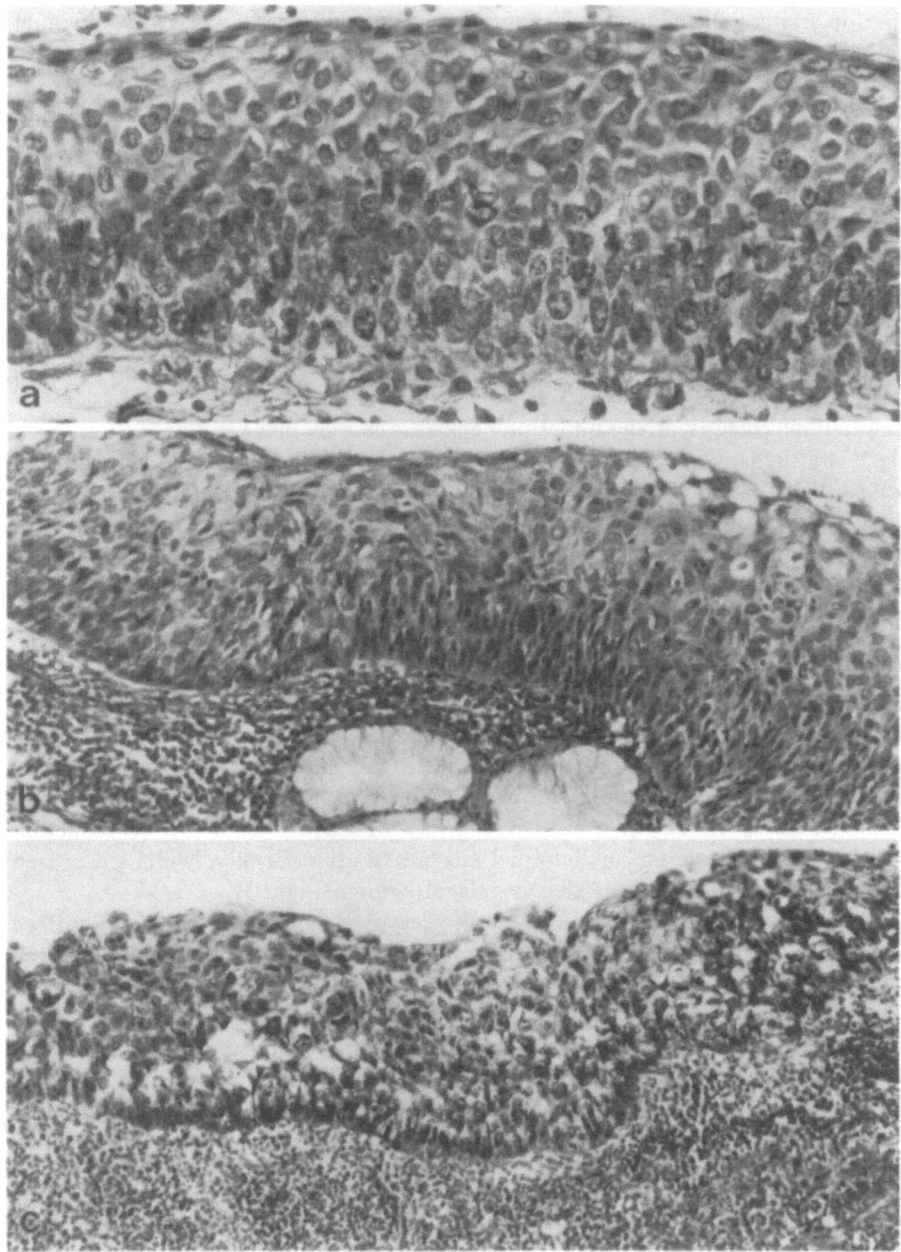

Fig. 6. a Dysplasia II of bronchial mucosa. × 350. **b** Dysplasia III of bronchial mucosa, × 180. **c** Carinoma in situ of bronchial mucosa. × 150

to the top strata. Cellular and nuclear atypia, as seen in dysplasia, reach a maximum in these proliferating metaplastic cells. As a rule, the stroma beneath a carcinoma in situ shows severe inflammatory infiltration (Fig. 6c).

b) Electron Microscopy of Dysplasias

Ultrastructural findings enables us to distinguish consecutive stages of preneoplastic epithelial lesions, ranging from minor deviations from the norm to severe cellular atypia resembling that in true carcinoma.

α) Mild Dysplasia (Grade I)

Ultrastructural changes in the initial preneoplastic lesions that were defined as "dysplasia I" by light microscopy are expressed in slight structural deviations within the upper epithelial layers. Persisting kinocilia of ciliated cells show an alteration of the typical 9 + 2 structure of microtubules. Cross sections reveal varying numbers of atypically arranged microtubules. Longitudinal sections of these kinocilia show thickening and irregular outer borders (Fig. 7a, b). The ciliated cells, markedly reduced in number, may occasionally contain some compound cilia, i.e., ciliary structures, more or less numerous, embedded in the cytoplasmic matrix above the superficial cells (Fig. 7c). Between preserved or altered kinocilia, one may occasionally find coarse cytoplasmic protrusions of surface epithelia directed toward the bronchial lumen (Fig. 8). Some of the ciliated cells may show intracytoplasmic cilia whose ciliary microtubules appear within the cytoplasm of surface cells, below the luminal border and the row of kinopodia (Fig. 9a). Similar intracytoplasmic cilia are also found in the middle and basal epithelial layers of dysplastic areas (Fig. 9b). Along with the numerical reduction of cilia per cell unit, we see an abnormal increase of atypical microvilli characterized by a plush-like coating and associated vascular structures (Fig. 10).

Goblet cells of regular structure are also less frequent in the course of surface degeneration, but abnormal cells with the criteria of secretory activity are found more often, characterized by an electron-dense cytoplasm with many ribosomes and electron-dense granules, partly surrounded by membranes (Fig. 10).

The surface cells facing the bronchial lumen are interconnected by terminal bars. The nuclei of the upper epithelial layers fail to show recognizable atypia in mild dysplasia. Within the cytoplasm of altered ciliated cells, the number and localization of mitochondria, slightly dispersed by the presence of secretory granules, fails to show any deviation from the norm.

Fig. 7. Lumen-adjacent (lumen-facing part of surface cell in mild dysplasia). a Atypical kinocilium in longitudinal section. The typical 9 + 2 array of microtubules is lost. The outer contour of the kinocilium is irregular, and thicker in its median part. *MT*, microtubule; *AK*, atypical kinocilium. × 22 000. b Two atypical kinocilia in cross section with an increased number of microtubules. *AK*, atypical kinocilium; *MT*, microtubule. × 22 000. c Compound cilia with cytoplasmic protrusion directed toward the lumen. *CC*, compound cilium; *CP*, cytoplasmic protrusion; *K*, kinocilium; *BB*, basal body. × 30 000

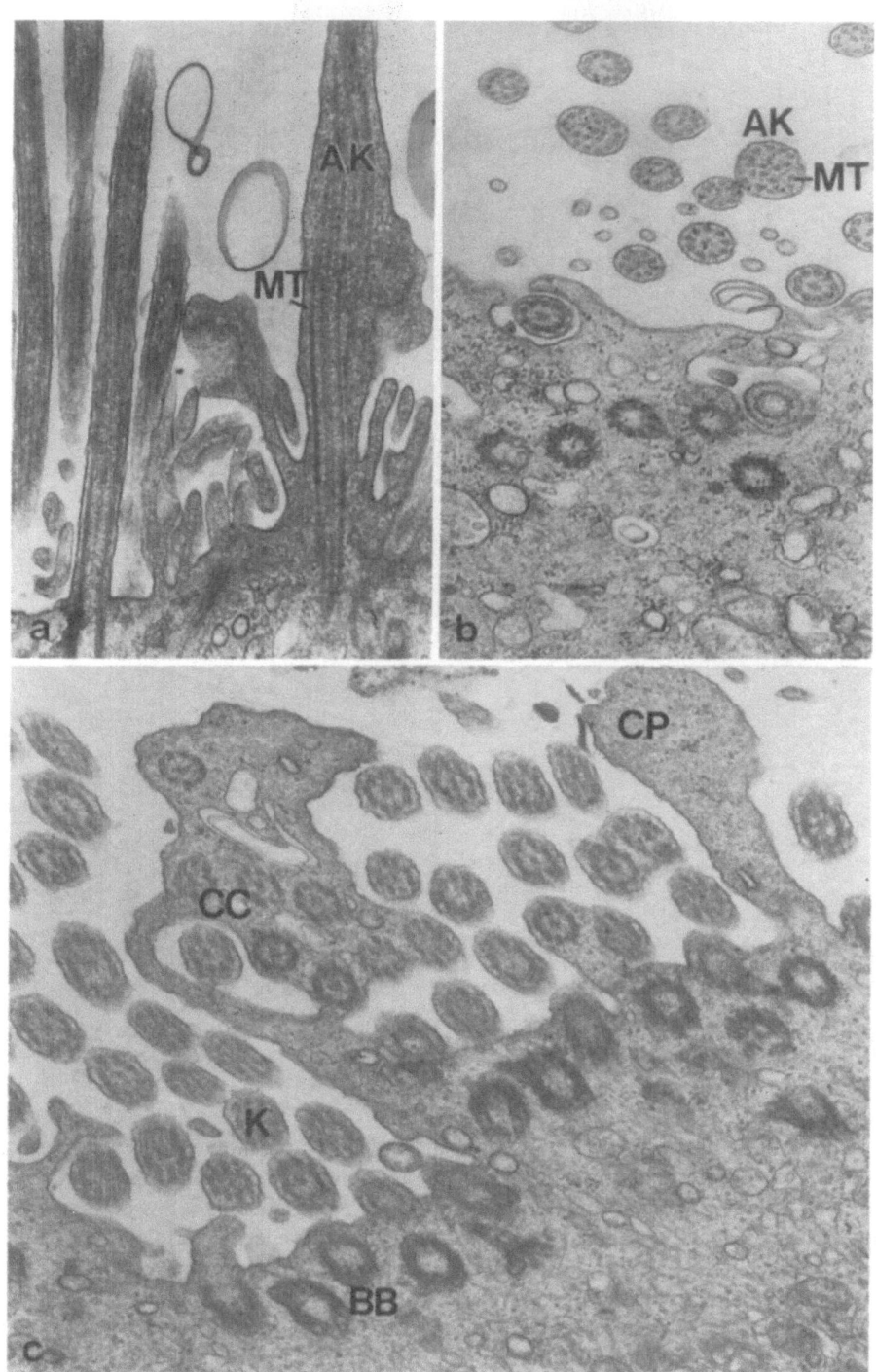

Fig. 7a–c

246

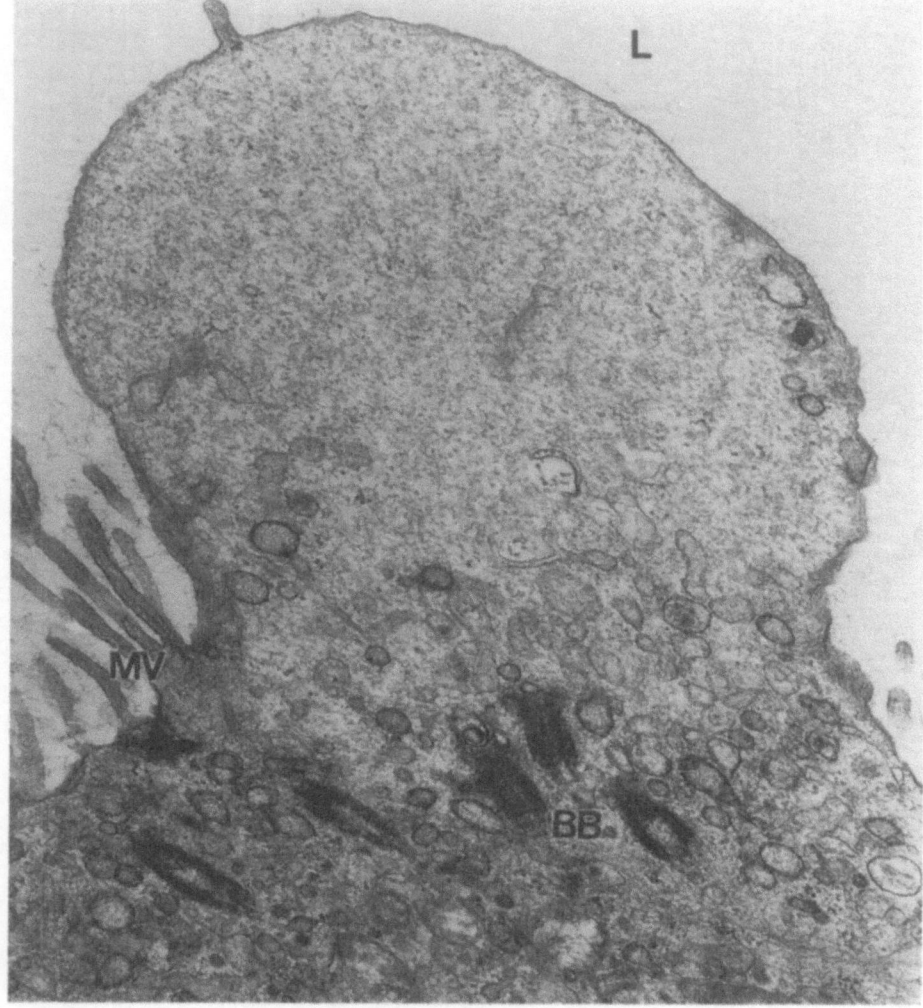

Fig. 8. Coarse cytoplasmic protrusion toward the lumen, from the surface cells of an epithelium in mild dysplasia. *L*, lumen; *MV*, microvilli; *BB*, basal bodies. × 25 500

The intermediate layers of epithelium in mild dysplasia show very few abnormal findings. Intercellular spaces in this region are rather narrow, crossed by a small number of cytoplasmic protrusions. Intercellular contacts are maintained by a few desmosomes. The texture of basal epithelial layers is somewhat loosened by wider intercellular spaces. Here, intercellular contacts are secured by a varying number of cytoplasmic protrusions with desmosomes or tonofilaments, single or bundled.

The cytoplasm of basal cells contains free ribosomes and polyribosomes. Granular and agranular endoplasmic reticulum and Golgi complexes are infrequent, however, nor is there an increased number of mitochondria. Even mild dysplasia shows enlarged

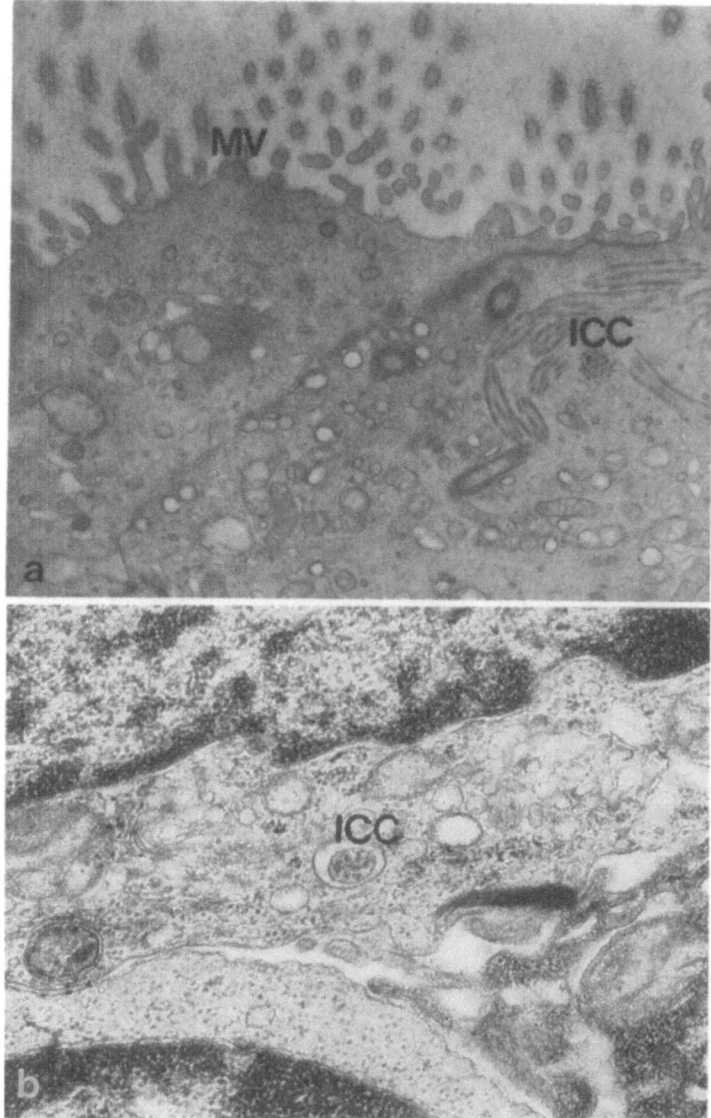

Fig. 9. a Longitudinal section of intracytoplasmic cilia in a surface cell of a mildly dysplastic area. Microvilli are only seen at the surface. × 16 500. **b** Cross section of an intracytoplasmic cilium in a basal cell of mildly dysplastic epithelium. *CC*, intracytoplasmic cilium; *MV*, microvilli. × 20 300

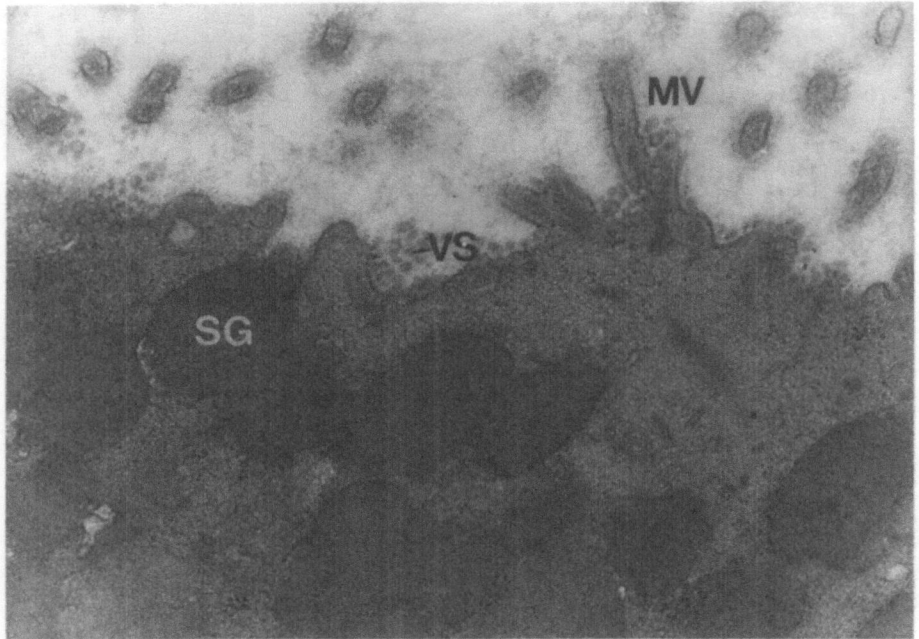

Fig. 10. Secretory cell at the surface of mildly dysplastic epithelium with electron-dense mucous granules. *SG*, mucous granules; *MV*, microvilli; *VS*, vesicular structures. × 19 300

nuclei in the basal epithelial layer; nuclear contours appear more or less lobulated by membrane invaginations. Chromatin distribution is peripheral, and nucleoli are often large and prominent and sometimes multiple, with mainly reticular structure. The zone of contact between basal cells and basement membrane shows smaller cytoplasmic protrusions oriented toward the basement membrane, and sometimes with visible filamentous structures (Fig. 11).

β) Advanced Stages of Dysplasia and Carcinoma In Situ

In parallel with the increasing severity of dysplastic changes in bronchial epithelium, kinocilia-bearing cells become less frequent and eventually disappear completely, even on electron microscopy. In moderate dysplasia there may be some occasional basal structures of kinocilia near the lumen, but they are never found in severe dysplasia or carcinoma in situ. In both these lesions we find two kinds of cells in the upper strata that are usually not present; abnormal mucus-producing cells, somewhat resembling those described in mild dysplasia (Fig. 10), and cells without mucus vacuoles but bearing numerous clear, droplet-like structures in their distended cytoplasm. In addition to some Golgi complexes, these cells contain a lot of granular endoplasmic reticulum.

All cells on the surface are interconnected by terminal bars, occasionally interspersed by larger cystic vacuoles. Greatly enlarged intercellular spaces with irregular

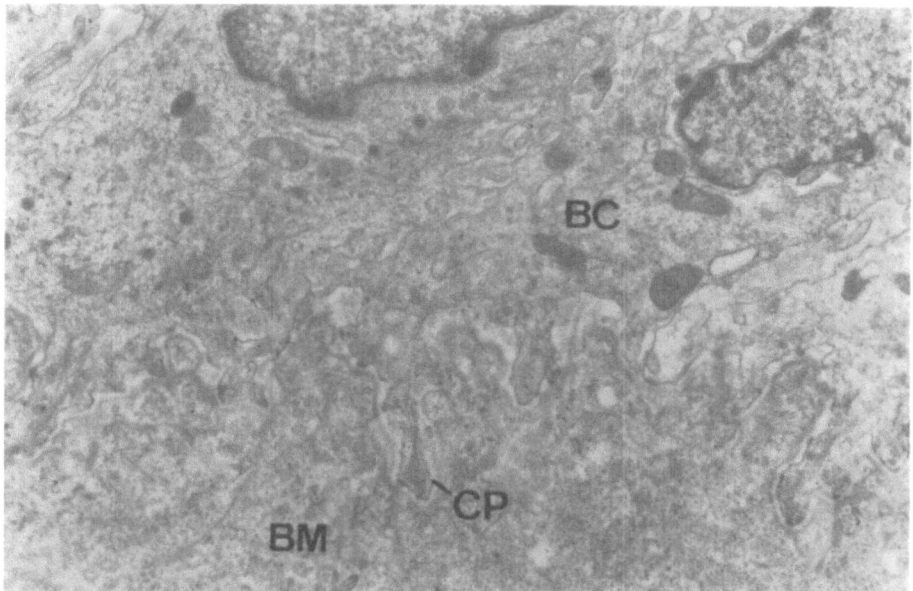

Fig. 11. Basal layer of mild dysplasia with small cytoplasmic protrusions toward the basement membrane. *BC*, basal cell; *BM*, basement membrane; *CP*, cytoplasmic protrusion. × 11 400

cytoplasmic protrusions reflect the increasing disintegration of texture in the intermediate zone of dysplastic epithelia that occurs in the higher grades of dysplasia and in carcinoma in situ (Fig. 12 b). The inhomogeneous texture is enhanced by vacuolization of the cytoplasm with droplet-like vesicles (Fig. 12a). Varying numbers of tentacle-like protrusions are stretched through these intercellular spaces. These protrusions may contain more or less distinct tonofilaments, single or bundled, ending in desmosomes (Fig. 12b).

In moderate and severe dysplasia, the cytoplasm of intermediate cells shows low electron density, but in carcinoma in situ some darker cells may also be found in this zone. The cytoplasm of these cells, which is rather poorly developed in relation to the size of nuclei, contains free ribosomes and polyribosomes, a few mitochondria, occasional lysosomal structures, and a growing number of tonofilaments.

The signs of atypia in this intermediate zone are less marked in moderate dysplasia than in severe dysplasia and carcinoma in situ. There are nuclear invaginations and an increasing number of nucleoli, often located peripherally with reticular structure and segregation of the nucleolar substance. So-called pseudoinclusion bodies are occasionally seen within the nuclei. Varying from one cell to the next, the arrangement of heterochromatin may be peripheral or diffusely dispersed over the whole nuclear matrix.

The basal zone of severe dysplasia and carcinoma in situ shows an even looser texture due to wider intercellular gaps interspersed with tentacles (Fig. 12b). The number of desmosomes varies from case to case (Fig. 13). We may distinguish two cell types: clear, and dark with electron-dense cytoplasm – both present in every case. The cyto-

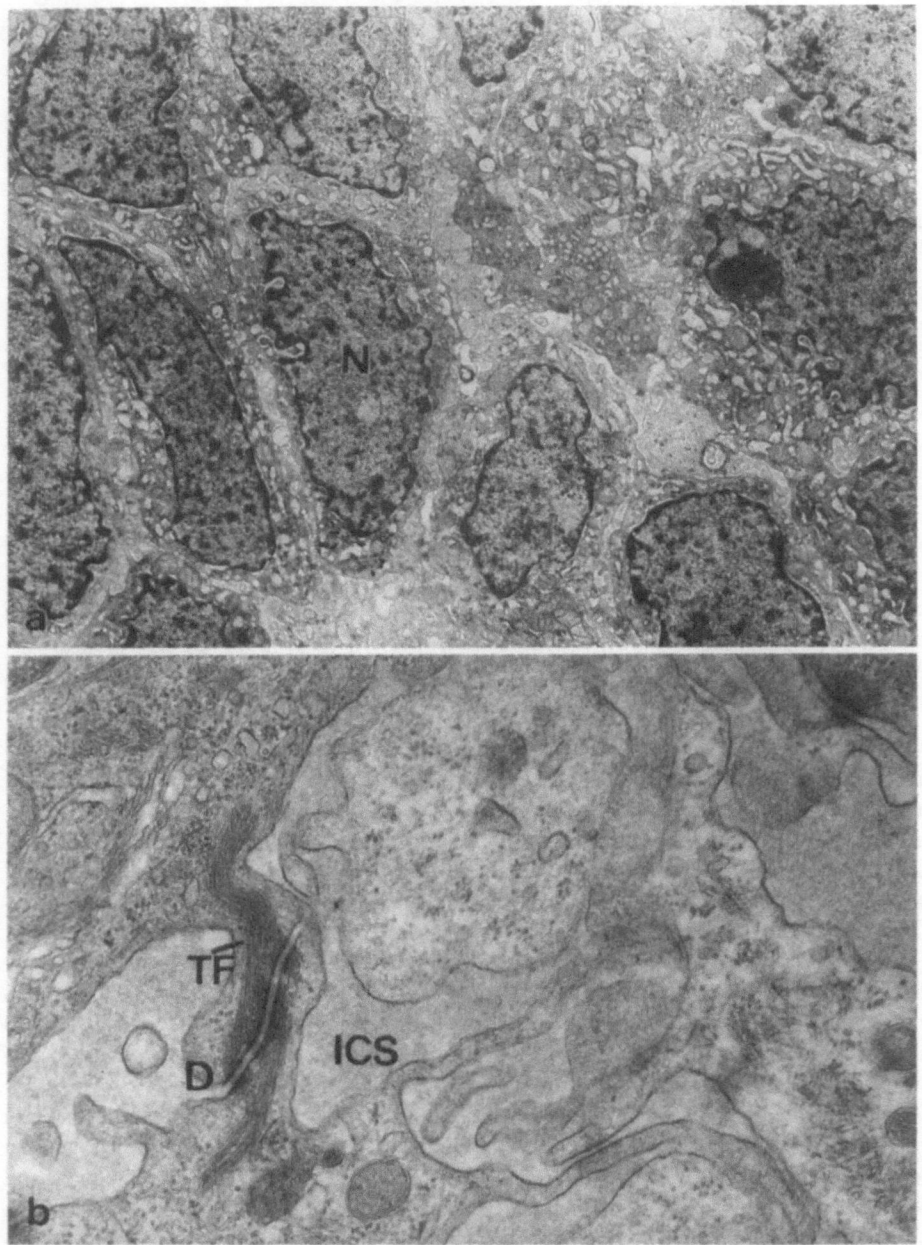

Fig. 12. a Intermediate layers in severe dysplasia. Cells with relatively large, partly lobated nuclei in vacuolar-disintegrated cytoplasm. *N*, nucleus. × 6000. **b** Desmosome with tonofilaments within a widened intercellular space. *D*, desmosome; *ICS*, intercellular space. *TF*, tonofilaments. × 22 300

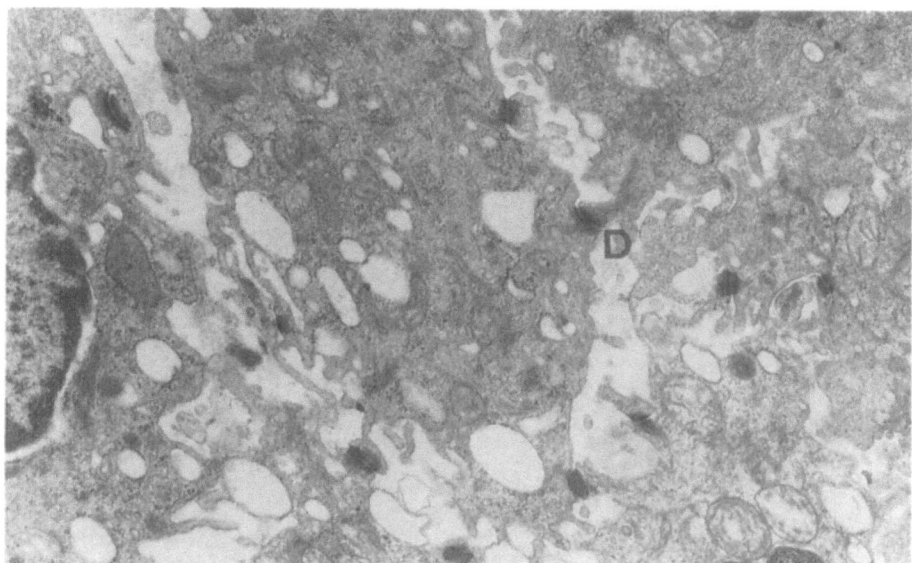

Fig. 13. Desmosomes more numerous in severe dysplasia. *D*, desmosomes. × 14 900

plasmic matrix contains mainly free ribosomes and polyribosomes. The clear cells may possess some granular endoplasmic reticulum; Golgi complexes and lysosomes occur in insignificant numbers. Isolated cells may show intracytoplasmic neurosecretory granules. In severely dysplastic areas one may find occasional intracytoplasmic cilia within basal cells.

Isolated or bundled tonofilaments, normally found in a typical perinuclear arrangement, are either completely lacking or distributed diffusely over the apical cytoplasm. In the basal zone these tonofilaments show a marked relationship with cytoplasmic protrusions oriented toward the basement membrane. Varying from cell to cell, the diameter of tonofilaments lies between 50 and 90 Å. Mitochondria may be abundant in these basal areas and are partly localized in basal cell protrusions, showing hydropic degeneration.

The nuclei of the darker cells found in the basal areas of severe dysplasia show an extreme polymorphism. The nucleoplasm—cytoplasm interface is enlarged by multiple nuclear invaginations (Fig. 14b). In contrast, the clear cells show lesser pleomorphism of nuclear shape. Patterns of chromatin distribution also differ in the two cell types. Whereas the clear cells of the basal layer in severe dysplasia differ only slightly from those seen in the intermediate zone, electron microscopy of the dark cells reveals heterochromatin clustering in an irregularly dispersed fashion over the nuclear matrix, with focal condensations and peripherally oriented complex condensations of heterochromatin (Fig. 14a). Nucleoli show the same peculiarities as those described in cells of the intermediate zone.

A very special feature is seen in the changing interfaces of the basal cell layer with the basement membrane in severe dysplasia and carcinoma in situ. This zone is subdivided by multiple tentacle-like cytoplasmic cellular protrusions, which vary consider-

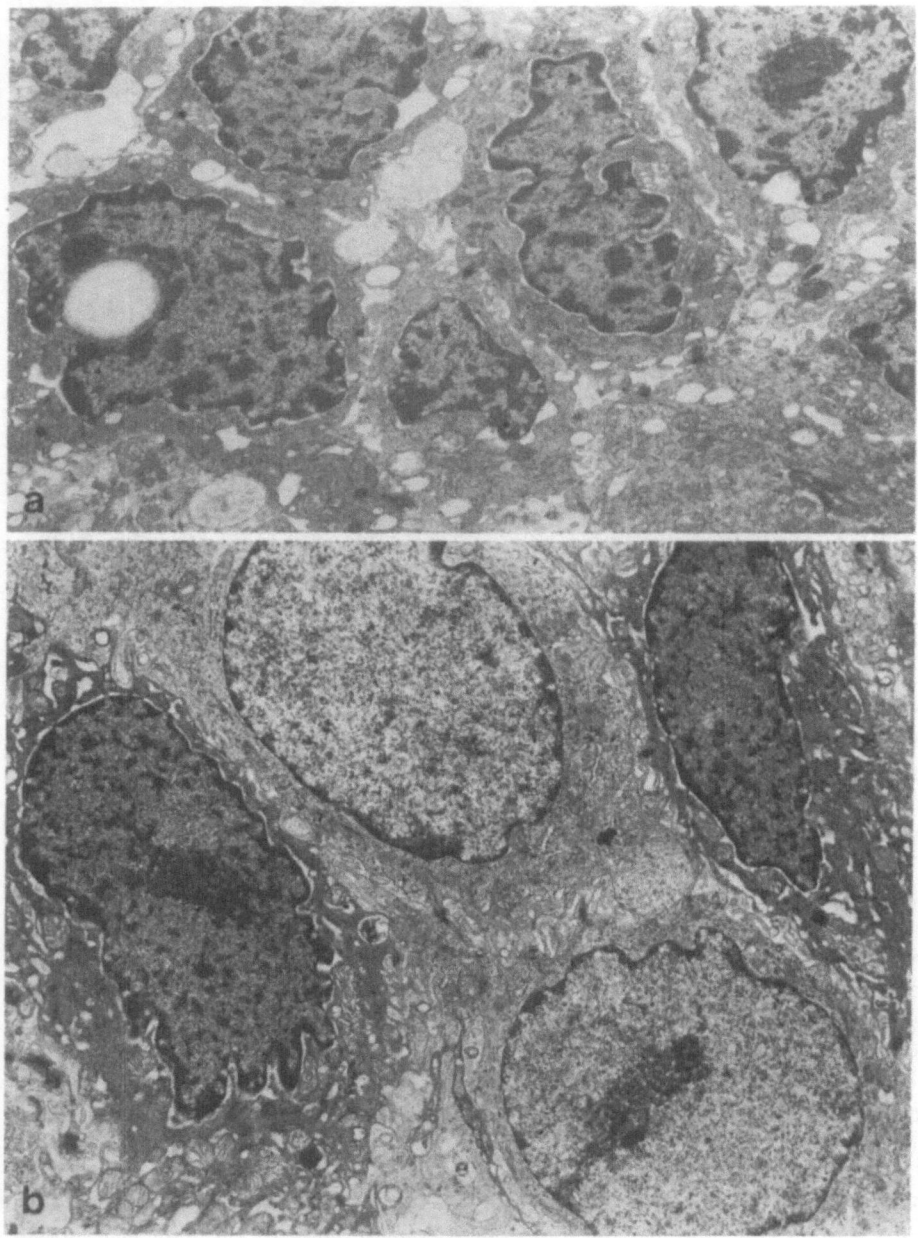

Fig. 14. a Basal layer of epithelium in dysplasia III. Cells with darker cytoplasm and strongly pleomorphic nuclei. Leopard-skin pattern of chromatin distribution (*Razzuk* 1970). × 4800. b Basal layers of carcinoma in situ. Two cells with dark cytoplasm, two others with clear cytoplasm. × 8400

Fig. 15a, b. Zone of contact between basal cell layers and the basement membrane in carcinoma in situ. Cytoplasmic protrusions directed toward the basement membrane, which they are entering diffusely. Tonofilaments and also mitochondria are seen within these protrusions. *BM*, basement membrane; *CP*, cytoplasmic protrusions; *HD*, hemidesmosomes; *TF*, tonofilaments. a × 10 200; b × 32 000

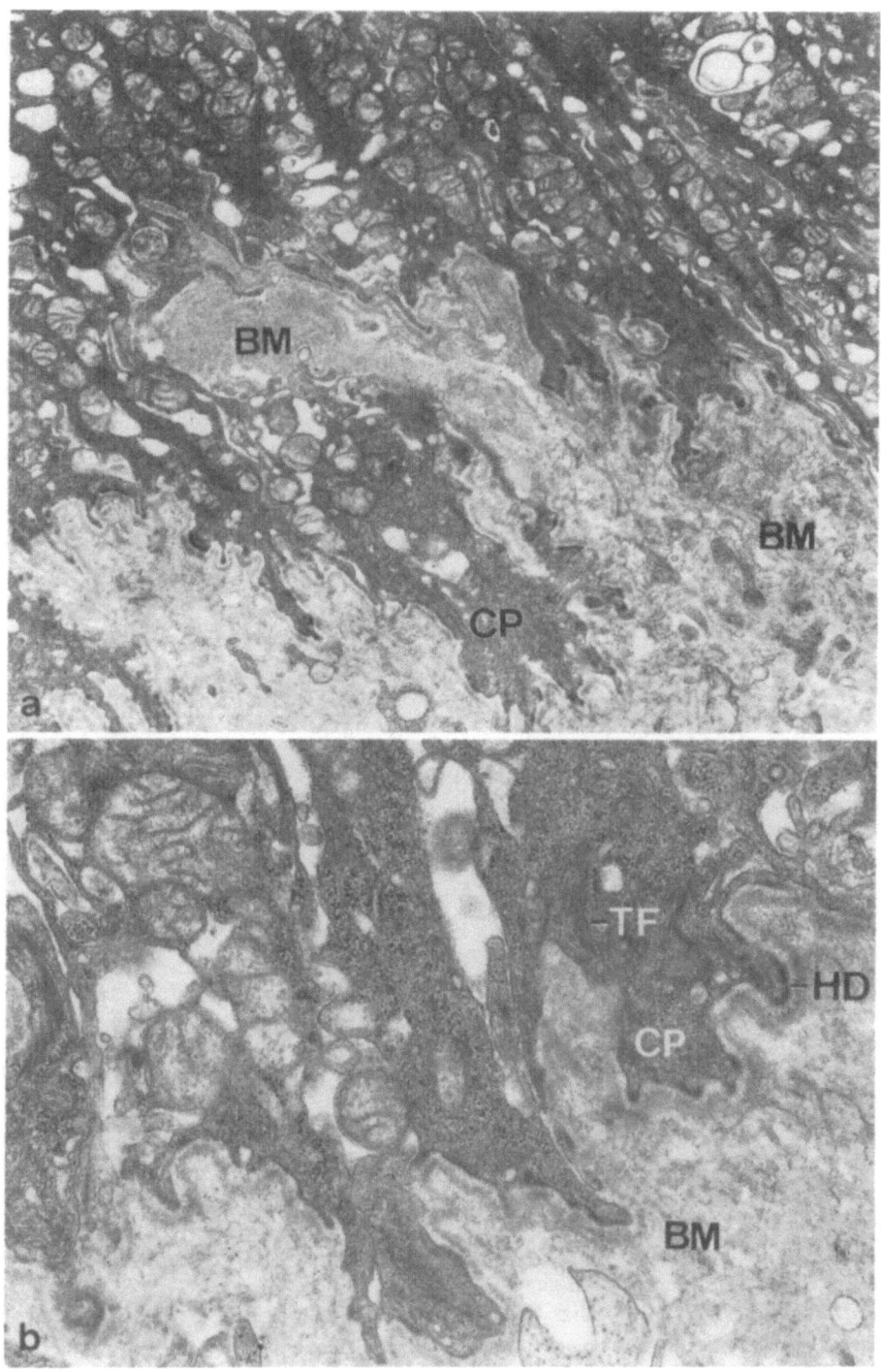

Fig. 15a, b

ably in size and shape but are always directed toward and between the fibrous structures of the basement membrane. The protrusions nearly always contain polyribosomes and some filamentous substance, partly bundled. Mitochondria, frequently swollen and sometimes tightly packed, appear in this zone. The cytoplasmic protrusions show a distribution of hemidesmosomes similar to that of basal cells in regular bronchial mucosa (Fig. 15a, b).

IV. Discussion

Using electron-microscopical studies of surgical biopsies from bronchial mucosa, we intended to find out whether and to what extent epithelial atypia and preneoplastic lesions of the bronchial mucosa, which are clearly identified and defined by light microscopy, could be similarly and reproducibly determined by their ultrastructural characteristics. The results of our investigations will be discussed in the following sections, and possible correlations and transitions from one state to another will be considered with particular reference to the problems of the pathogenetic steps in bronchial carcinogenesis.

1. Basal Cell Hyperplasia

The broader surface epithelium typical of basal cell hyperplasia is provoked by the multiplication of basal cells beyond their normal one or two layers. It appears in highly variable manifestations (*Ide* et al. 1959; *Auerbach* et al. 1956; *Ford* et al. 1961; *Carroll* 1961). The increased proliferative activities of the basal cells provide a source of new specific surface cells for bronchial epithelium. This may be evaluated with the aid of autoradiography and cytophotometry. An increasing number of DNA-synthesizing cells was found in this way within the hyperplastic epithelium in basal cell hyperplasia (*Sandritter* et al. 1965; *Lesch* and *Oehlert* 1966).

In the etiology of basal cell hyperplasia, damage by carcinogenic materials must be considered in addition to inflammatory factors (*Kotin* et al. 1966). For instance, the incidence of basal cell hyperplasia correlates closely with the amount of tobacco consumed (*Auerbach* et al. 1956, 1961, 1979; *Hamilton* et al. 1957; *Cunningham* and *Winstanley* 1959; *Kierszenbaum* 1965).

The high incidence of these epithelial alterations in the lungs of bronchial cancer patients and their regular, if transitory, occurrence in experimental chemically induced carcinogenesis suggests a correlation between basal cell hyperplasia and the development of certain types of bronchial carcinoma (*Mohr* 1979; and others).

The reversible nature of basal cell hyperplasia in the course of transitory inflammatory changes in the mucosa is generally assumed (*Otto* and *Wagner* 1956; *Otto* 1957, 1970). To date, however, it has been impossible to distinguish, by light or electron microscopy, the reversible regeneratory from the irreversible, possibly precancerous, basal cell hyperplasias.

2. Goblet Cell Hyperplasia

In diseases of the bronchial mucosa associated with hypersecretion, particularly chronic catarrhal bronchitis, typical morphological findings included not only glandular hypertrophy of the bronchial wall, but also goblet cell hyperplasia of surface epithelia (*Giese* 1967; *Hartung* 1968; *Müller* 1973). The frequent combination of goblet cell and basal cell hyperplasia suggests that both reflect an increased cell turnover. The presence of opaque granules in the goblet cells at the climax of the secretory cycle may be the morphological correlate of the changed texture of bronchial mucus observed in hypersecretory diseases; the altered appearance of mucous vacuoles may also reflect a change in the interciliary liquids necessary for adequate mucociliary function (*Iravani* and *Melville* 1978). The presence of promucin granules, which *Gieseking* (1971) was the first to identify, is the morphological feature interpreted in terms of accelerated secretion of immature mucus. Goblet cell hyperplasia is often observed as the first reaction of the bronchial mucosa to the inhalation of irritants (*Lamb* and *Reid* 1969; *Passey* and *Blackmore* 1967). Some facts indicate that this epithelial atypia may be the facultative, transitory, and reversible stage between normality and metaplasia or dysplasia. Goblet cell hyperplasia was observed more frequently in patients with bronchial carcinoma (*Nasiell* 1963a); other authors later interpreted the proliferation of mucus-producing cells in bronchial epithelium as the basic step in the development of precancerous epithelial lesions (*Trump* et al. 1978).

3. Metaplasia

Stratification (transitory metaplasia) differs from squamous metaplasia only by the lack of microscopically visible intercellular bridges and/or the absence of keratinization. Clear differentiation of the two types is possible by electron microscopy (*Gould* et al. 1971). Significant criteria are seen in certain epidermal features typical of squamous metaplasia: membrane-coating granules (MCG), multiple desmosomes and tonofilaments, and the presence of bundled tonofilaments even in the middle epithelial layer. According to our electron-microscopic studies, surface cells show similar features in both types of metaplasia, namely, isolated cytoplasmic mucus granules, secretory droplets, and lumen-oriented microvilli. None of our specimens of squamous metaplasia have shown keratinization in the superficial area. In the intermediate zone, however, stratification seems to exhibit more cells with secretory droplets, which probably correspond to the SMG cells described by *Trump* et al. (1978) in normal epithelium and in metaplastic and dysplastic alterations of bronchial mucosa, attributing a particular proliferative potential to this cell type.

The absence of the specific surface functions of bronchial epithelium provoked by loss of ciliated and goblet cells characterizes stratification and epidermoid metaplasia (*Kotin* et al. 1966). Experimental follow-up studies conducted on carcinogenic and noncarcinogenic damage revealed a sequence of changes developing from basal and goblet cell hyperplasia to stratification and squamous metaplasia. Under the influence of carinogenic stimuli, metaplasia has been defined by many authors (*Wong* and *Buck*

1971; *Gould* et al. 1971; *Harris* et al. 1973a, b; *Reznik-Schüller* and *Mohr* 1974; *Kobayashi* et al. 1978; *McDowell* et al. 1978; *Mohr* 1979) as a transitionàl stage on the way to dysplasia.

Squamous metaplasia is seen in a significant histogenetic association with squamous cell bronchial carcinoma (*Nasiell* 1963b; *Kotin* et al. 1966; *Coalson* et al. 1970; *Inoue* and *Dionne* 1977; *Trump* et al. 1978). The recent studies by *Becci* et al. (1978a, b) have, nevertheless, provided evidence for the reversibility of both squamous and transitional metaplasia (stratification).

4. Micropapillomatosis

Our specimens of mucosa showing micropapillomatosis with typical subepithelial vessel proliferation comprised all forms of metaplastic change in addition to cellular and nuclear atypia like that found in dysplastic areas. Light- and electron-microscopical findings in the epithelia of micropapillomatosis correspond to those seen in stratification an epidermoid metaplasia, in dysplasia of all grades, and even in carcinoma in situ. The interpretation of micropapillomatosis as a preneoplastic lesion is supported by the increasing incidence of such changes in the bronchial epithelium of patients with manifest bronchial carcinoma (*Nasiell* 1963a; *Müller* 1979). Remembering the changing pattern of vascularization in the early phases of bronchial carcinoma, we may interpret these vascular proliferations as the earliest change in the stroma of a future carcinoma. These capillaries are supplied by branches of the bronchial arteries which would supply the nutritive vessels in fully developed tumors (*Müller* and *Meyer-Schwickerath* 1978).

5. Dysplasia and Carcinoma In Situ

The terms "dysplasia" and "carcinoma in situ", universally accepted for preneoplastic lesions of the uterine cervix and larynx (*Grundmann* 1973), have been applied to conditions of the bronchial mucosa in recent years. When the WHO classification of pulmonary tumors was revised in October 1977, dysplasia and carcinoma in situ were introduced as separate entities between benign and malignant tumors of the lung. Dysplasia is now defined as "less severe epithelial changes than those seen in carcinoma in situ, typically not involving the full thickness of the epithelium" (*Sobin* 1979).

The definition of gradual differences in dysplasia relies in particular on criteria developed by cytological investigations (*Saccomano* et al. 1965, 1974; *Kato* et al. 1976; *Nasiell* et al. 1978). Whether these preneoplastic changes are classified as one of the three grades of dysplasia or as carcinoma in situ, depends on the presence and number of cellular and nuclear atypias in the different layers of an unusually metaplastic epithelium. Variables for the assessment of cellular and nuclear atypia are based largely on the criteria adopted for the identification of carcinoma cells. Classification according to nuclear atypia is supported by the cytomorphometry of sputum cells. Graded differences between squamous metaplasia, dysplasias I–III, and carinoma in situ may be quantified very exactly by the DNA content of the cells (*Nasiell* et al. 1978).

In light-microscopically assessed dysplasia I, surface epithelia show ultrastructural changes reflecting a more or less severe loss of the specific functions in ciliated and goblet cells. One of these signs is the presence of atypical kinocilia with altered substructures, often in great number and irregularly arranged. Moreover, such cilia may be thicker, with irregular contours. The term "compound cilia" describes certain abnormal structures assembled in one cytoplasmic matrix showing ciliar components and a partly atypical array of microtubules (*McDowell* et al. 1976). It is unlikely that such abnormal kinocilia are able to keep up the ciliary clearance function of bronchial mucosa (*Ghadially* 1978). In fact, these compound cilia may be interpreted as the early morpological counterpart of cellular functions impaired by external damage (*Mohr* 1979). Pathological reactions of ciliated surface epithelia were also observed in the bronchial mucosa of smokers (*Ailsby* and *Ghadially* 1973; *McDowell* et al. 1976).

Intracytoplasmic cilia in superficial cells are indicative of dysplasia (*Wong* and *Buck* 1971). They have been observed in all grades of dysplasia and in carcinoma in situ, even in the basal layers of epithelia. Similar findings were reported following experimental application of carcinogens to the bronchial lumen (*Mohr* 1979). Larger coarse cytoplasmic protrusions of surface epithelia into the bronchial lumen represent one of the very early signs of cellular alterations produced by carcinogenic substances in animal experiments (*Harris* et al. 1973b). Similarly, the numerical decrease of ciliated cells and of cilia per cell must be seen as an early manifestation of the degenerative impairment of specific cellular functions.

The quantitative reduction or complete loss of typical goblet cells is a feature common to all preneoplastic changes of the epithelium. However, we may observe certain cell types in which ultrastructurally visible, sparse secretory granules, osmiophilic and surrounded by a membrane, suggest an abnormal secretory function. These granules show a certain resemblance to the promucin granules of goblet cells seen in the early phases of accelerated mucus production, e.g., in chronic bronchitis (*Gieseking* 1971).

In advanced dysplasia and carcinoma in situ the superficial layer shows atypical cells that are ultrastructurally characterized by small droplet-like intracytoplasmic structures devoid of mucous vacuoles. This cell type recorded in our studies very likely corresponds to the "small mucous granule cells" described by other authors (*Trump* et al. 1978; *Becci* et al. 1978a, b). Severely dysplastic areas show an atypical array of organelles in all the cells, and it is no longer possible to classify them into definite cell types, such as ciliated cells, etc.

The altered ciliogenesis and mucus production observed in preneoplastic epithelial lesions reflect degenerative processes within the surface epithelium. Similar reactions were observed in the development of stratification under Vitamin A deficiency, without additional application of carcinogens. The signs of marked degenerative changes in surface epithelia documented in our findings have been repeatedly reported in experimental studies with chemical carcinogens, and in human lungs after carcinogen exposure (*Ailsby* and *Ghadially* 1973; *Harris* et al. 1973a, b; *Becci* et al. 1978a, b; *Trump* et al. 1978).

To be evaluated in the context of a possible development of bronchial carcinoma, however, the loss of specific cell functions must be correlated with the behavior of cells with proliferative capacity. The pathogenetic significance of the findings depends on the decrease of specific cellular functions and on the loss of differentiation or increase of cellular and nuclear atypia. Another sign is the disorderly arrangement of epithelial layers, starting from basal and intermediate strata, but eventually affecting all the layers. The electron-microscopic criteria of tissue disorganization are seen in irregularly widened intercellular spaces and strongly invaginated cell borders. These ultrastructural findings in the intercellular spaces differ variably, showing extreme expression in severe dysplasia and in carcinoma in situ and probably reflecting the impaired coherence of cells. Apparently the imperfect intercellular contact is maintained by cytoplasmic protrusions which are tipped with desmosomes and bridge the wider intercellular spaces (*Watson* et al. 1966; *Harris* et al. 1971, 1973a, b; *Kobayashi* et al. 1978). The mean number of desmosomes counted in preneoplastic areas varies from case to case. In these cellular protrusions, single and bundled tonofilaments are usually associated with desmosomes (*Konradova* et al. 1977). This picture of altered intercellular connections found in preneoplastic lesions was also observed in very similar manifestations in bronchial carcinoma, especially in squamous carcinoma (*Bensch* et al. 1968; *Razzuk* et al. 1970; *Coalson* et al. 1970; *Inoue* and *Dionne* 1977). The development of altering intercellular contacts is currently discussed as a primary process in carcinogenesis (*Ghadially* 1978).

Another characteristic ultrastructural feature in advanced grades of dysplasia is the presence of two cell types, termed "dark" or "clear" according to the electron density of their cytoplasm. The dark cells predominate basally but also occur in intermediate and occasionally in surface epithelial layers of carcinoma in situ. Cellular and nuclear polymorphism are more marked in those cells with electron-dense cytoplasm. Comparable findings in cells with differing cytoplasmic density have also been described in bronchial carcinoma (*Hattori* et al. 1967). Preneoplastic cells frequently showed an increase of free ribosomes and decrease of endoplasmic reticulum; similar findings were reported in bronchial carcinoma, except in adenocarcinoma (*Stoebner* et al. 1967; *Obiditsch-Mayer* and *Breitfellner* 1968; *Coalson* et al. 1970; *Fasske* 1970). The basal layers of dysplastic lesions show an increase of tonofilaments in basal cells; in this case these tonofilaments, normally arranged around the nucleus, are spread diffusely all over the cytoplasm, although maintaining their affinity to cytoplasmic protrusions and desmosomes.

Severe dysplasia and carcinoma in situ specimens show ultrastructural cell alterations ranging from the basal to the topmost cell layers and correlating with the light microscopy observations. Atypical enlarged nuclei appear pleomorphic with numerous invaginations, a feature typical of the carcinoma cell and explained as an increased interface between nucleus and cytoplasm, reflecting the increased metabolic activity within the cell (*Ghadially* 1978). Many nuclei of the less electron dense cells show a marginal distribution of heterochromatin. In contrast, the more electron dense cells possess larger islets of chromatin at the periphery as well as in random distribution over the nuclear matrix. The picture strongly resembles the chromatin pattern seen in small-cell bronchial carcinoma, where it is described as "leopard skin" (*Razzuk* et al. 1970). Enlarged nucleoli in a marginal position observed in preneoplastic cells seem to indicate increased protein synthesis. Our findings of nuclear and nucleolar atypia in dysplastic epithelia correspond, to a considerable extent, to the findings in manifest bronchial carcinoma.

The relevant light-microscopic criterion for differentiating preneoplastic epithelial lesions from invasive carcinoma is the pattern found at the epitheliostromal border. Our electron-microscopical studies have shown that ultrastructurally, marked deviations from the normal pattern may occur at a light-microscopically intact basement membrane under more or less dysplastic epithelium. In mild dysplasia the basal cell layer is found to extend small cytoplasmic protrusions toward the basement membrane; during the subsequent grades of preneoplastic change, these protrusions enter more deeply into the membrane material, at least focally. The zone of contact between basal cells and basement membrane, smooth and poorly structured in normal mucosa, shows considerably discontinuity in severe dysplasia and carcinoma in situ, but the basement membrane is not yet fully penetrated nor destroyed. Pictures like those documented in our findings in milder dysplasia have been recorded in experimental studies of chemically induced bronchial carcinoma (*Harris* et al. 1971, 1973a, b; *Reznik-Schüller* and *Mohr* 1975), and comparable alterations were assessed in preneoplastic changes in organs other than the lung and bronchi (epidermis, breast) (*Frei* 1962; *Tarin* 1969; *Siegismund* et al. 1979; and others).

In the cytoplasmic protrusions directed toward the basement membrane, we found, as very characteristic features, ribosomes and other organelles and also filamentous structures, often arranged in parallel to the orientation of cytoplasmic protrusions.

The formation of pseudopodal cytoplasmic protrusions is a frequently described activity of carcinoma cells at the stromal border (*Frei* 1962; *Tarin* 1969; *Erlandson* and *Carstens* 1972). Contractile proteins, i.e., structures of cell-deforming potential, are discussed in this context, assuming that cellular motility is a prerequisite for invasion of adjacent connective tissues (*Inoue* and *Dionne* 1977). The microfilaments and tonofilaments of tumor cells, observed in great number within the growth zone of carcinomas, could be regarded as an expression of the cell-deforming potential (*Malech* and *Lentz* 1974; *Gabbiani* et al. 1976; *Macartney* et al. 1979). The filaments directed toward the basement membrane, which were observed inside the cytoplasmic protrusions of basal cells, might possibly be interpreted as a similar expression of the early invasive potential inherent in preneoplastic epithelium.

In view of extensive experimental follow-up studies of bronchial carcinogenesis, the correct classification of the dysplasias and carcinoma in situ into a sequence of carcinogenesis seems to present no problems. Experimental studies have regularly recorded the development of metaplastic epithelium toward initially mild and then severe atypias leading to carcinoma in situ and manifest carcinoma. The predominant precursors of later tumors are epithelial hyperplasia and epithelial metaplasia (*Harris* et al. 1971, 1973a, b; *Nettesheim* and *Schreiber* 1975; *Becci* et al. 1978a, b; *Kobayashi* et al. 1978; *Mohr* 1979; and others).

To date we have been unable to assess the rate of incidence of preneoplasia or its predisposition to turn into invasive carcinoma in man. Reversibility of preneoplastic changes is assumed in mild and moderate dysplasia (*Auerbach* et al. 1961, 1979; *Nasiell* et al. 1977; *Trump* et al. 1978). Clinical experience and the extent of morphologically verified alterations in dysplasia III and in carcinoma in situ suggest that these two lesions with high invasive potential are most likely to turn into carcinoma (*Carter* 1978).

References

Ailsby RL, Ghadially FN (1973) Atypical cilia in human bronchial mucosa. J Pathol 109:75–78

Auerbach O, Petrich TG, Stout AP, Statsinger AL, Muehsam GE, Foran JB, Gore JB (1956) The anatomical approach to the study of smoking and bronchogenic carcinoma. Cancer 9:76–83

Auerbach O, Stout AP, Cuyler-Hammond E, Garfinkel L (1961) Changes in bronchial epithelium in relation to cigarette smoking and in relation to lung cancer. N Engl J Med 265:253–267

Auerbach O, Cuyler-Hammond E, Garfinkel L (1979) Changes in bronchial epithelium in relation to cigarette smoking, 1955–1960 versus 1970–1977. N Engl J Med 300:381–386

Basset F, Porier J, Le Crom M (1971) Etude ultrastructurale de l'épithelium bronchiolaire humain. Z Zellforsch Mikrosk Anat 116:425–442

Becci PJ, McDowell EM, Trump BF (1978a) The respiratory epithelium. VI. Histogenesis of lung tumors induced by benzo(a)pyrene ferric oxide in the hamster. J Natl Cancer Inst 61:607–618

Becci PJ, McDowell EM, Trump BF (1978b) The respiratory epithelium. IV. Histogenesis of epidermoid metaplasia and carcinoma in situ in the hamster. J Natl Cancer Inst 61:577–586

Bensch KG, Corrin B, Pariente R, Spencer H (1968) Oat cell carcinoma of the lung; its origin and relationship to bronchial carcinoid. Cancer 22:1163–1172

Carroll R (1961) Changes in the bronchial epithelium in primary lung cancer. Br J Cancer 15:215–219

Carter D (1978) Pathology of early squamous cell carcinoma of the lung. Pathol Annu 13:131–147

Clara M (1937) Zur Histobiologie des Bronchialepithels. Z Mikrosk Anat Forsch 41:321–347

Coalson JJ, Mohr JA, Pirtle JK, Dee AL, Rhoades ER (1970) Electron microscopy of neoplasms of the lung with special emphasis on the alveolar cell carcinoma. Am Rev Respir Dis 101:181–197

Cunningham GJ, Winstanley DP (1959) Hyperplasia and metaplasia in the bronchial epithelium. Ann R Coll Surg Engl 24:323–330

Cutz E, Conen PE (1970) Ultrastructure and cytochemistry of Clara cells. Am J Pathol 62:127–141

David H (1978) The respiratory system. In: David H (ed) Ortho- and pathomorphology of human and animal cells in drawing, diagrams and constructions. VEB Fischer, Jena, pp 213–226

Erlandson RA, Carstens PHB (1972) Ultrastructure of tubular carcinoma of the breast. Cancer 29:987–995

Fasske E (1970) Die Histo- und Cytomorphologie der Lungencarcinome. Internist 11:318–327

Feyrter F (1969) Das bronchiale (bronchopulmonale) Helle-Zellen-Organ. In: Kaufmann E (ed) Spezielle pathologische Anatomie, vol I/1. de Gruyter, Berlin, (Supplement, pp 673–678)

Ford DK, Filder HK, Lock DR (1961) Dysplastic lesions of the bronchial tree. Cancer 14:1226–1234

Frei JV (1962) The fine structure of the basement membrane in epidermal tumors. J Cell Biol 15:335–342

Gabbiani G, Csank-Brassert GJ, Schneeberger JC, Kapanci Y, Trenchev P, Holborow EJ (1976) Contractile proteins in human cancer cells: Immunofluorescent and electron microscopic study. Am J Pathol 83:457–474

Ghadially FN (1978) Ultrastructural pathology of the cell. Butterworths, London Boston

Giese W (1967) Pathologische Anatomie der chronischen Bronchitis. Beitr Klin Tuberk 136:155–172

Gieseking R (1968) Elektronenmikroskopische Befunde bei chronischer Bronchitis. In: Bopp KP, Hertle FH (eds) Chronische Bronchitis. Schattauer, Stuttgart New York, pp 67–77

Gieseking R (1971) Elektronenmikroskopie der Bronchialsekretion. In: Chronic inflammation of the bronchi. Prog Respir Res 6:43–50

Gieseking R (1973) Oberflächenzellen aus Atmungsorganen. In: Hirsch GC, Ruska H, Sitte P (eds) Grundlagen der Cytologie. VEB Fischer, Jena, pp 633–645

Gould VE, Wenk R, Sommers (1971) Ultrastructural observations on bronchial epithelial hyperplasia and squamous metaplasia. Cancer 28:426–436

Greenberg SD, Smith MN, Spjut HJ (1975) Bronchiolo-alveolar carcinoma – cell of origin. Am J Clin Pathol 63:153–167

Grundmann E (1973) Die Bedeutung der präcancerösen Zell- und Gewebsveränderungen in Experiment und Klinik. Arch Ohren Nasen Kehlkopfheilkd 205:55–67

Hamilton JD, Sepp A, Brown TC, McDonald FW (1957) Morphological changes in smokers lungs. Can Med Assoc J 77:177–182

Harris CC, Spron MB, Kaufman DG, Smith JM, Baker MS, Saffiotti U (1971) Acute ultrastructural effects of benzo(a)pyrene and ferric oxide on the hamster tracheobronchial epithelium. Cancer Res 31:1977–1989

Harris CC, Kaufman DG, Sporn MB, Saffiotti U (1973a) Histogenesis of squamous metaplasia and squamous cell carcinoma of the respiratory epithelium in an animal model. Cancer Chemother Rep 4/2:43–54

Harris CC, Kaufman DG, Sporn MB, Smith JM, Jackson F, Saffiotti U (1973b) Ultrastructural effects of N-methyl-N-nitrosourea on the tracheobronchial epithelium of the Syrian golden hamster. Int J Cancer 12:259–269

Hartung W (1968) Pathologisch-anatomische Befunde bei chronischer Bronchitis. In: Bopp KP, Hertle FH (eds) Chronische Bronchitis. Schattauer, Stuttgart New York, pp 49–59

Hartung W (1979) Anatomie der Lunge. In: Ulmer WT, Reichel G (eds) Bronchitis, Asthma, emphysem. Springer, Berlin Heidelberg New York (Handbuch der Inneren Medizin, vol IV/2, pp 1–24

Hattori S, Matsuda M, Tateishi R, Terazawa T (1967) Electron microscopic studies on human lung cancer cells. Gan 58:283–290

Hayek H von (1970) Die menschliche Lunge. Springer, Berlin Heidelberg New York

Heitz PH (1977) Endokrines System des Magen-Darm-Traktes und der Respirationsorgane. Verh Dtsch Ges Pathol 61:24–34

Ide G, Suntzeff V, Cowdry EV (1959) A comparison of the histopathology of tracheal and bronchial epithelium of smokers and nonsmokers. Cancer 17:475–484

Inoue S, Dionne GP (1977) Tonofilaments in normal bronchial epithelium and in squamous cell carcinoma. Am J Pathol 88:345–353

Iravani J, Melville GN (1978) Physiologie und Pathophysiologie des mucociliären Klärsystems. In: Kaik G, Hitzenberger G (eds) Die medikamentöse Behandlung der obstruktiven Atemwegserkrankungen. Symposion Wien. Schnetztor, Konstanz, pp 225–228

Kato H, Nasiell M, Auer G, Zetterberg A (1976) Cytophotometric DNA analysis in atypical squamous metaplasia of bronchial epithelium. In: Outline of principal research projects. Department of Surgery, Tokyo Medical College

Kierszenbaum AL (1965) Bronchial metaplasia. Observations on its histology and cytology. Acta Cytol (Baltimore) 9:365–371

Kobayashi N, Kanisawa M, Okamoto T, Okita M, Katsuki H (1978) Sequential cytologic study of the development of squamous cell carcinoma induced in subcutaneously implanted bronchial autograft of dog. Acty Cytol (Baltimore) 22:99–104

Konradova V, Hlouskova Z, Tomanek A (1977) Pathologische ultrastrukturelle Befunde im Epithel der Luftwege bei Kindern und Erwachsenen mit wiederholten und chronischen respiratorischen Erkrankungen. Z Erkr Atmungsorgane 147:270–280

Kotin P, Courington D, Falk HL (1966) Pathogenesis of cancer in a ciliated mucus-secreting epithelium. Am Rev Respir Dis 93:115—124

Lamb D, Reid L (1969) Goblet cell increase in rat bronchial epithelium after exposure to cigarette and cigar tobacco smoke. Br Med J I:33—35

Lesch R, Oehlert W (1966) Regeneration und Fehlregeneration im menschlichen Bronchialepithel. Verh Dtsch Ges Pathol 50:155—160

Macartney JC, Roxburgh J, Curran RC (1979) Intracellular filaments in human cancer cells: A histological study. J Pathol 129:13—30

Malech HL, Lentz TL (1974) Microfilaments in epidermal cancer cells. J Cell Biol 60:473—482

McDowell EM, Barrett LA, Harris CC, Trump BF (1976) Abnormal cilia in human bronchial epithelium. Arch Pathol Lab Med 100:429—436

McDowell EM, McLaughlin JS, Merenyl DK, Kieffer RF, Harris CC, Trump BF (1978) The respiratory epithelium. V. Histogenesis of lung carcinomas in the human. J Natl Cancer Inst 61:587—606

Mohr U (1979) Etiology and pathogenesis of early neoplastic lesions in an experimental model. Verh Dtsch Krebsges 2:165—174

Müller KM (1973) Chronische Bronchitis und Emphysem. Fischer, Stuttgart New York (Veröffentlichungen aus der morphologischen Pathologie, vol 93)

Müller KM (1979) Krebsvorstadien der Bronchialschleimhaut. Verh Dtsch Ges Pathol 63:112—131

Müller KM, Meyer-Schwickerath M (1978) Bronchial arteries in various stages of bronchogenic carcinoma. Pathol Res Pract 163:34—46

Nasiell M (1963a) The general appearance of the bronchial epithelium in bronchial carcinoma. Acta Cytol (Baltimore) 7:97—106

Nasiell M (1963b) Die Bedeutung der Epithelmetaplasie für die Frage des Bronchialkarzinoms. Bericht 1. Tagung d. Dtsch. Ges. f. angewandte Cytologie, 5.—7.9.1963 München, pp 40—47

Nasiell M, Sinner W, Tornvall G, Vogel B, Enstadt I (1977) Clinically occult lung cancer with positive sputum cytology and primary negative roentgenologic findings. Scand J Respir Dis 58:134—144

Nasiell M, Kato H, Auer G, Zetterberg A, Roger V, Karlen L (1978) Cytomorphological grading and Feulgen DNA analysis of metaplastic and neoplastic bronchial cells. Cancer 41:1511—1521

Nettesheim P, Schreiber H (1975) Advances in experimental lung cancer research. 3. Histogenesis of bronchogenic carcinoma. In: Grundmann E (ed) Geschwülste/Tumors III. Springer, Berlin Heidelberg New York (Handbuch der allgemeinen Pathologie, vol VI/7, pp 659—669)

Obiditsch-Mayer I, Breitfellner G (1968) Electron microscopy in cancer of the lung. Cancer 21:945—971

Otto H (1957) Die Bewertung des metaplastischen Bronchialregenerates. Beitr Pathol Anat 117:397—424

Otto H (1970) Bronchialepithelregeneration. In: Meessen H, Roulet F (eds) Die Organe. Springer, Berlin Heidelberg New York (Handbuch der allgemeinen Pathologie, vol III/4, pp 114—115)

Otto H, Wagner H (1956) Beiträge zur Frage der Regeneration des Bronchialepithels. Beitr Pathol Anat 116:436—460

Passey RD, Blackmore M (1967) Some experimental biological effects of cigar and cigarette smoke. Thorax 22:290—296

Pearse AGE, Polak JM (1974) Endocrine tumours of neural crest origin: Neurolophomas, APUDomas and the APUD concept. Med Biol 52:3—18

Razzuk MA, Race GJ, Lynn JA, Martin JA, Urschel HC, Paulson DL (1970) Observations on ultrastructural morphology of bronchogenic carcinoma. J Thorac Cardiovasc Surg 59:581—587

263

Reznik-Schüller H, Mohr U (1974) Investigations on the carcinogenic burden by air pollution in man. X. Morhological changes of the tracheal epithelium in Syrian golden hamsters during the first 20 weeks of benzo(a)pyrene instillation: an ultrastructural study. Zentralbl Bakteriol [B] 159:503–525

Reznik-Schüller H, Mohr U (1975) Investigations on the carcinogenic burden by air-pollution in man. XII. Early pathological alterations of the bronchial epitehlium in Syrian golden hamsters after intratracheal instillation of benzo(a)pyrene. 2. Further ultrastructural studies. Zentralbl Bakteriol [B] 160:108–129

Rhodin JAG (1966) Ultrastructure and function of the human tracheal mucosa. Am Rev Respir Dis 93:1–15

Saccomanno G, Saunders PR, Archer VE, Auerbach O, Kuschner M, Bechler PA (1965) Cancer of the lung: the cytology of sputum prior to the development of carcinomas. Acta Cytol (Baltimore) 9:613–623

Saccomanno G, Archer VL, Auerbach O, Saunders RP, Brennan L (1974) Development of carcinoma of the lung as reflected in exfoliated cells. Cancer 33:256–270

Sandritter W, Seidel A, Kleinhans D, Paddags I, Dontenwill W (1965) Cytophotometrische Messungen des DNS-Gehaltes an menschlichen und tierexperimentellen Bronchialmetaplasien. Z Krebsforsch 67:69–79

Schulz H (1959) Die submikroskopische Anatomie und Pathologie der Lunge. Springer, Berlin Göttingen Heidelberg

Siegismund G, Gorka T, Löblich HJ (1979) Vergleichende elektronenmikroskopische Untersuchungen von Keratoakanthomen und Plattenepithelcarcinomen der Haut. Verh Dtsch Ges Pathol 63:318–321

Sobin LH (1979) The WHO histological classification of lung tumours. In: Muggia FM, Rosencweig M, Lung cancer. Raven Press, New York (Progress in therapeutic research, pp 93–107

Stoebner P, Cussac Y, Porte A, Le Gal Y (1967) Ultrastructure of anaplastic bronchial carcinomas. Cancer 20:286–294

Tarin D (1969) Fine structure of murine mammary tumours: the relationship between epithelium and connective tissue in neoplasms induced by various agents. Br J Cancer 23:417–425

Terzakis JA, Sommers SC, Andersson B (1972) Neurosecretory appearing cells of human segmental bronchi. Lab Invest 26:127–132

Trump BF, McDowell EM, Glavin F, Barrett LA, Becci PJ, Schürch W, Kaiser HE, Harris CC (1978) The respiratory epithelium. III. Histogenesis of epidermoid metaplasia and carcinoma in situ in the human. J Natl Cancer Inst 61:563–575

Watson JHL, Brinkman GL (1964) Electron microscopy of the epithelial cells of normal and bronchitic human bronchus. Am Rev Respir Dis 90:851–866

Watson JHL, Bryant V, Brinkman GL (1966) The ultrastructure of epithelium of human bronchus in epidermoid carcinomas. 6th International Congress of Electron Microscopy, Kyoto. Maruzen, Nihonbushi, Tokyo

Wong YC, Buck RC (1971) An electron microscopic study of metaplasia of the rat tracheal epithelium in vitamin A deficiency. Lab Invest 24:55–66

Pulmonary Blastoma

D. FRANCIS and M. JACOBSEN

Pulmonary blastoma has been considered a very rare primary lung tumor. Since the first report in 1945 by *Barrett* and *Barnard*, an increasing number of cases have been recognized and reported. The true incidence is difficult to ascertain because the histological appearance of pulmonary blastomas is so variable that it may lead to various other tumor diagnoses. This survey is based on 11 cases from the author's own experience and 72 cases collected from the literature.

The amount of information from reported cases varies considerably, and several cases were published shortly after the diagnosis was confirmed by surgical resection. New information elicited by personal correspondence with the authors of reports of surviving pulmonary blastoma patients has been incorporated in the present investigation.

I. Definition

Pulmonary blastoma (PB) is a primary lung tumor consisting of a mixture of immature embryonal-like mesenchymal and epithelial components (Fig. 1). The tumor may in some areas resemble embryonal lung tissue of up to 3–4 months gestational age.

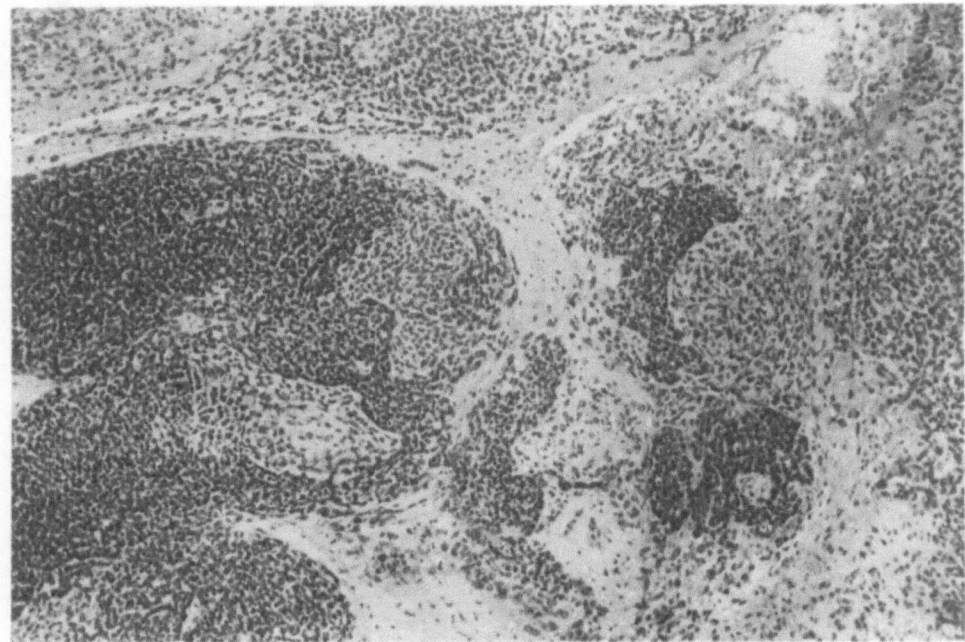

Fig. 1. Pulmonary blastoma: A mixture of immature-looking mesenchymal and epithelial components. Surgical specimen from a 58-year-old man. H & E, × 63

Heterotopic organoid structures are not found. Tumors showing an exclusively monotypic histological appearance in accordance with areas of an otherwise typical PB should, in our opinion, be accepted as PBs.

II. Historical Aspects

The tumor was first described in 1945 by *Barrett* and *Barnard* and again in 1952 by *Barnard*, who named it an embryoma of the lung.

In 1961 *Spencer* added three further cases and defined the tumor entity. He drew attention to the similarities to nephroblastoma and suggested the commonly used term, pulmonary blastoma. So far, our studies have revealed 83 reported cases, including 11 from the author's personal observations. A number of cases of PB have previously been published under various diagnoses such as embryoma (*Barnard* 1952), carcinosarcoma of peripheral origin (*Peabody* 1959), malignant teratoid tumor (*Schiødt* and *Jensen* 1960), adenosarcoma (*Campesi* and *Sommariva* 1961), mixed embryonic tumor (*Boss* 1962), embryonal sarcoma (*Chitambar* et al. 1969), malignant mixed tumor (*Davis* et al. 1972), and blastomatous tumor (*Meinecke* et al. 1976).

However, it has not been our intention to judge whether other reported cases of carcinosarcoma or other mixed tumors of the lung could in fact have been PB.

III. Histogenesis

Barnard (1952) suggested that the tumor developed from a part of lung which remained dormant and undeveloped or that the tumor was recapitulating its own life history.

Based on *Waddell's* investigation (1949), *Spencer* (1961) presumed that the PB develops from the pulmonary blastema, i.e., from a pluripotent cell of a single germ layer, similar to what is thought to be the genesis of nephroblastoma. Other authors (*Stackhouse* et al. 1969; *McCann* et al. 1976; *Roth* and *Elguezabal* 1978) regard PB as a subgroup of carcinosarcomas, which hence develops from two germ layers.

Embryologic transplantation experiments (*Dameron* 1969) and electron-microscopic studies (*McCann* et al. 1976; *Fung* et al. 1977) have hitherto not clarified whether PB develops from one or two germ layers. Several authors have found histological similarities between hamartoma and blastoma (*Spencer* 1977; *Stone* and *Churg* 1977) or transition between blastoma and carcinosarcoma (*Souza* et al. 1965; *Davis* et al. 1972; *Kern* and *Stiles* 1976; *Peacock* and *Whitwell* 1976; *Roth* and *Elguezabal* 1978). Morphological similarities between hamartoma, PB, and carcinosarcoma may point toward the tumors being variants of mixed mesodermal tumors of the lung (*Motlik* and *Triska* 1968; *Jacobsen* and *Francis* 1980).

IV. Epidemiology

1. Age and Sex Distribution

PB has been reported in infants of a few months of age (*Pacharee* and *Parichatikanond* 1972; *Blair* and *Al-Doroubi* 1976; *Jayet* et al. 1977), but are more often found in adults, in contrast to nephroblastoma, where the adult form is regarded as very rare. However, recently 167 cases of the latter tumor were collected from the world literature by *Babaian* et al. (1980).

Sex and age at the time of diagnosis for the 83 cases of PB are shown in Fig. 2. There were 60 males and 23 females (ratio 2.6:1). The mean age was 43 years (males

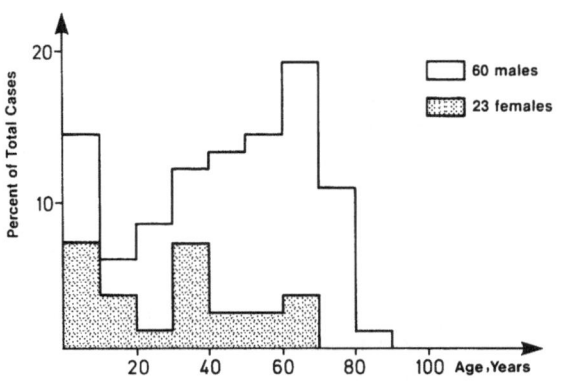

Fig. 2. Pulmonary blastoma: Sex and age at the time of diagnosis. *n* = 83

48.2 years, females 29.2 years). Twenty percent of the cases appeared before the age of 20 years, and 40% before 40 years. A possible explanation for the differences in age distribution in PB and nephroblastoma was given by *Spencer* (1961), who drew attention to differences in the adult maturation of the organ systems involved.

2. Geographical and Racial Distribution

PB has been reported in patients from all continents: 44 from Europe (including one African and one native Australian), 32 from the United States (six of whom were black, one Japanese, and one Puerto Rican), and seven from Asia.

3. Frequency

PB is regarded as a very rare tumor. From the Mayo Clinic files, a survey covering the period 1915–1965 disclosed four cases (*Stackhouse* et al. 1969). Recently the frequency was found to be 0.25%–0.5% among malignant primary lung tumors (*Motlik* and *Triska* 1968; *Cornet* et al. 1975; *Jacobsen* and *Francis* 1980).

4. Heredity

Familial accumulation has not been reported, nor has PB been linked to any specific syndrome, as is the case with nephroblastoma (*Bennington* and *Beckwith* 1975). In three cases of PB, coexistence with other malignant tumors has been reported: large cell carcinoma of the lung (*Karcioglu* and *Someren* 1974), breast cancer (*Kern* and *Stiles* 1976), and adenocarcinoma of the large intestine (*Stackhouse* et al. 1969).

V. Clinicopathological Features

1. Clinical Features

Based on the 83 cases, the most frequent or first-mentioned symptoms other than radiological evidence of a lung infiltrate (23%) were pneumonia or fever (17%), dyspnea (16%), cough (13%), hemoptysis (13%), pain (13%), or neurological symptoms (4%). Hemoptysis appeared in 24 cases (29% of all cases); pain, dyspnea, fever, or cough each appeared in 18–20 cases (20%–23%).

Except for radiological evidence of an intrathoracic mass, the preoperative diagnostic investigation has so far not been encouraging. Of the 83 cases, a positive microscopic diagnosis was preoperatively achieved in 27 cases (33%). Exfoliative cytology was reported positive for malignant tissue in 11 cases, needle biopsies in eight cases, and bronchoscopic biopsies in 14 cases. The presence of both mesenchymal and epithelial

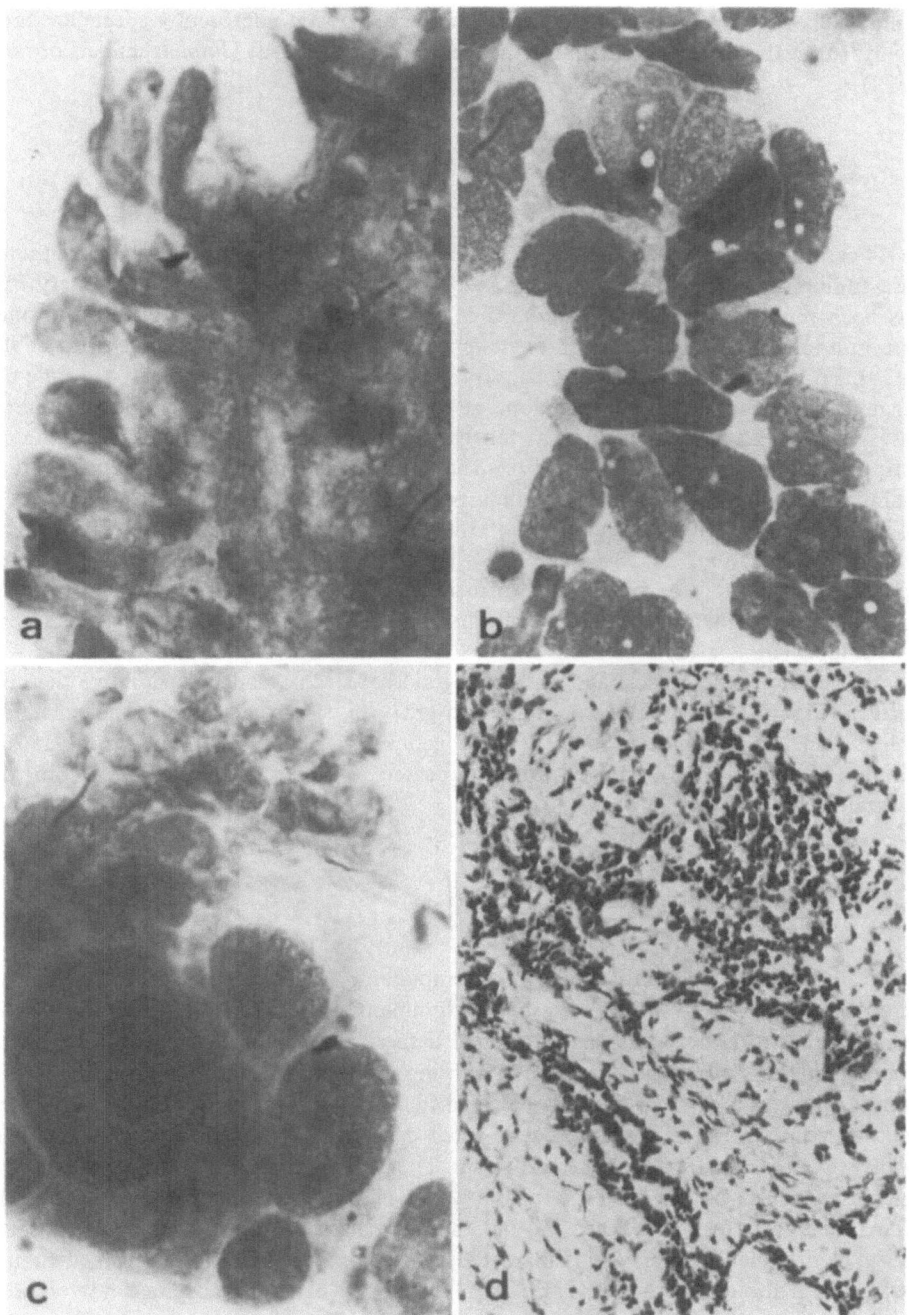

Fig. 3a—d. Pulmonary blastoma: Preoperative diagnostic specimens. **a** Tumor cells with mesenchymal differentiation. **b** Undifferentiated tumor cells. **c** Tumor cells with epithelial differentiation. **a—c** Fine needle aspiration biopsy from a 59-year-old woman. Air-dried smear. May-Grünwald-Giemsa stain, × 1000. **d** Immature stroma with areas showing epithelial-like differentiation. Bronchial biopsy from a 73-year-old man. H & E, × 150

tumor cells or tumor tissue in the preoperative diagnostic microscopy specimens are highly suggestive of a mixed tumor, hence a PB (Fig. 3a–d) (*Francis* and *Jacobsen* 1979).

2. Gross Features

In 44 cases the tumors were located in the right lung in 38 cases in the left lung; in one case tumors were found in both lungs (*Wiechowski* et al. 1975). Extrapulmonary PB has been reported twice (*RayChaudhuri* et al. 1972; *Valderrama* et al. 1978), in one case in a lung lobe sequestered from an apparently normal left lung (*Valderrama* et al. 1978). PB showed no predilection for any particular lobe of the lungs. At the time of diagnosis, the tumors affected one lobe in 62 cases (73%), two adjacent lobes in nine cases (11%), and the whole lung in ten cases (12%). Based on the macroscopic description, or in the absence thereof, on the radiological findings, the PB was located mainly in the peripheral part of the lung tissue in 28 cases (34%), whereas in 39 cases (47%) the tumors involved all parts of the lung parenchyma. Intrabronchial tumor growth was described in 23 cases (28%), in 17 of which the intrabronchial growth appeared as polypoid or finger-like protrusions. The size ranged from 1.5 to 26 cm. A pseudocapsule consisting of compressed lung tissue or bronchial wall was a characteristic finding (Fig. 4a–d).

On section, the typical PB was soft, grayish to pink, and bulged above the cut surface (Fig. 4b). A few PBs were hard and gritty in consistency due to the considerable stromal differentiation. A few were genuinely cystic (*Kern* and *Stiles* 1976; *Valderrama* et al. 1978), whereas others appeared to be cystic because of bleeding or central necroses.

3. Histopathological Features

Typically there is a mixture of three components – blastomatous, epithelial, and stromal – any one of which may be predominant. Gradual transitions from blastomatous areas to either epithelial or stromal tissues are often observed (Fig. 5a, b). The components are mixed and present in varying amounts in different sections of the tumor and may show varying degrees of differentiation and maturation. The blastomatous components are composed of small cells with dark oval nuclei and with a scanty, poorly demarcated, light cytoplasm. The cells are arranged without orientation and often appear as rosettes around thin-walled endothelium-lined vessels (Fig. 5a, b). The reticulin pattern is delicate and indistinct. A slight change in this picture is seen as small, rounded, rather well-demarcated areas, composed of closely packed tumor cells, which though of the same size as in the clearly blastomatous areas now appear epithelial (Fig. 6a). In some instances the cells are oriented around a central defect or lumen. Reticulin-positive fibers surround such cell groups but are not seen within them (Fig. 6b). Slightly further differentiated epithelial tumor cells appear with a light and sometimes well-demarcated cytoplasm. In solid islands and cords, the cells are poly-

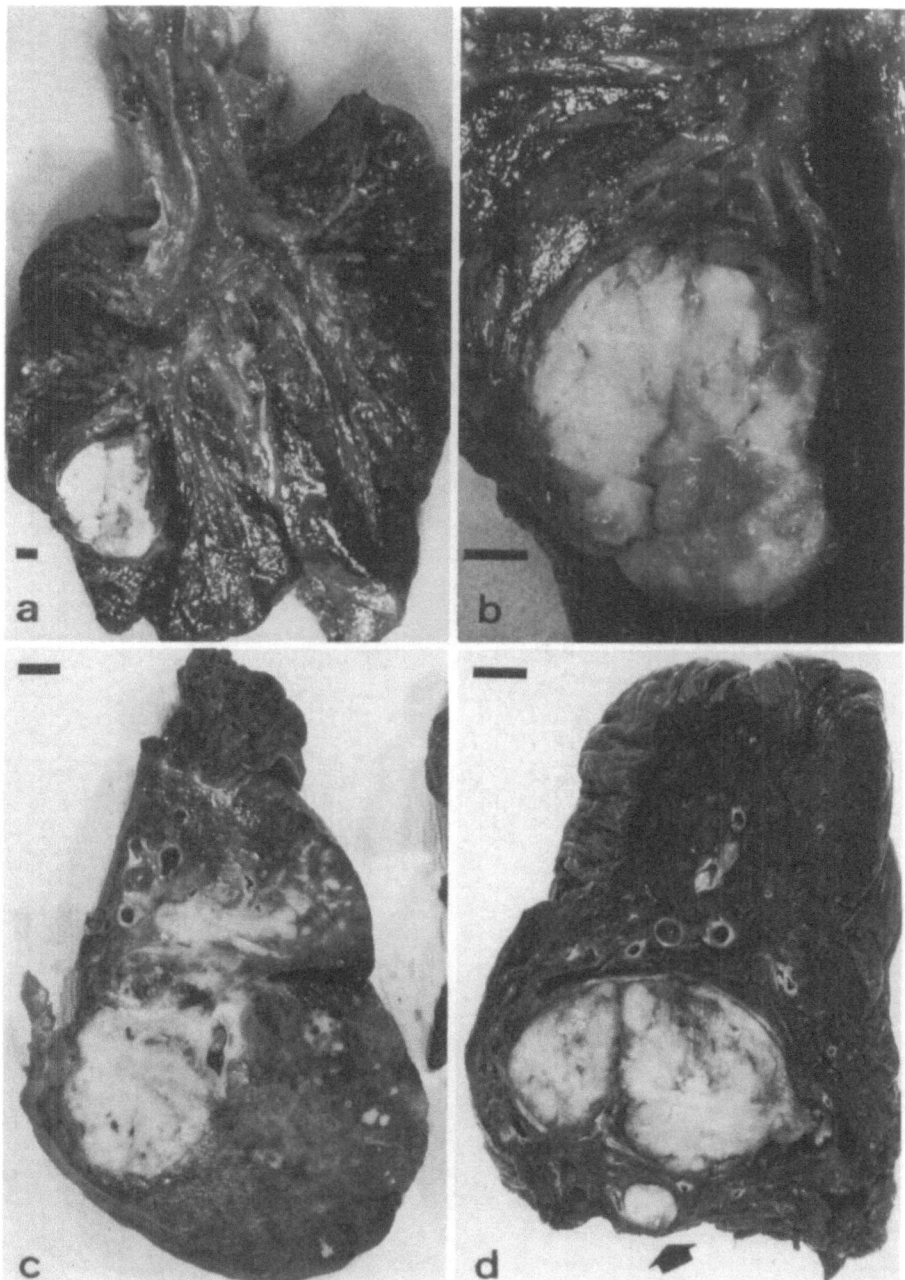

Fig. 4a–d. Pulmonary blastoma: Gross features. **a, b** The tumor is located in the peripheral part of the left lower lobe and is surrounded by a pseudocapsule consisting of compressed lung tissue and a bronchial wall. Autopsy specimen from a 68-year-old man. 1-cm scale indicated. **c** Tumor undemarcated, surrounded by carcinomatous growth. Surgical specimen from a 64-year-old woman. 1-cm scale indicated. **d** Tumor well-demarcated with a pseudocapsule and intrabronchial growth *(arrow)*. Surgical specimen from a 58-year-old man. 1-cm scale indicated

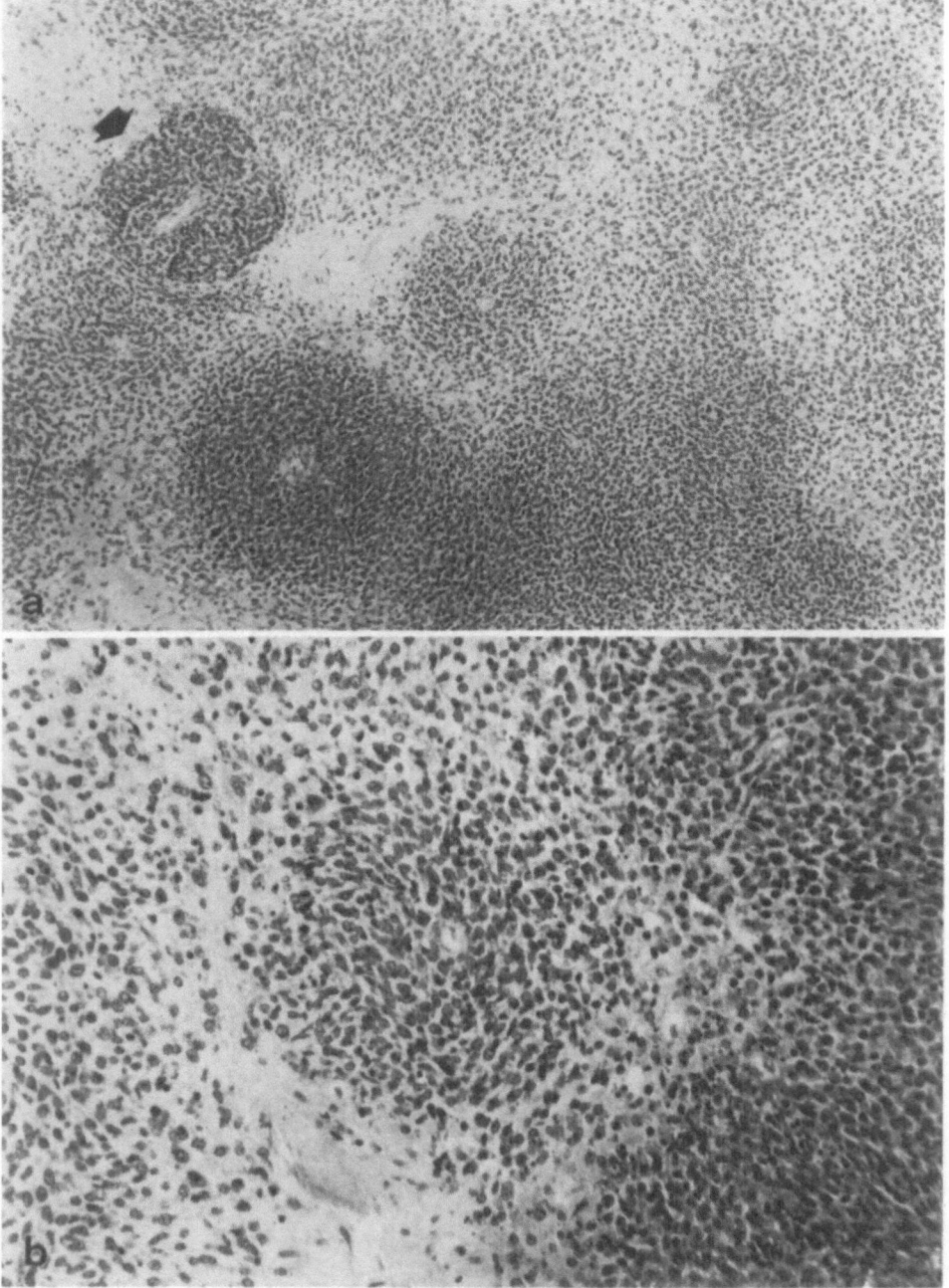

Fig. 5a, b. Pulmonary blastoma proper: The blastomatous component. The cells are arranged around thin-walled vessels. One area *(arrow)* reveals the earliest possible epithelium-like differentiation. Surgical specimen from a 58-year-old man. **a** H & E, × 63; **b** H & E, × 150

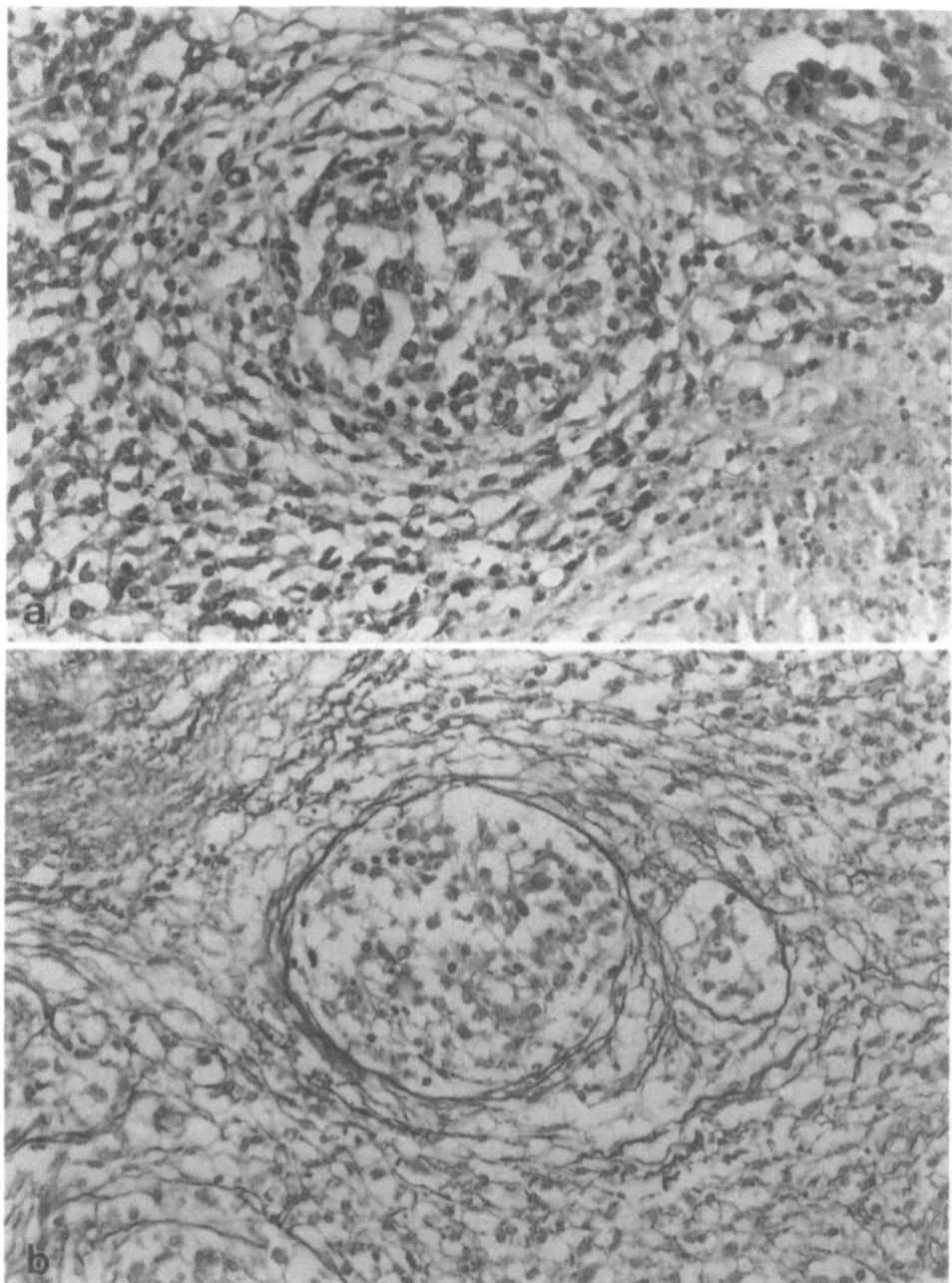

Fig. 6a, b. Pulmonary blastoma proper. **a** Blastomatous area containing island of tumor cells with epithelium-like differentiation. H & E, × 150. **b** Same area as **a**. Reticulin-positive fibers surround the islands. Autopsy specimen from a 66-year-old man. Silver impregnation, × 150

gonal, sometimes arranged in a cribriform or basaloid pattern (Fig. 7a, b). In areas showing tubular and gland-like formations, the tumor cells are more box-shaped or cylindrical and both cilia and secretory droplets can be demonstrated (Fig. 7c, d). In some cases the well-demarcated branching cords show signs of epidermoid differentiation, seen as flattening of the tumor cells and keratin pearl formation (Fig. 7e, f). Epithelial differentiation may be barely apparent or may be dominant. Stromal constituents of PB most often enclose fibroblastic and myxoid regions (Fig. 8a, b). The tumor cells are elongated and arranged in fascicles or stellate and located in a more abundant alcian-positive intercellular ground substance. Collagenous fibers are sparse; some may be present due to secondary changes. Myogenic differentiation is quite often seen but cross-striation is demonstrated in only a few cases. Other stromal constituents of PB include immature or well-differentiated cartilage and bone (Fig. 8c, d). Table 1 shows the frequency of the different types of epithelial and mesenchymal differentiations.

A few tumors are structurally sterotypic throughout, composed of a loose immature undifferentiated stroma containing branching tubular formations, imitating fetal lung tissue of 3—4 months gestational age (*Spahr* et al. 1979). However, the histological pattern in most cases differs from area to area, and quite often there are transitions into anaplastic elements that defy classification (Fig. 8e).

In some cases there are areas in which the epithelial and/or mesenchymal components reveal a rather mature histological appearance. Such areas may be dominated by a monotypic tumor tissue resembling primary or secondary monotypic sarcoma (Fig. 9a), in other areas or cases, the components may resemble ordinary primary bronchogenic carcinoma (Fig. 9b, c) (*Jacobsen* and *Francis* 1980). The compressed lung tissue or the dilated bronchial wall composing the tumor pseudocapsule is often partly invaded by tumor tissue.

Local recurrences (Fig. 10a, b) are usually more dedifferentiated in appearance than the corresponding primary tumor (*Schiødt* and *Jensen* 1960; *Jacobsen* and *Francis* 1980). The histological appearance of *metastatic lesions* is extremely variable. Table 2 contains all cases of PB known to us, special attention being focused on the distribution of secondaries and their histological components. Furthermore, the last known status and the survival in months are given. Previously unpublished information elicited by our correspondence with the authors is underlined.

In 37 of the collected cases the microscopic appearance of the metastases has been described. In 19 of these the metastases were monotypic (Fig. 11a, b) (monotypic

Table 1. Pulmonary blastoma: 83 cases. Frequency of the different types of epithelial and mesenchymal differentiation

Tubules or gland-like formations	90%
Myxoid differentiation	31%
Cartilage formations	24%
Epidermoid differentiation	23%
Myogenic differentiation	20%
Cross-striation	5%
Bone formation	5%

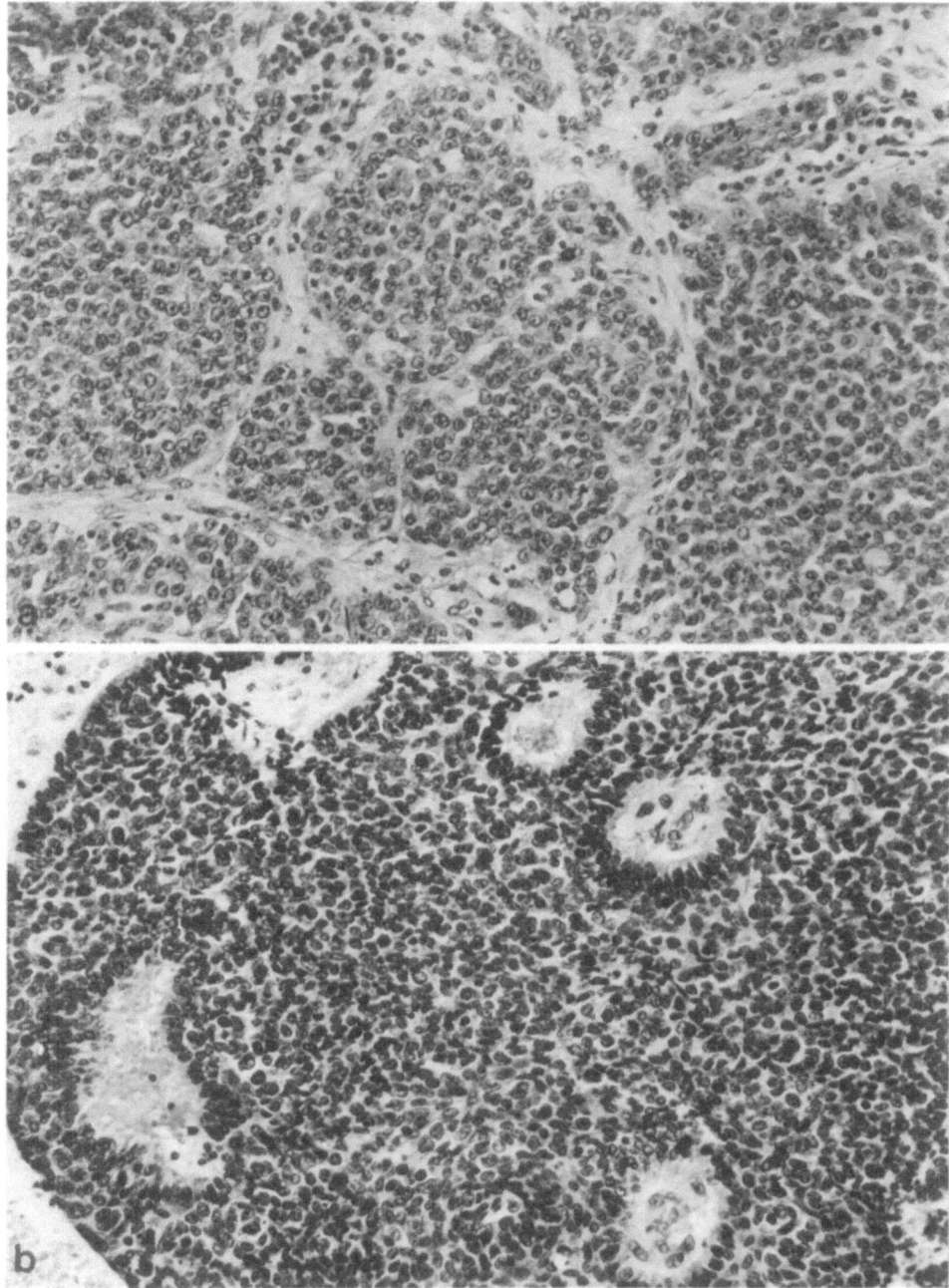

Fig. 7a–f. Pulmonary blastoma: Different types of epithelial differentiation. **a** Well-demarcated islands of monomorphic epithelial tumor cells. Surgical specimen from a 64-year-old woman. **b** Area with basaloid pattern, same case as **a**

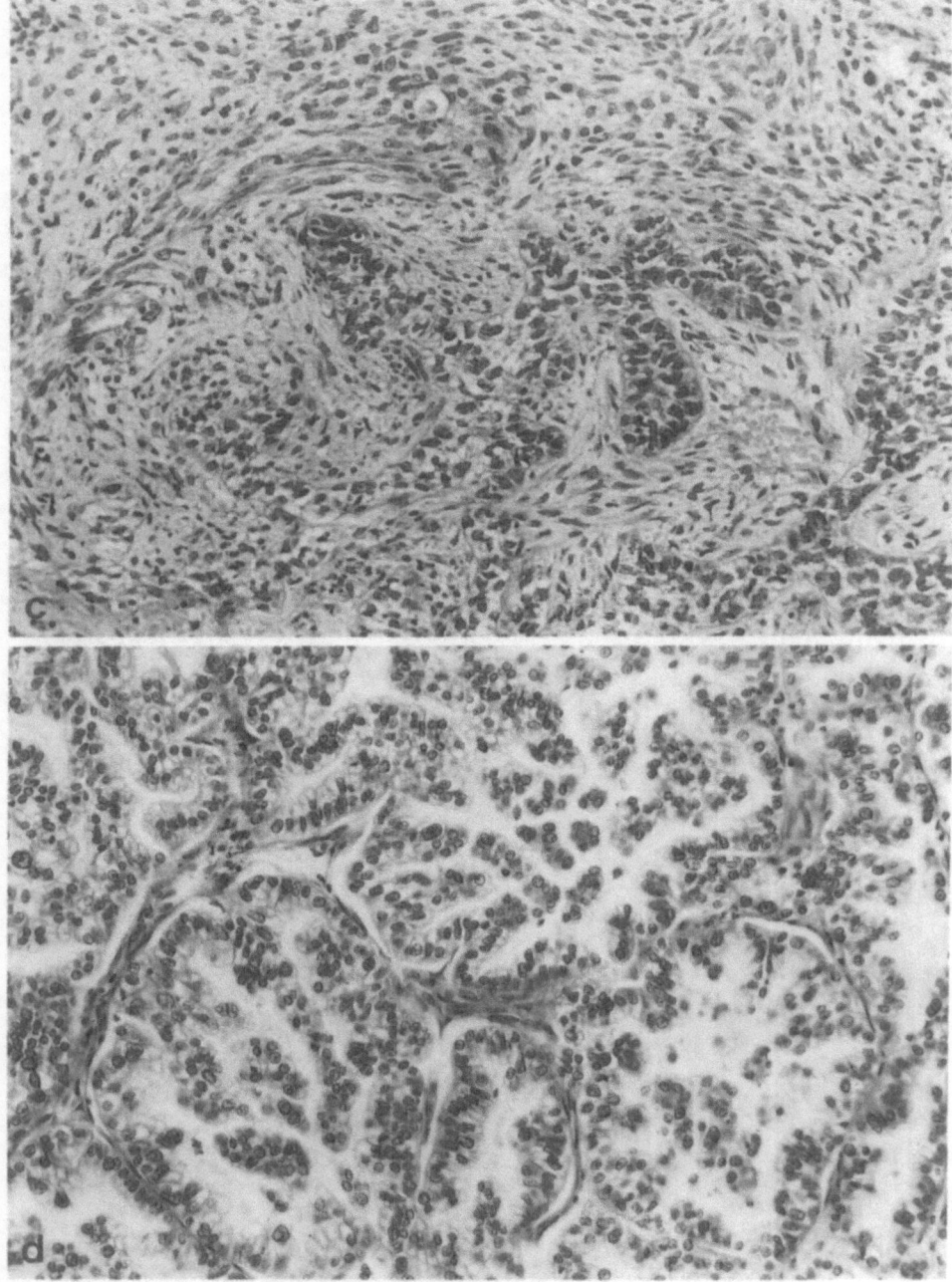

Fig. 7c. Epithelial cells arranged in branching cords, some of which show beginning tubular formation. Surgical specimen from a 67-year-old man. **d** Monomorphic adeno-carcinoma, showing small box-shaped cells with dark nuclei and a well-demarcated light cytoplasm. Surgical specimen from a 59-year-old woman

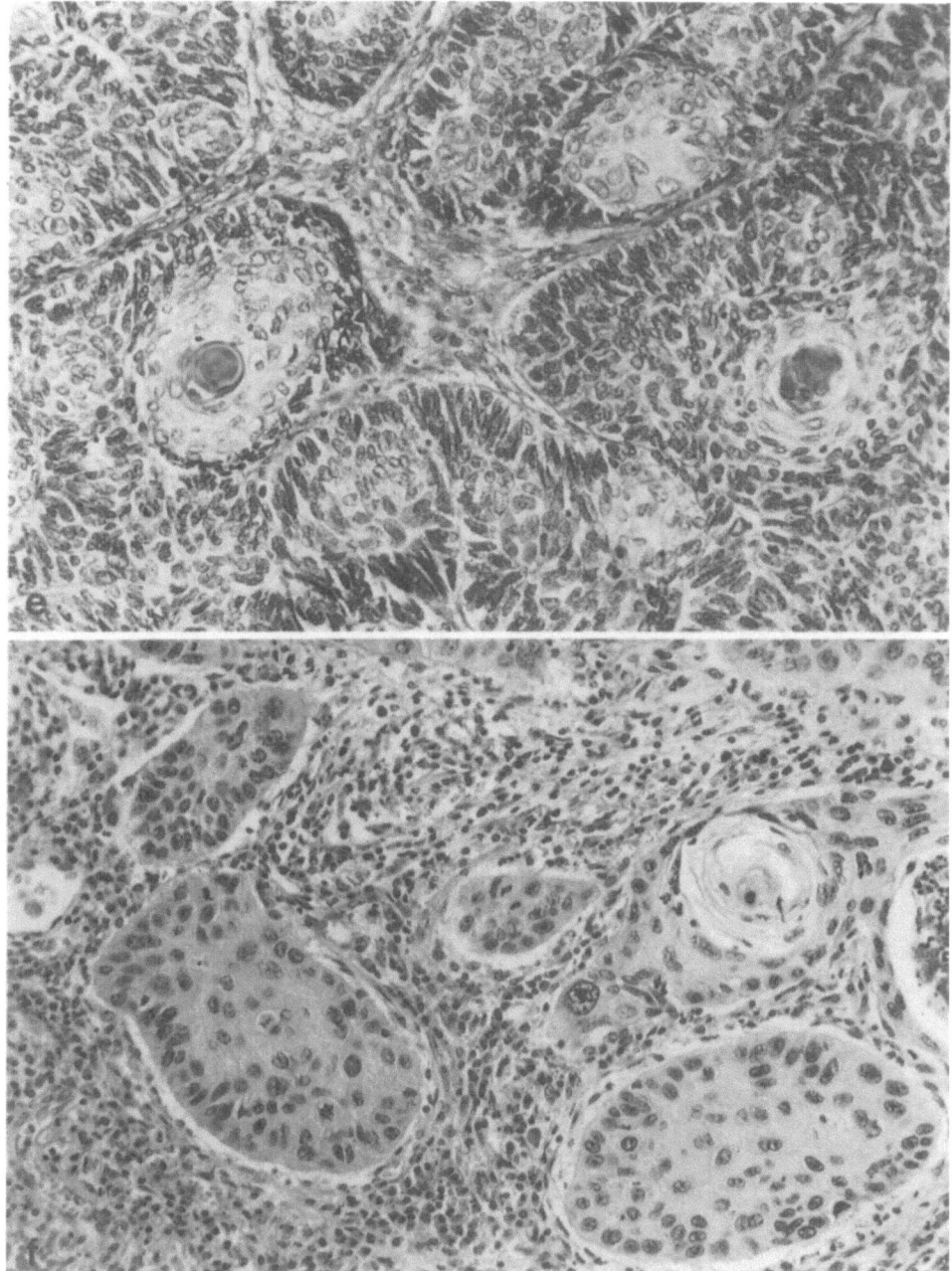

Fig. 7e. Epidermoid differentiation. Well-demarcated cords with abrupt differentiation into keratin pearls. Same case as Fig. 3d. Surgical specimen from a 73-year-old man. f Epidermoid carcinoma, showing cellular pleomorphism and keratinization. Surgical specimen from a 66-year-old man. a—f H & E, × 150

278

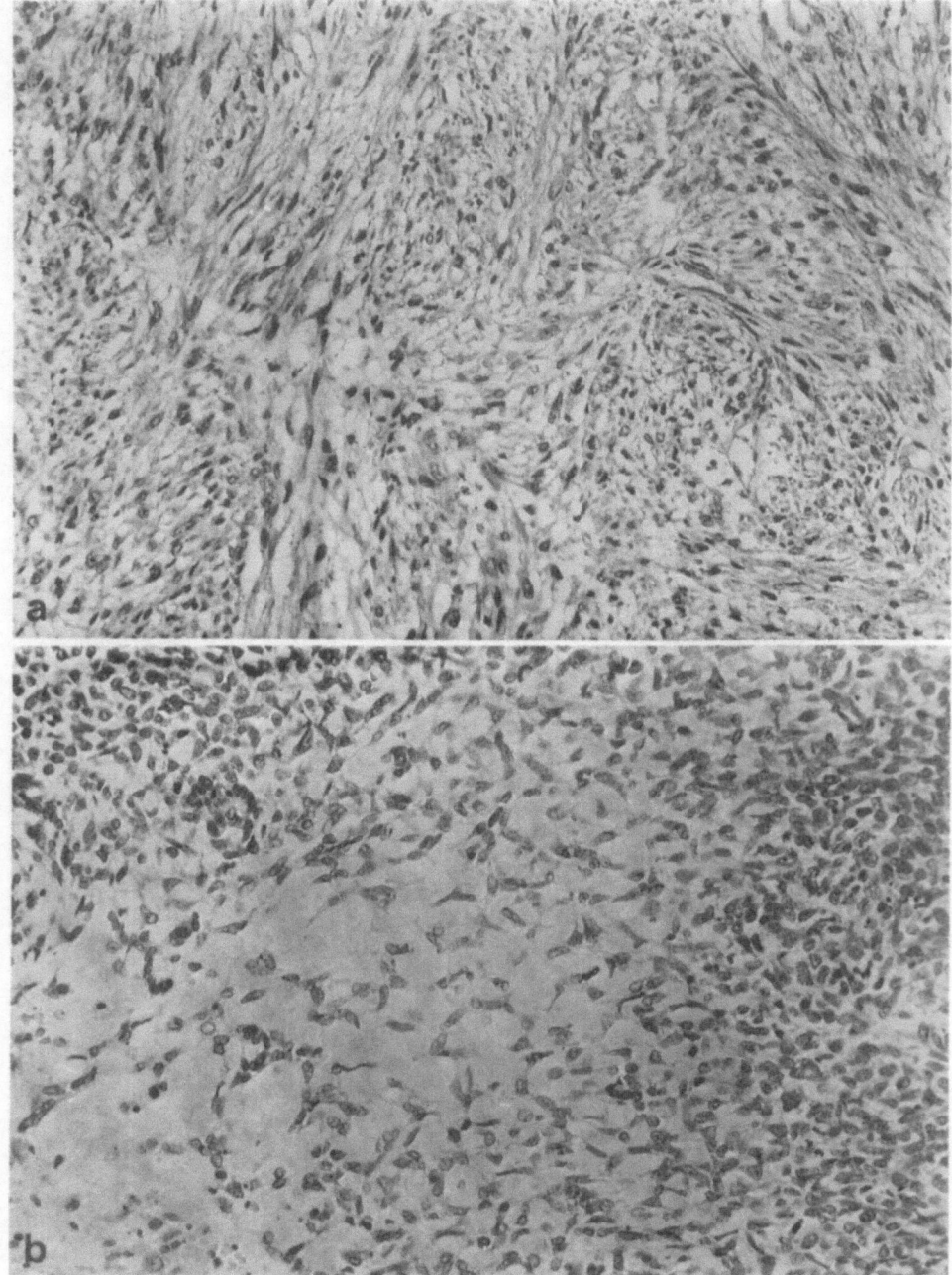

Fig. 8a—e. Pulmonary blastoma: Different types of mesenchymal differentiation.
a Elongated tumor cells arranged in fascicles. Autopsy specimen from a 69-year-old
man. **b** Myxoid area. Stellate cells in an abundant myxomatous ground substance.
Same case as Figs. 1 and 5a, b. Surgical specimen from a 58-year-old man.

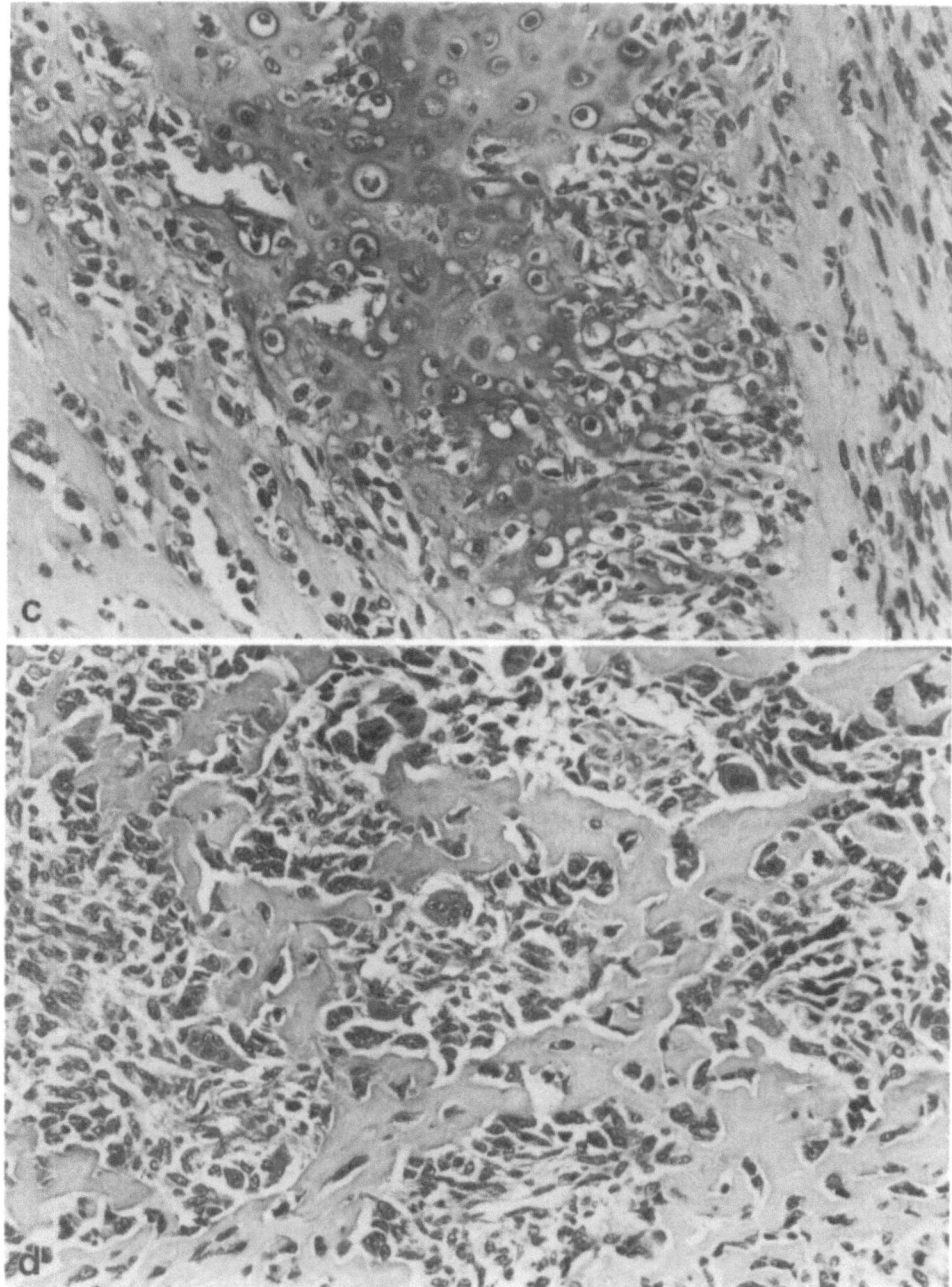

Fig. 8c. Chondromatous differentiation. Same case as Figs. 3d, 7e, and 8d. Surgical specimen from a 73-year-old man. **d** Osteoid differentiation. Osteoclasts and osteoblasts are lining bony trabeculae. Same case as Figs. 3d, 7e, and 8c

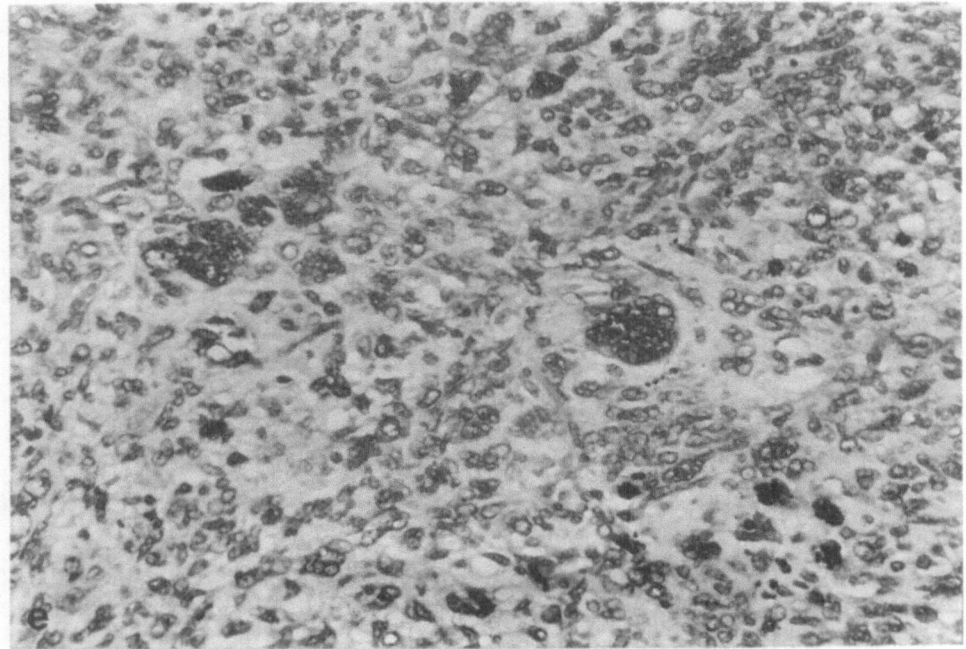

Fig. 8e. Pleomorphic mesenchymal component, with tumor giant cells. Same case as Figs. 3a—c and 7d. Surgical specimen from a 59-year-old woman. a—e H & E, × 150

epithelial metastases in six cases, monotypic mesenchymal metastases in 11 cases, and both types in two cases). Mixed metastases (Figs. 11c, d) were recorded in 18 cases, five of which also revealed metastases of monotypic appearance.

In our studies we experienced that it was impossible to conclude whether a surgically resected PB would show malignant biological behavior or not. Likewise, it was impossible in a single case to tell which histological components of the PB would turn out to be the most aggressive or malignant, resulting in secondaries of a similar histological structure or morphology.

Differential diagnoses will include other lung tumors consisting of a mixture of epithelial and mesenchymal tumor components. Tumors such as epidermoid carcinoma with a spindle cell component, mixed bronchial mucosa gland tumor, and teratoma should be reasonably easy to recognize. Metastases from primary embryonal tumors of the kidney, testis, etc. should be ruled out. In certain cases, difficulties may arise in distinguishing PB from mesothelioma, hamartoma, and carcinosarcoma.

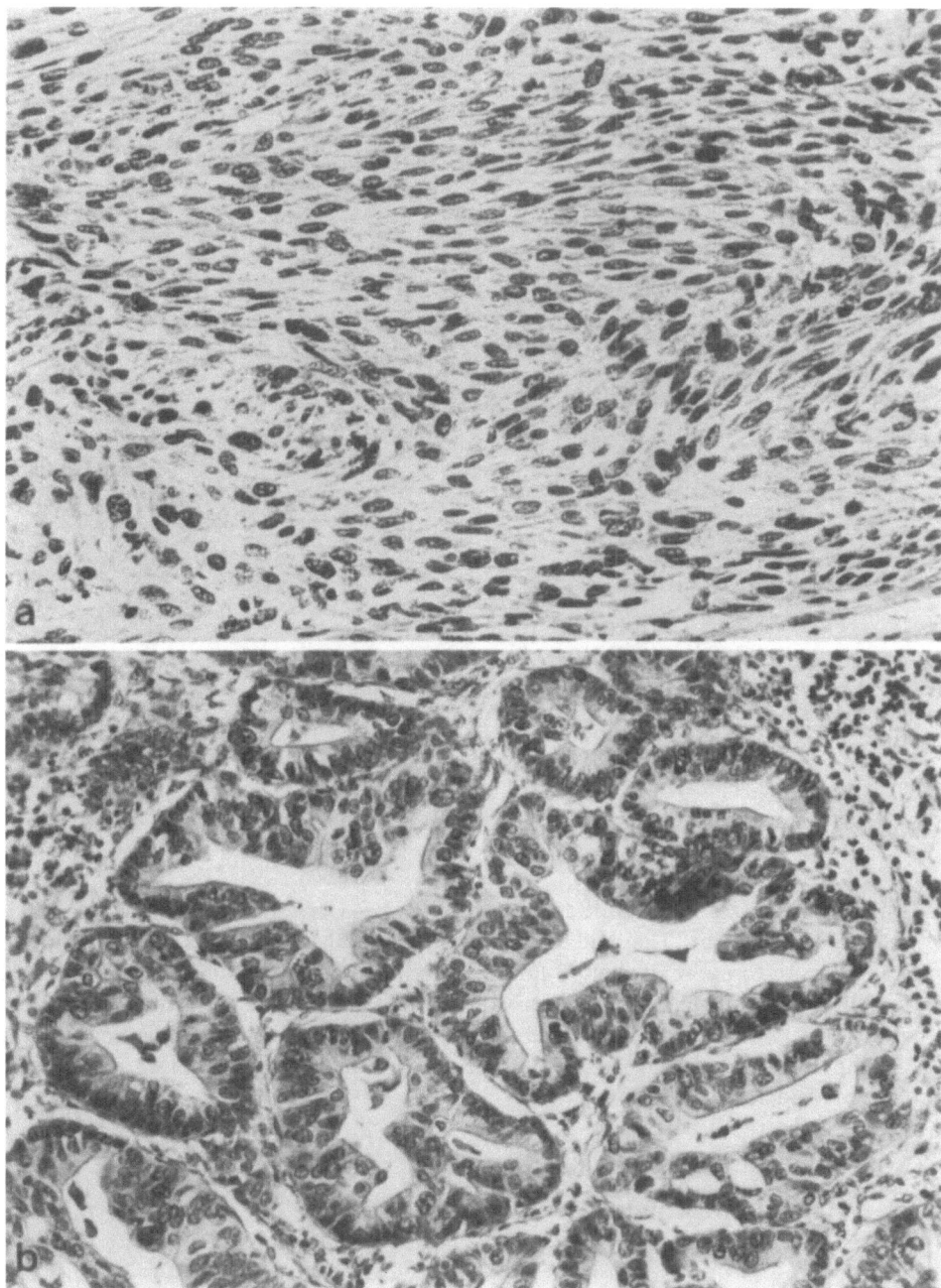

Fig. 9a–c. Pulmonary blastoma: Mesenchymal and epithelial component resembling ordinary malignant lung tumors. **a** Sarcomatous component with spindle cells arranged in fascicles. The tumor cells are pleomorphic. Surgical specimen from a 69-year-old man. **b** Adenocarcinoma of mature type. Same case as Fig. 7f. Surgical specimen from a 66-year-old man

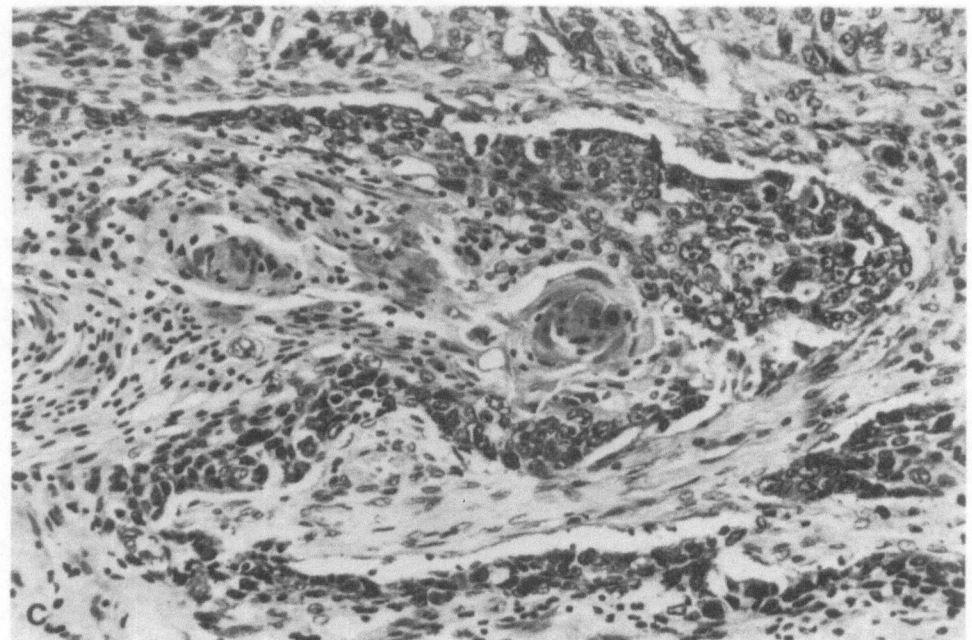

Fig. 9c. Epidermoid carcinoma of mature type. Same case as Fig. 7a, b. Surgical specimen from a 64-year-old woman. a—c H & E, × 150

4. Ultrastructural Findings

In only a few cases has the ultrastructure of PB been investigated (*Fung* et al. 1977; *McCann* et al. 1976). The studies have emphasized the similarities of this tumor to fetal lungs up to approximately 3 months gestational age (*Hage* 1973), and epithelial as well as mesenchymal elements have been recognized. The ultrastructural studies have as yet afforded little additional insight into the histogenesis and pathogenesis of PB. Intranuclear particles believed to be of viral origin were reported in one case (*Marsden* and *Scholtz* 1976).

VI. Natural History and Pattern of Metastases

Though surrounded by a pseudocapsule, PB shows local invasive growth. Among 66 surgically resected specimens, tumor growth into the bronchial lumina was seen in 28%, and involvement of the pleura and the mediastinum in 25% and 8% of the cases, respectively. Apparently neither of these types of involvement affected the postoperative survival significantly (McWhitney test). Local recurrences occurred in 38% of the

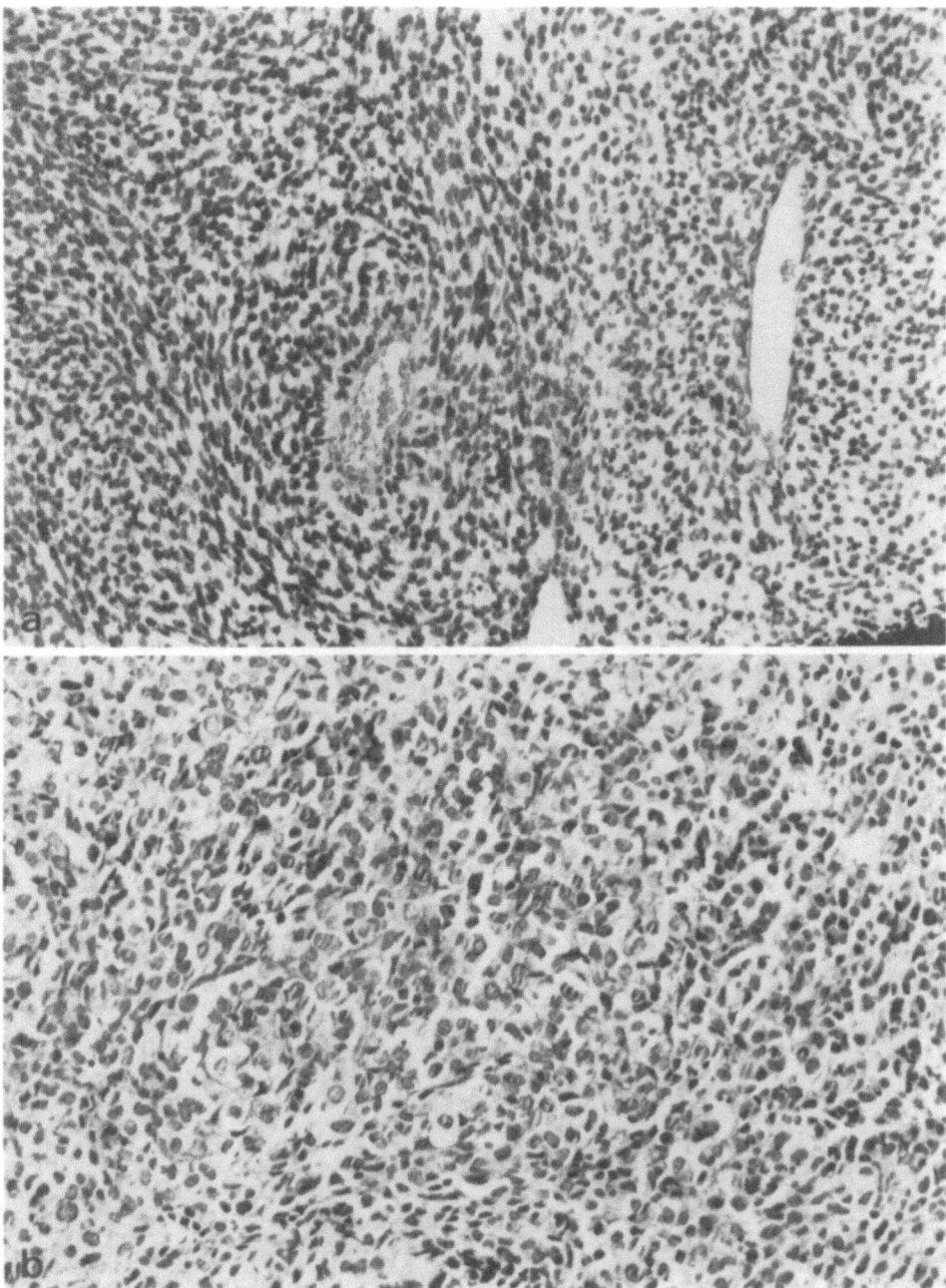

Fig. 10a, b. Pulmonary blastoma: Recurrences. **a** Undifferentiated tumor cells arranged around thin-walled vessels. Same case as Figs. 1, 5a, b, and 8b. Surgical biopsy from the chest wall of a 58-year-old man. **b** Undifferentiated tumor cells without organization. To be compared with the primary tumor in Fig. 9a. Surgical biopsy from the chest wall of a 69-year-old man. **a, b** H & E, × 150

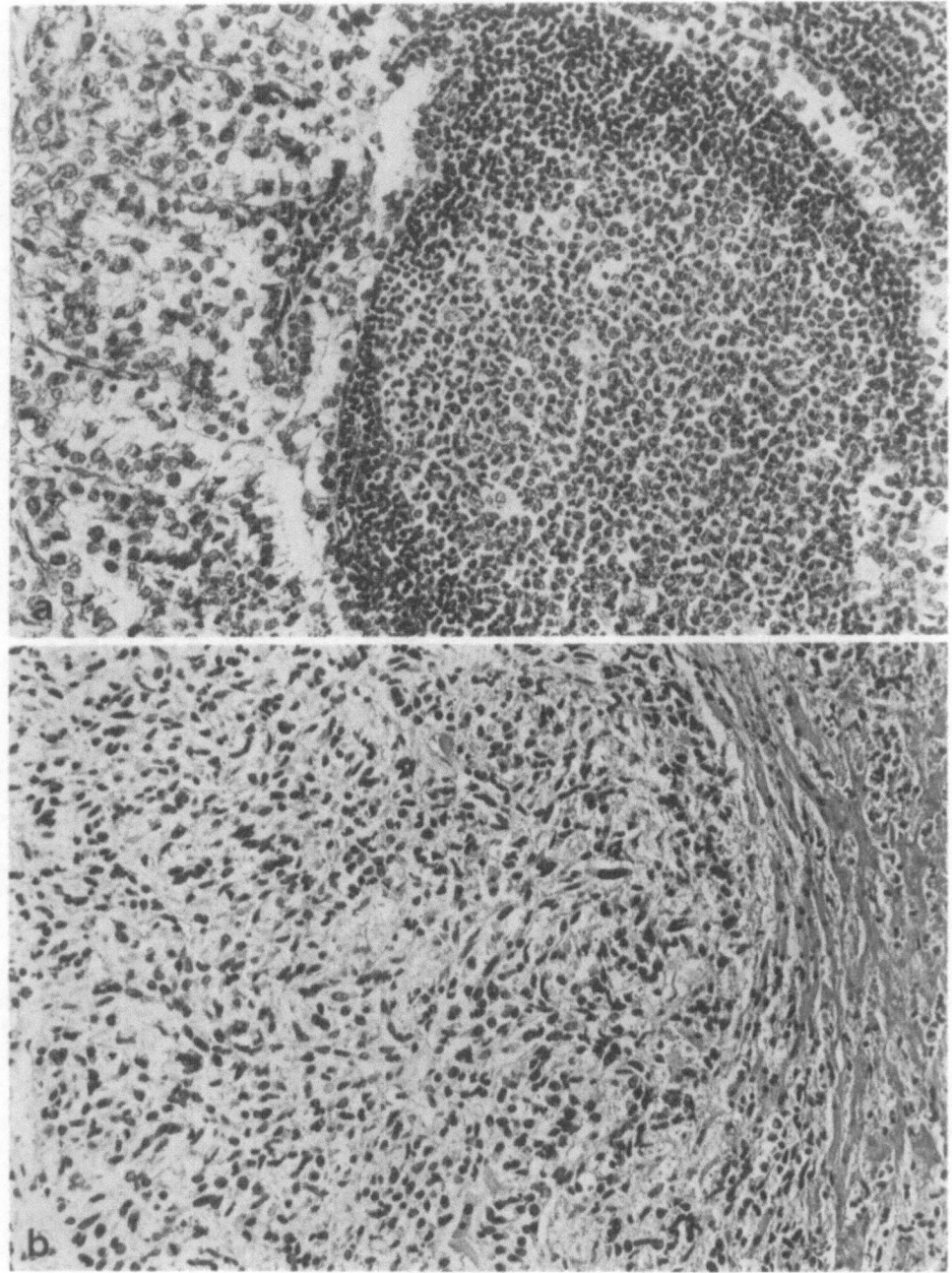

Fig. 11a—d. Pulmonary blastoma: Different types of appearances in the metastases.
a Lymph node metastasis. Box-shaped tumor cells with a well-demarcated light cytoplasm arranged in adenomatous formations appearing in the marginal sinus. Same case
as Figs. 7f and 9b. Surgical specimen from a 66-year-old man. b Liver metastasis.
Elongated tumor cells arranged in fascicles of mesenchymal appearance. Same case as
Fig. 8a. Autopsy specimen from a 69-year-old man

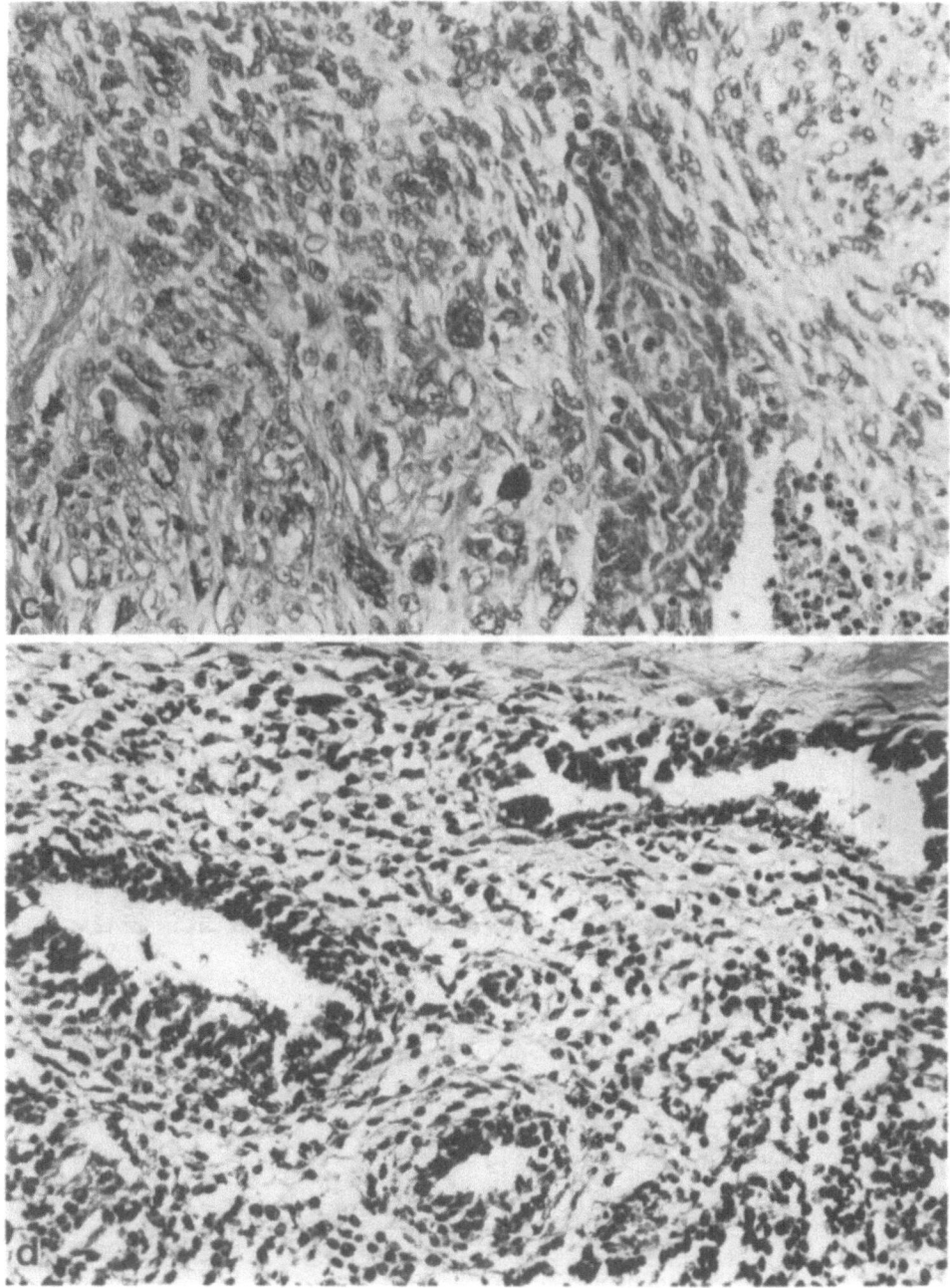

Fig. 11c. Satellite tumor in the lung. Island of epithelial tumor cells surrounded by a pleomorphic mesenchymal tumor component. Same case as Figs. 3a—c, 7d, and 8e. Surgical specimen from a 59-year-old woman. **d** Kidney metastasis. Biphasic differentiation with tubular formations in an undifferentiated stromal component. Same case as Fig. 6a, b. Autopsy specimen from a 66-year-old man. **a—d** H & E, × 150

Table 2. Pulmonary blastoma: All known cases. Previously unpublished information is underlined

Author(s)	Age and Sex	Secondaries Location	Components	Last known status	Follow-up (months)
Barrett and Barnard (1945)	40 ♀	Wide spread	Mixed	<u>Alive and well (1963)</u>	<u>240</u>
Peabody (1959)	74 ♂	Recur.	Mesench.	Dead	5
Schiφdt and Jensen (1960)	66 ♂	Local		Dead	10
Spencer (1961)	59 ♂	Local	Mixed	Dead, pyopneumothorax	5
Spencer (1961)	55 ♂	Brain		Autopsy diagnosis	0
Spencer (1961)	19 ♀			<u>Alive (1958), no further follow-up</u>	12
Campesi and Sommariva (1961)	36 ♂	Recur.		Dead, cachexia	3
Boss (1962)	3 ♀	Recur., local	Mesench.	Dead	6
Souza et al. (1965)	48 ♂			Alive and well (1975)	<u>144</u>
Bauermeister et al. (1966)	59 ♂	<u>Recur., wide spread</u>	<u>Mixed, epith.</u>	<u>Dead</u>	<u>72</u>
Henry and Keal (1966)	77 ♂	Local	Mesench.	Autopsy diagnosis	0
Parker et al. (1966)	68 ♂	Wide spread	Mixed	Dead	7
Parker et al. (1966)	33 ♀	Local	Mixed	Dead	122
Motlik and Triska (1968)	68 ♂			Dead	12
Motlik and Triska (1968)	78 ♂	None		Autopsy diagnosis	0
Motlik and Triska (1968)	70 ♂	Local, spermatic cord	Epith., mesench.	Autopsy diagnosis	0
Minken et al. (1968)	50 ♂			<u>Alive, no further follow-up</u>	36
Barson et al. (1968)	50 ♂	Recur., wide spread	Mixed	Dead	5
RayChaudhuri and Winstanley (1969)	45 ♂	Recur., wide spread	Mixed epith.	Dead	6
Chitambar et al. (1969)	20 ♂	Recur., wide spread	Mesench.	Dead	12
Stackhouse et al. (1969)	32 ♀	Local		Dead	7
Stackhouse et al. (1969)	60 ♂	Local, wide spread	Mesench.	<u>Dead</u>	<u>16</u>
Cox et al. (1970)	58 ♂			Alive	2
Danzinger (1970)	72 ♂	None		Autopsy diagnosis	0
Dumon et al. (1970)	35 ♂	<u>Recur., liver</u>		<u>Dead</u>	<u>17</u>
Bates (1971)	32 ♀			<u>Alive and well</u>	<u>72</u>
Nazari et al. (1971)	15 ♂	<u>Local, spine</u>	<u>Mixed, mesench.</u>	Dead, medullary compression	<u>17</u>
Davis et al. (1972)	58 ♂			Dead, heart disease	11
Davis et al. (1972)	40 ♂			Dead, postoperative hemorrhage	0

Reference	Age/Sex	Location	Type	Status	No.
Davis et al. (1972)	58 ♂	Recur., wide spread	Mesench.	Dead	18
Davis et al. (1972)	65 ♂			Dead, respiratory failure	0
Davis et al. (1972)	61 ♀			Alive	3
RayChaudhuri et al. (1972)	32 ♂			No information	
Thompson (1972)	72 ♂	Local		Dead, respiratory failure	1/2
Scheffer (1972)	20 ♂	Local		Dead	6
Pacharee and Parichatikanond (1972)	1/6 ♂	None		Autopsy diagnosis	0
Dixon and Breslow (1973)	42 ♀	Wide spread		Dead	3
Iverson and Straehley (1973)	11 ♂			Alive and well (1978)	169
Iverson and Straehley (1973)	1 ♀	Wide spread		Dead	2
Vila et al. (1973)	50 ♂	Recur., local	Mixed	Dead	3
Herzog and Putman (1974)	63 ♀			Alive	12
Karcioglu and Someren (1974)	48 ♂	None		Autopsy diagnosis	0
Rao et al. (1974)	30 ♀	Chest wall	No biopsy	Alive, no further follow-up	3
Cornet et al. (1975)	2 ♀	Recur.		Dead	9
Cornet et al. (1975)	45 ♂			Alive and well	42
Ghaffar et al. (1975)	9 ♂	Recur., wide spread		Dead	10
Ghaffar et al. (1975)	48 ♂			Alive, no further follow-up	36
Willnow and Hofmann (1974)	5 ♂	Local		Alive and well	120
Willnow and Hofmann (1974)	3 ♀	Wide spread		Dead	4
Patil et al. (1975)	25 ♂	Local	Mixed	Autopsy diagnosis	0
Wiechowski et al. (1975)	39 ♀	Wide spread		Dead	12
McCann et al. (1976)	40 ♂	Recur., wide spread		Dead	5
Non et al. (1976)	73 ♂	Recur.		Dead	1
Meinecke et al. (1976)	80 ♂	Wide spread	Epith. mesench.	Dead	11
Kern and Stiles (1976)	29 ♂	Recur., wide spread	Mixed	Dead	108
Kern and Stiles (1976)	55 ♀	Recur., lung	Mixed	Dead, metastatic breast cancer	252
Peacock and Whitwell (1976)	30 ♀	Local		Alive	6
Peacock and Whitwell (1976)	23 ♂	Recur., local		Dead	4
Kennedy and Prior (1976)	29 ♀	Breast, armpit	Mixed	Alive	192
Kennedy and Prior (1976)	27 ♂	Recur.		Dead	26
Marsden and Scholtz (1976)	4 ♂	Local, bone	Mixed	Dead	9
Blair and Al-Doroubi (1976)	1 ♀	Brain	Mixed	Dead	2
Kodaira et al. (1976)	10 ♀			Alive	1/2

Table 2 (continued)

Author(s)	Age and Sex	Secondaries Location	Components	Last known status	Follow-up (months)
Fung et al. (1977)	19 ♀	Wide spread		Dead	6
Jayet et al. (1977)	1/2 ♂	None		Autopsy diagnosis	0
Jayet et al. (1977)	43 ♂	Wide spread	Mixed	Dead	5
Dressner et al. (1977)	31 ♂			Alive and well (1978)	60
Lieutaud et al. (1978)	61 ♂			Alive, no further information	
Roth and *Elguezabal* (1978)	66 ♂	Recur., bone	Mesench.	Dead	8
Valderrama et al. (1978)	3 ♂	Lung	Mesench.	Alive	34
Valderrama et al. (1978)	4 ♀			Alive	26
Spahr et al. (1978)	47 ♂	Chest wall		Dead	3
Present series	59 ♀	Wide spread	Mixed	Dead	1
Present series	64 ♂	Local	Epith., mesench. Epith.	Dead, respiratory failure	1/2
Present series	58 ♂	Chest wall	Mesench.	Dead	16
Present series	66 ♂	Recur., local	Epith.	Dead	12
Present series	73 ♂	Recur., local	Epith.	Dead	24
Present series	67 ♂	Recur.	Epith.	Dead	82
Present series	69 ♂	Recur., local	Mesench.	Dead	6
Present series	66 ♂	Wide spread	Mixed	Dead	9
Present series	68 ♂	Lung, local	Epith., mesench. Epith.	Dead	1/2
Present series	69 ♂	Wide spread	Mesench.	Dead	6
Present series	77 ♂	Local	Epith.	Autopsy diagnosis	0

Table 3. Pulmonary blastoma: 83 cases. Distribution of secondaries among all cases of pulmonary blastoma, among cases with metastatic disease, and among surgically resected cases

Location of secondaries	n	Percentage of all cases	Percentage of cases with metastatic lesion	Percentage of operated cases
Hilar lymph nodes with or without mediastinal involvement	31	37.3	54.4	30.3
Recurrent tumor growth	25	30.1	43.8	37.9
Focal lung metastases or satellites	17	20.4	29.8	21.2
Growth in the chest wall and/or in the operation scar	13	15.6	22.8	19.7
Liver	9	10.8	15.8	9.1
Extrathoracic lymph nodes	9	10.8	15.8	10.6
Central nervous system	7	8.4	12.3	7.6
Bones	7	8.4	12.3	6.1
Gastrointestinal canal or peritoneum	4	4.8	7.0	3.0
Adrenal gland	4	4.8	7.0	4.5
Kidney	3	3.6	5.2	1.5
Pancreas	2	2.4	3.5	3.0
Spleen	2	2.4	3.5	3.0
Breast	1	1.2	3.7	1.5
Spermatic cord	1	1.2	1.7	–
Unspecified or wide spread	4	4.8	7.0	6.1

cases, half of which showed involvement of the thoracic wall. Twelve cases (19%) had tumor tissue in the operation scar. Among all reported cases, 57 (66%) showed recurrent tumor tissue and/or metastases. The metastases most often appeared in the hilar lymph nodes with mediastinal involvement (31 cases). Focal lung metastases or satellites (new primaries?) were reported in 17 cases. The secondaries were confined to the thoracic cavity in 50% of the 57 cases. The most frequent extrathoracic locations of metastases were liver, central nervous system and bones. The distribution of the secondaries is shown in Table 3.

The recurrences and the metastases most often appeared within one year after the primary resection. Only in two cases (*Bauermeister* et al. 1966; and one personal case) was a late recurrence fatal; in four cases, however, recurrences were successfully resected over a period of many years (*Parker* et al. 1966; *Kennedy* and *Prior* 1976; *Kern* and *Stiles* 1976).

In 26 cases no secondaries were reported; four of these patients were alive and well 20, 14, 12 and 10 years after the resection (*Barnard* 1952; *Souza* et al. 1965; *Iverson* and *Straehley* 1973; *Willnow* and *Hofmann* 1974). Six patients had a recurrence-free observation period of 2–8 years (*Minken* et al. 1968; *Bates* 1971; *Cornet* et al. 1975; *Ghaffar* et al. 1975; *Dressner* et al. 1977; *Valderrama* et al. 1978). Of the remaining 16 patients, eight are dead and eight were followed for 12 months or less.

VII. Treatment

Surgical resection was performed in 66 cases (80%), with a mean survival time of 33 months, compared with 2 months in the 17 nonresected cases.

Radiation therapy was given after resection in 15 patients and in combination with chemotherapy in three patients.

In recent years various chemotherapeutic agents have been used singly or in combination in the treatment of recurrent disease after surgery, or in inoperable cases.

Twenty-two patients received chemotherapy alone or in combination with resection and/or radiation therapy, and their mean survival time was 16 months. Alkylating agents (cyclophosphamide, chlorambucil, triethylmethiophosphoramide, and lomustine), antibiotics (dactinomycin, doxorubicin, and bleomycin), antimetabolites (fluorouracil and methotrexate), and antimitotics (vincristine, vinblastine, and podophyllotoxin) have all been tried. A recent recommendation is to supplement resection — if complete — by irradiation and in all cases to employ chemotherapy consisting of vincristine, dactomycin, and cyclophosphamide in addition to surgery (*Valderrama* et al. 1978).

VIII. Prognosis

The prognosis of PB is not as encouraging as previously believed. Thirteen patients (15.7%) have survived 5 years and seven (8.4%) have survived 10 years. This is similar to what is reported for the prognosis of adenocarcinomas and large-cell undifferentiated carcinoma of the lung (*Mountain* et al. 1974).

Based on clinical information and information obtained from microscopic examination of the (therapeutically) resected specimens, 64 PBs (resected cases with at least 1 month follow-up) were stratified according to stage (*Mountain* et al. 1974; *Carr* 1980). Because of the small number of patients, stages 2 and 3 were pooled.

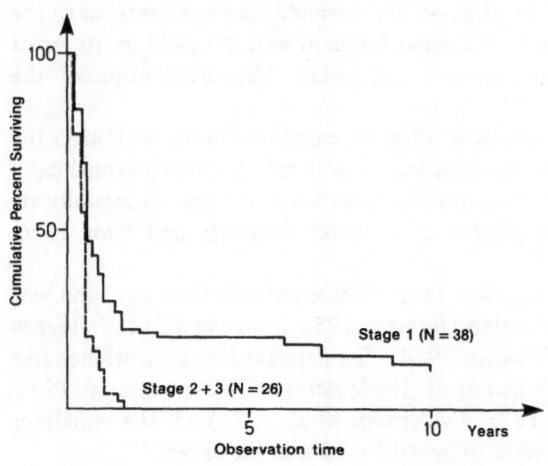

Fig. 12. The cumulative survival in 64 cases of pulmonary blastoma stratified according to postsurgical treatment—pathological stage

Figure 12 demonstrates the cumulative survival (calculated according to *Peto* et al. 1977) in PB stratified according to the postsurgical treatment—pathological stage. The prognosis in stage 1 is significantly better than the prognosis in stage 2 + 3 ($P = 0.0003$). The survival in PB is not significantly influenced by single factors such as sex, age, or location of the tumor (McWhitney test).

The biological behavior of PB remains unpredictable, as there are no reliable histological criteria by which the few relatively benign PBs can be distinguished from the more malignant ones.

The use of cyclic chemotherapy applied in combination with surgery might show an improved survival rate in the future.

IX. Conclusion

Pulmonary blastoma is a primary lung tumor consisting of a mixture of blastomatous and immature-looking epithelial and mesenchymal components. The histogenesis is not clarified, although it is the author's view that the tumor is a variant of mixed mesodermal tumor and hence developed from *one* germ layer.

The mean age at PB diagnosis is 43 years (range 2 months to 80 years). The male/female ratio is 2.6:1. PB has been described from all continents. The frequency among malignant primary lung tumors is 0.25%–0.5%. No familial accumulation has been reported. Hemoptysis, pain, dyspnea, fever, and cough are the most common symptoms. Preoperative diagnosis is difficult to achieve. Needle biopsies seem to be the most fruitful diagnostic method. PB shows no predilection for any particular lobe or location in the lung. In 20% of cases, polypoid intrabronchial growth is described. The size ranges from 1.5 to 25 cm in diameter. The tumor is surrounded by a pseudocapsule, often invaded by tumor tissue.

A characteristic microscopic feature is a blastomatous component, in addition to the more obvious epithelial and mesenchymal differentiation. The components are mixed and present in varying amounts and show varying degrees of differentiation and maturation.

Two-thirds of PBs reveal recurrences and/or metastases. Local recurrences are usually more dedifferentiated than the corresponding primary tumor, whereas the appearance of the metastases is extremely variable. The prognosis is poor; the 5-year-survival rate is only 16%.

With an increasing number of PBs being recognized and reported, it should be possible in the near future to gain more knowledge about this interesting lung tumor with its unpredictable biological behavior.

Acknowledgment. We wish to thank Mrs. Bodil Tjellesen and Mrs. Lisbet Ørgaard Nielsen for their careful typing of the manuscript and Mr. Aksel Ankerstjerne for his technical assistance.

References

Babaian RJ, Skinner DG, Waisman J (1980) Wilm's tumor in the adult patient. Diagnosis, management, and review of the world medical literature. Cancer 45:1713–1719

Barnard WG (1952) Embryoma of lung. Thorax 7:299–301

Barrett NR, Barnard WG (1945) Some unusual thoracic tumours. Br J Surg 32:447–457

Barson AJ, Jones AW, Lodge KV (1968) Pulmonary blastoma. J Clin Pathol 21:480–485

Bates HR (1971) Pulmonary blastoma (embryonal sarcoma of the lung). Va Med Mon 98:249–251

Bauermeister DE, Jennings ER, Beland AH, Judson HA (1966) Pulmonary blastoma, a form of carcinosarcoma. Am J Clin Pathol 46:322–329

Bennington JL, Beckwith JB (1975) Tumors of the kidney, renal pelvis, and ureter. Armed Forces Institute of Pathology, Washington, pp 50–51

Blair JD, Al-Doroubi QI (1976) Pulmonary blastoma in an infant. Am J Pathol 82:90a

Boss JH (1962) Mixed embryonic tumor of the lung in a three-year-old girl. Am Rev Respir Dis 85:735–740

Campesi G, Sommariva V (1961) Rarissima neoformazione polmonare di tipo adeno-sarcomatoso. Sua possibile interpretazione in rapporto a nuove vedute embriogenetiche. Arch "De Vecchi" Anat Pathol Med Clin 36:109–128

Carr DT (1980) Diagnosis and staging. In: Hansen HH, Rørth M (eds) Lung cancer 1980. Excerpta Medica, Amsterdam, pp 49–70

Chitambar IA, Gujral JS, Aikat BK (1969) Embryonal sarcoma of the lung. A case report with a discussion regarding its morphogenesis. J Thorac Cardiovasc Surg 57:657–662

Cornet E, Mussini-Montpellier J, Michaud JL, Lenne Y, de Lajartre AY (1975) Le pneumoblastome. A propos de deux cas, revue de la littérature. Rev Fr Mal Respir 3:143–156

Cox JL, Fuson RL, Daly JT (1970) Pulmonary blastoma. A case report and review of the literature. Ann Thorac Surg 9:364–371

Dameron F (1969) Phénomènes d'induction dans l'organogenèse du poumon chez l'embryon de poulet. In: Wolff E (ed) Les interactions tissulaires au cours de l'organogenese. Dunod, Paris, pp 153–171

Danziger H (1970) Pulmonary blastoma. Can Med Assoc J 102:146–147

Davis PW, Briggs JC, Seal RME, Storring FK (1972) Benign and malignant mixed tumours of the lung. Thorax 27:657–673

Dixon DS, Breslow A (1973) Pulmonary blastoma. Am Rev Respir Dis 108:968–971

Dressner SA, Okinaka AJ, Smith JP, Gray GF (1977) Pulmonary blastoma. NY State J Med 77:1953–1954

Dumon JF, Garbe L, Lebreuil G, Dor V, Payan H, Dumon G (1970) Tumeur du blasteme pulmonaire. J Fr Med Chir Thorac 25:75–84

Francis D, Jacobsen M (1979) Pulmonary blastoma. Preoperative cytologic and histologic findings. Acta Cytol (Baltimore) 23:437–442

Fung CH, Lo JW, Yonan TN, Milloy FJ, Hakami MM, Changus GW (1977) Pulmonary blastoma. An ultrastructural study with a brief review of literature and a discussion of pathogenesis. Cancer 39:153–163

Ghaffar A, Vaidynathan SV, Elguezabal A, Levowitz BS (1975) Pulmonary blastoma: report of two cases. Chest 67:600–602

Hage E (1973) The morphological development of the pulmonary epithelium of human foetuses studied by light- and electron microscopy. Z Anat Entwicklungsgesch 140:271–279

Henry K, Keal EE (1966) Pulmonary blastoma with a striated muscle component. Br J Dis Chest 60:87–92

Herzog KA, Putman CE (1974) Pulmonary blastoma. Br J Radiol 47:286–288

Iverson RE, Straehley CJ (1973) Pulmonary blastoma; long-term survival of juvenile patient. Chest 63:436–440

Jacobsen M, Francis D (1980) Pulmonary blastoma. A clinico-pathological study of eleven cases. Acta Pathol Microbiol Scand [A] 88:151–160

Jayet A, Bosic C, Saegesser F (1977) Pneumoblastomes. A propos de deux observations. Schweiz Med Wochenschr 107:349–352

Karcioglu ZA, Someren AO (1974) Pulmonary blastoma. A case report and review of the literature. Am J Clin Pathol 61:287–295

Kennedy A, Prior AL (1976) Pulmonary blastoma: a report of two cases and a review of the literature. Thorax 31:776–781

Kern WH, Stiles QR (1976) Pulmonary blastoma. J Thorac Cardiovasc Surg 72:801–808

Kodaira Y, Akiyama H, Morikawa M, Shimizu K (1976) Pulmonary blastoma in a child. J Pediatr Surg 11:239–241

Lieutaud R, Chrestian MA, Vague D, Jacquemier J, Choux R (1978) Tumeurs malignes bi-tissulaires du poumon. A propos de deux observations. Arch Anat Cytol Pathol 26:158–163

Marsden HB, Scholtz CL (1976) Pulmonary blastoma. Virchows Arch [Pathol Anat] 372:161–165

McCann MP, Fu Y-S, Kay S (1976) Pulmonary blastoma. A light and electron microscopic study. Cancer 38:789–797

Meinecke R, Bauer F, Skouras J, Mottu F (1976) Blastomatous tumors of the respiratory tract. Cancer 38:818–823

Minken SL, Craver WL, Adams JT (1968) Pulmonary blastoma. Arch Pathol 86:442–446

Motlik K, Triska J (1968) Bronchopulmonary carcinosarcomas. Acta Univ Carol [Med] (Praha) 14:3–25

Mountain CF, Carr DT, Anderson WAD (1974) A system for the clinical staging of lung cancer. AJR 120:130–138

Nazari A, Amir-Mokri E, Sarram A, Yaghmai I (1971) Pulmonary blastoma. Chest 60:187–189

Non DP, Lang WR, Patchefsky A, Takeda M (1976) Pulmonary blastoma: cytopathologic and histopathologic findings. Acta Cytol (Baltimore) 20:381–386

Pacharee P, Parichatikanond P (1972) Pulmonary blastoma. A case report in an infant and review of the literature. J Med Assoc Thai 55:43–48

Parker JC, Payne WS, Woolner LB (1966) Pulmonary blastoma (embryoma). Report of two cases. J Thorac Cardiovasc Surg 51:694–699

Patil SD, Talib VH, Kotwal SE, Deshpande MS (1975) Pulmonary blastoma (embryoma lung). A case report with review of literature. Indian J Cancer 12:348–353

Peabody CN (1959) Carcinosarcoma of lung of peripheral origin. J Thorac Surg 37:766–770

Peacock MJ, Whitwell F (1976) Pulmonary blastoma. Thorax 31:197–204

Peto R, Pike MC, Armitage P, Breslow NE, Cox DR, Howard SV, Mantel N, McPherson K, Peto J, Smith PG (1977) Design and analysis of randomized clinical trials requiring prolonged observation of each patient. Br J Cancer 35:1–39

Rao KM, Gupta RP, Das PB, John S, Walter A (1974) Pulmonary blastoma: a case report. Thorax 29:138–141

RayChaudhuri M, Winstanley DP (1969) Pulmonary blastoma with diverse metastases. J Pathol 98:81–82

RayChaudhuri M, Eastham WN, Frederiksz PA (1972) Pulmonary blastoma with diverse mesenchymal proliferation. Thorax 27:487–491

Roth JA, Elguezabal A (1978) Pulmonary blastoma evolving into carcinosarcoma. A case study. Am J Surg Pathol 2:407–413

Scheffer E (1972) Longblastoom. Ned Tijdschr Geneeskd 116:906–907

Schiødt T, Jensen KG (1960) Malignant teratoid tumour of the lung: malignant hamartoma? Thorax 15:120–123

Souza RC, Peasley ED, Takaro T (1965) Pulmonary blastomas. A distinctive group of carcinosarcomas of the lung. Ann Thorac Surg 1:259–268

Spahr J, Draffin RM, Johnston WW (1979) Cytopathologic findings in pulmonary blastoma. Acta Cytol (Baltimore) 23:454–459

Spencer H (1961) Pulmonary blastomas. J Pathol Bacteriol 82:161–165

Spencer H (1977) Hamartomas, blastoma and teratoma of the lung. In: Spencer H (ed) Pathology of the lung, 3rd edn. Pergamon Press, Oxford, pp 973–997

Stackhouse EM, Harrison EG, Ellis FH (1969) Primary mixed malignancies of lung: Carcinosarcoma and blastoma. J Thorac Cardiovasc Surg 57:385–399

Stone FJ, Churg AM (1977) The ultrastructure of pulmonary hamartoma. Cancer 39: 1064–1070

Thompson TT (1972) Roentgen manifestations of pulmonary blastoma. Chest 62: 104–105

Valderrama E, Saluja G, Shende A, Lanzkowsky P, Berkman J (1978) Pulmonary blastoma. Report of two cases in children. Am J Surg Pathol 2:415–422

Vila R, McCoy JJ, McCall RE (1973) Pulmonary blastoma, report of a case. JSC Med Assoc 69:251–256

Waddell WR (1949) Organoid differentation of the fetal lung. A histologic study of the differentiation of mammalian fetal lung in utero and in transplants. Arch Pathol 47:227–247

Wiechowski S, Czerniak B, Marzymska G, Stankiewicz-Borkiel D (1975) Blastoma pulmonis. Gruzlica 43:743–749

Willnow U, Hofmann V (1974) Zu Morphologie und Histogenese der primären Lungentumoren des Kindes. Helv Paediatr Acta 29:425–438

Subject Index

The numbers set in *italics* refer to those pages on which the respective catch-word is discussed in detail

298

Index of Volumes 67–72 Current Topics in Pathology

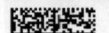